A Political Practice of Occupational Therapy

For Elsevier:

Commissioning Editor: **Rita Demetriou-Swanwick/Dinah Thom**

Development Editor: **Catherine Jackson**

Project Manager: **Emma Riley**

Designer: **Stewart Larking**

Illustration Buyer: **Kirsteen Wright**

Illustrator: **Cactus**

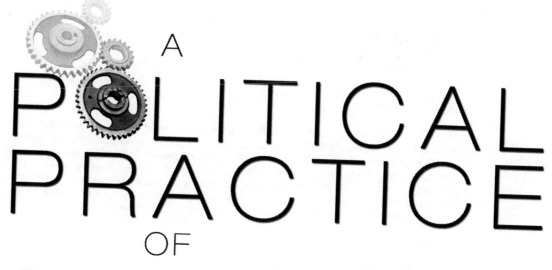

A POLITICAL PRACTICE OF OCCUPATIONAL THERAPY

EDITED BY

Nick Pollard BA PGCE DipCOT MA MSc
Senior Lecturer in Occupational Therapy,
Sheffield Hallam University,
Sheffield, UK

Dikaios Sakellariou MSc BSc(OT)
Lecturer in Occupational Therapy,
Cardiff University,
Cardiff, UK

Frank Kronenberg BSc BA
International Guest Lecturer
in Occupational Therapy without Borders;
Part-time Lecturer, Zuyd University,
The Netherlands; Co-founder and Director,
Shades of Black Productions

FOREWORD BY
Hanneke van Bruggen DipOT Honorary Degree of
Doctor of Science
Executive Director, European Network of Occupational Therapy,
Hogeschool van Amsterdam, NL

EDINBURGH LONDON NEW YORK OXFORD PHILADELPHIA ST LOUIS SYDNEY TORONTO 2009

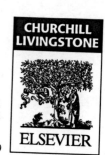

CHURCHILL
LIVINGSTONE

ELSEVIER

CHURCHILL
LIVINGSTONE
ELSEVIER

© 2008, Elsevier Limited. All rights reserved.
First published 2009

ISBN: 978 0 443 10391 9

British Library Cataloguing in Publication Data
A catalogue record for this book is available from the British Library.

Library of Congress Cataloging in Publication Data
A catalog record for this book is available from the Library of Congress.

Note

Neither the Publisher nor the Editors assume any responsibility for any loss or injury and/or damage to persons or property arising out of or related to any use of the material contained in this book. It is the responsibility of the treating practitioner, relying on independent expertise and knowledge of the patient, to determine the best treatment and method of application for the patient.

The Publisher

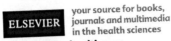
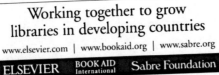
Transferred to Digital Printing in 2012

Contents

v

List of contributors

Brendan Abel
BA

Graduate, Syracuse University, New York, USA

Karin J. Barnes
PhD OTR

Associate Professor, Occupational Therapy Department, University of Texas Health Science Center at San Antonio, San Antonio, Texas, USA

Rani Bechar
MA OTR/L

Occupational Therapist, Department of Rehabilitation, Cedars Sinai Medical Center, Los Angeles, California, USA

Alison J. Beck
PhD OTR

Associate Professor, Occupational Therapy Department, University of Texas Health Science Center at San Antonio, San Antonio, Texas, USA

Amber Bertram
MA OTR/L

Renown Rehabilitation Hospital, Reno, Nevada, USA

Jeanine Blanchard
PhD (candidate) OTR

Project Coordinator, Division of Occupational Therapy and Occupational Science at the School of Dentistry, University of Southern California, USA

Tiffany Boggis
MBA OTR/L

Assistant Professor, School of Occupational Therapy, Pacific University, Oregon, USA

Shana Boltin
BOT

Paediatric Occupational Therapist, Victoria, Australia

Melodie Clarke
Bachelor(Anthropology)

Julie Coleman
BA PgDip UnivDip(OT) SROT

Lecturer in Occupational Therapy, Sheffield Hallam University, Sheffield, UK

Richard Davies
BSc(Hons)

Occupational Therapist, Sheffield, UK

Medea Despotashvili
PhD

Psychologist, SOS Children's Village International, Vienna, Austria

Gelya Frank
PhD

Professor, Division of Occupational Science and Occupational Therapy at the School of Dentistry and Department of Anthropology, University of Southern California, USA

Peggy J. Goetsch
MS LMSW

Executive Director, Racing Industry
Charitable Foundation, Illinois, USA

Colleen Harvey Martin
MA OTR/L

Occupational Therapist,
Munich, Germany

Maggie M. Heyman-Hotch
MOT OTR/L

Occupational Therapist, Salem,
Oregon, USA

Linsey Howie
PhD MA BA DipOT AccOT

Deputy Dean, Faculty of Health Sciences,
and Associate Professor and Head, School
of Occupational Therapy, Faculty of Health
Sciences, La Trobe University, Victoria,
Australia

Allison Joe
MA OTR/L

Occupational Therapist,
Department of Rehabilitation,
Stanford University Hospital,
Palo Alto, California, USA

Maria Kapanadze
PhD student PsyMA OYBSc

Georgian Occupational Therapy Association,
NGO NADI (National Advocacy on Disability
Issues)

Captain Jeff Kirby
CA

Community Development Worker – Christ
Church, Pittsmoor, Sheffield, UK

Sister Vanessa Kirby
CA

Community Development Worker – Christ
Church, Pittsmoor, Sheffield, UK

Heather J. Kitching
MA OTR(L)

Doctoral Student, Division of Occupational
Science and Occupational Therapy, School
of Dentistry, Department of Anthropology,
University of Southern California, USA

Frank Kronenberg
BSc BA

Director and Co-founder, Shades
of Black Productions, Cape Town,
South Africa; International Guest
Lecturer, Occupational Therapy
Without Borders; and Lecturer,
Zuyd University, The Netherlands

Shannon K. Lizer
PhD APN/CPN

Director of Nursing,
Highland Community Village,
Freeport, Illinois, USA

Catherine McNulty
BHSc(OT) PGTharn Diploma

Senior Occupational Therapist, Sleaford
Recovery Team, Sleaford Community Mental
Health Team, Sleaford, Lincolnshire, UK

Andrina Mitchell
BSc DipVET

Fieldwork Supervisor, Occupational Science
and Therapy, School of Health
and Social Development, Deakin University;
Health Promotion Officer, South West
Primary Care Partnership, Victoria,
Australia

Karin J. Opacich
PhD MHPE OTR/L FAOTA

Opacich Consultative Services, Chicago
Illinois, USA

Tamar Paluch
BOT

Master's Student, La Trobe University;
Occupational Therapist, Melbourne,
Australia

x

Stephen Parks
PhD

Associate Professor of Writing and Rhetoric, Writing Program, College of Arts and Sciences, Syracuse University, New York, USA

Nick Pollard
BA PGCE DipCOT MA MSc

Senior Lecturer in Occupational Therapy, Sheffield Hallam University, Sheffield, UK

Dikaios Sakellariou
MSc BSc(OT)

Lecturer in Occupational Therapy, Department of Occupational Therapy, School of Healthcare Studies, Cardiff University, UK

Nino Skhirtladze
MA BSc

Occupational Therapist, Psychologist, Tbilisi Youth House Foundation, Tbilisi, Georgia

Jaynee Taguchi-Meyer
OTD OTR/L

Assistant Professor and Academic Coordinator of Fieldwork Education, Division of Occupational Science and Occupational Therapy at the School of Dentistry, University of Southern California, USA

Clarissa Wilson
BOT

Education and Development Co-ordinator, Queensland Transcultural Mental Health Centre (QTMHC), Queensland Health, and Co-ordinator of Occupational Opportunities for Refugees and Asylum Seekers (OOFRAS), Queensland, Australia

Ruth Zemke
PhD OTR FAOTA

Professor Emerita, Division of Occupational Science and Occupational Therapy, University of Southern California, USA

Foreword

There is no better moment to produce this book than in the European Year of Equal Opportunities for All (European Commission 2007) and at the end of the African Decade of Persons with Disabilities (1999–2009), which proclaims the full participation, equality and empowerment of people with disabilities in Africa.

Occupational therapy should contribute to the four key objectives of the European Year (2007):

* **Right:** raising awareness on and enhancing the rights to occupations of those who continue to experience inequality in spite of equality legislation
* **Representation:** facilitating underrepresented groups, such as persons with disabilities, migrants, etc., to participate more in society
* **Recognition:** facilitating and celebrating diversity and equality
* **Respect:** promoting social cohesion and good relations between different groups.

And to the main objectives of the African Decade:

* To promote the participation of persons with disabilities in the process of economic and social development
* To ensure and improve access to rehabilitation, education, training, employment, sports, the cultural and physical environment
* To prevent causes of disability
* To support the development of and strengthen disabled persons' organizations
* To advocate and raise disability awareness in general, and awareness of the African Decade of Persons with Disabilities in particular.

In this book there is no sign that occupational therapists were involved in the World Programme of Action Concerning Disabled Persons (UN decade 1983–1992): just like many other disciplines they failed to implement that programme. That decade did not bring any noticeable improvement in the quality of life of people with disabilities in Africa; only countries in the northern hemisphere appeared to have benefited from the decade. This is what prompted the African disability movement to lobby and gain UN support for the African Decade of Persons with Disabilities. A plan of action has been promulgated by the African heads of state, but will it again be just a 'talk show'? 'We need to urge governments to redirect resources away from conflict to more meaningful issues of development... During the African Decade we want to see a change of attitude at local, national and international level that will enable people with disabilities to assert their political, social and economic rights' (Phiri 2003). At the last Occupational Therapy African Regional Group (OTARG) meeting in September 2007, the decision was taken that African occupational therapists should write their own occupational therapy book, with case studies from different African countries, which can contribute to the African Decade of Persons with Disabilities.

Several times this book mentions a movement towards political practice in occupational therapy since 2004, when the World Federation of Occupational Therapists (WFOT) confirmed that occupational justice and occupational apartheid were valid problems for occupational therapy (Ch. 7). The contribution of the European Network of Occupational Therapy in Higher Education (ENOTHE) to inclusively building occupational therapy is mentioned in the same chapter; however, in Europe awareness and changes in occupational therapy practice and education became quite obvious in 1995 because of the enlargement of

Europe and its policy concerning social rights, a fact that is underestimated here. In 1996, in the general assembly of ENOTHE in Madrid, the decision was taken that one place in the board was in principle reserved for the eastern European countries and that one of the priorities of ENOTHE should be to support eastern European countries in their endeavour to establish occupational therapy in order to facilitate the participation of persons with disabilities in their society. In 2003 (the European Year of Persons with Disabilities) ENOTHE managed, in close collaboration with many disability organizations, to secure two big projects from the European Commission that have contributed to social reform in Bulgaria, Hungary and Romania and, in the Caucasus, Georgia and Armenia, and the establishment of three occupational therapy educational programmes that have embraced the idea of occupational justice as an inclusive vision for their curricula. Identifying the right chances for occupational therapy at the right time with the right partners and in the right political context made these projects successful. Here the word politics has connotations with the original meaning of Plato and Aristotle to create the 'ideal' society or a community (*polis*). Politics implies measures that could and should be implemented in the hope of developing a better community than that which is already present.

In Europe the lack of focus in the profession (Ch. 2) changed halfway through the 1990s. Some educational institutions became aware of the necessity to include more social and political perspectives of occupational therapy in their curricula. Yet even today most occupational therapists will say, 'It is too early to tell whether or not the profession per se will move in the direction of political engagements and social transformation. Perhaps these areas will remain outside mainstream practice' (Ch. 7, p. 112). However, if, as Frank and Zemke further suggest, 'the ideas motivating the movement are important enough to be introduced to occupational therapy students', and they form a core of our curricula, then a strong future political focus will become much more likely.

This book can contribute to the four above-mentioned key objectives towards a diverse society with equal opportunities for all:

- **Rights:** 'This book is part of a recent re-examination and reconceptualization of occupational therapy to recognize a broader global and social responsibility and acknowledge a need for the profession to realize the goals of occupational justice by addressing inequality and poverty' (Ch. 2, p. 27). Accordingly, the effectiveness of occupational development interventions and outcomes should be measured by their ability to respond to the complex nature of poverty. Once framed in these terms, occupational rights become a constitutive element of occupational development and occupational injustice, and occupational deprivation becomes both a cause and a symptom of poverty. The rights-based approach contributes to making poverty approaches more politically sensitive (Koonings 2007).
- **Representation:** Most of the occupational practice examples advocate listening more closely to the voices of disadvantaged groups and demonstrate how to break the cycle of exclusion, deprivation and occupational apartheid or how to engage politically with indigenous communities, refugees or street children. A common understanding of needs and wishes, constraints, resources and construction of the conflict and cooperation situation needs to be reached before solutions can be negotiated (Ch. 1). It is of great importance that the clients or target groups are involved in all phases of the process; occupational therapists, clients or the (deprived) communities should all learn to work with the pADL tool and 3P archaeological processes and analyse their own situation. There will be a chance of success only when there is a common analysis, strategy for development and impact analysis together with all actors or true partners (Lynn & Oyeyinka 2003).
- **Recognition:** Do occupational therapists work with a diversity of clients? Do all clients have access to our practice? And how do we reach those groups who are excluded? This book offers some quite critical questioning. Demonstrating 'community involvement' should mean a little more than demonstrating the assent of local people to the plans of the local authority. Finding ways of joint working should put deprived communities in the lead and ensure that all local (national and international) authorities and service providers play their role. The only way forward is acknowledgement, acceptance and taking responsibility. The profession itself has a problem with recognizing diversity. As Sakellariou and Pollard argue in their chapter about class and gender (Ch. 5), in the USA, the UK and several west European countries the profession consists mainly of white, middle-class women. Ethnic

minorities and persons with disabilities are notoriously underrepresented in European occupational therapy education. Students of different migrant or ethnic minority backgrounds often feel excluded by teachers and fellow students and are not attracted to occupational therapy programmes. Furthermore, there is a high dropout rate (van Bruggen 2007). It is quite difficult to find good practice about successfully implemented diversity policy in occupational therapy practice and education. The American Occupational Therapy Association has made diversity one of its centennial goals and WFOT and ENOTHE are in the process of developing projects on diversity. Research shows that increasing diversity in the health care professions (Sullivan 2004) will improve health care access and quality for minority patients and assure a health care system for all.

- **Respect:** 'The welfare state tells persons with disabilities not to worry because even if we are a burden on carers, we will still be cared for by that vast professional army or our loved ones who work tirelessly on our behalf rather than allowing us the dignity to work for ourselves and indeed to become ourselves' says Mike Oliver of the Independent Living Institute (Oliver 1999). Contributing to an occupationally just society is not just the responsibility of policy-makers and governments but is a challenge to every one of us, whether we live in a welfare state or a developing country. As Kronenberg and Pollard say (2005) 'everybody is responsible for everything'.

Furthermore the book reveals some significant dilemmas in the achievement of political practice in the profession. Paluch, Boltin and Howie demonstrate that their education was not sufficient for the new areas of occupational therapy; 'Having used this tool [pADL] at an earlier stage would have enriched our learning and comprehension of the political complexities of Indigenous health'(Ch. 10, p. 157), while different educators do not see how they can fit a new subject in their already overloaded curriculum. It is questionable whether this should just be a matter of fitting in one subject or developing a different vision on which to base a totally new curriculum.

The great added value of the book comes from the debates covering an enormous diversity of political aspects within the profession, its performance and the tools it provides. If occupational therapists are more aware of the power of their discipline they can realize the enormous wealth it can offer to health, well-being, community development and research through collaboration with various scientific disciplines such as women's, disability and developmental studies, and the social and political sciences.

'The concern of the profession to work with people towards autonomous goals or toward community participation is connected with enabling active citizenship and achieving a reciprocated sense of value. This is an occupational goal but it cannot be realized without political initiatives'(Ch. 2, p. 34). Not dealing with the political aspects of the profession could harm and limit the core values of occupational therapy, which are embedded in the occupational engagement of citizens.

December 2007

Hanneke van Bruggen

References

African Decade of Persons with Disabilities: http://www.africandecade.org/

European Commission 2007 European Year of Equal Opportunities for All. Available online at: http://ec.europa.eu/employment_social /eyeq/index.cfm?cat_id=SPLASH; accessed 2 January 2008

Koonings K 2007 Bringing politics into poverty: the political dimensions of poverty alleviation, Utrecht University. In: A rich menu for the poor. Effectiveness and Quality Department (DEK), Ministry of Foreign Affairs, The Hague, p 8

Kronenberg F, Pollard N 2005 Introduction, a beginning… In: Kronenberg F, Simó Algado S, Pollard N (eds) Occupational therapy without borders. Elsevier/Churchill Livingstone, Edinburgh, p 1–13

Lynn K M, Oyeyinka B 2003 Competence building and policy impact through the innovation review process: a commentary. UNESCO, Paris

Oliver M 1999 Disabled people and the inclusive society: or the times they really are changing. Independent Living Institute. Available online

at: http://www.independentliving.org/docs4/
oliver.html; accessed 2 January 2008

Phiri A M 2003 The challenge of the decade.
Southern Africa Federation of the Disabled.
Available online at: http://www.safod.org/
African%20Decade/african_decade.html;
accessed 2 January 2008

Sullivan L W 2004 Missing persons: minorities in
the health professions. Sullivan Commission.

Washington, DC. Available online at: http://
www.aacn.nche.edu/
Media/pdf/SullivanReport.pdf; accessed 2
January 2008

Van Bruggen J E 2007 Unpublished grant
application

Preface

There is a growing awareness in occupational therapy of the need to address the political contexts in which practice, education and research take place. Occupational therapists are discussing and developing forms of transformational practice with the aim of effecting occupational justice, questioning existing roles within traditional health and social care services and asserting new ones that are oriented to wider community needs. A key element in this is an emerging political understanding and reframing of the concept of occupation.

The authors have been engaged in some of the discussions and developments around this issue at a global and local level, through the World Federation of Occupational Therapists, the European Network of Occupational Therapists in Higher Education, a series of conference presentations and publications, and the development of educational modules. However, our contributions to this discussion have mostly been exploratory, aiming to open aspects of a debate that seems to have been gathering pace through the end of the last century and the early years of this one.

This book presents a more developed set of views. If it marks a new stage in the understanding of occupational therapy in its political contexts this can offer only a partial discussion: it offers some navigational tools but not solutions. Of course, there are questions about the validity of these, coming from three white men from European backgrounds in a profession that is predominantly female, and arguing about contexts of disability, socioeconomic and political disadvantage far away from where we live and work. These issues have been problematized. The theory chapters in this book often rely on the practical engagements and experiences of others rather than our own, and therefore we have included a number of practice-based chapters that explore applications and adaptations of the ideas we have explored. Consequently this book should be read as a voice in a continuing debate – we welcome your critical engagement, whether as students, researchers, educators or practitioners.

This book is intended for all occupational therapists who have an interest in developing a political understanding of their engagements with clients. To facilitate the use of the concepts we have cross-referenced the chapters so that the reader can follow arguments through their interconnections. We have set out definitions of specific terms used in the discussions, and each theory chapter is prefaced with an abstract to aid the reader. Politics is sometimes regarded as an unsavoury, complex, irrelevant and dismissible subject, one that is beneath true professional considerations. Whether you are a student, educator, practitioner or researcher, we hope that you will find material here to employ and enjoy!

Sheffield, 2008

Nick Pollard, Dikaios Sakellariou and Frank Kronenberg

Acknowledgements

Nick

For my father, Michael Pollard.

Many thanks and love to my wife Linda, and Emma, Sally, Molly, Joshua and Daisy, and brother Simon, for their support.

Many thanks are also due to my colleagues and students at Sheffield Hallam University. Many of the authors here have also been around to bounce ideas with at various stages of writing. Frank and I had some useful early e-mail engagements with Zofia Kumas-Tan and Elelwani Ramugondo, among others.

Thanks are also due to the continuing inspiration of numerous comrades from the Federation of Worker Writers and Community Publishers (1976–2007).

Dikaios

My early debts are due to the late Professor Tsuyoshi Sato and the late Professor Gurpal Sandhu for unfailing support. Professors Yuji Sawada and Sadako Tsubota were always there to discuss and challenge ideas. Special thanks are reserved for Kit Sinclair, who, during a visit to Hong Kong back in December 2004, invited me to get involved with the WFOT-CBR (World Federation of Occupational Therapists – Community-based Rehabilitation) data collection project. It was through this involvement that I was introduced to Nick and Frank. As a late entrant to this journey, I am grateful to both for inviting me aboard.

Nick and I had several meetings in Chapeltown. Linda and the kids all provided support and doughnuts – thank you to all! Many friends and colleagues were by my side to provide support and a listening ear or accompany me to the pub when all else failed! Many thanks to all.

My parents, Vagelio and Nikos, and my brother Aris provided, as always, unending support and understanding through the long process of developing this book – thank you.

Frank

For my mom Nelly Kronenberg, who first taught me about small 'p' politics, and my dad Theo Kronenberg, who first got me interested in big 'P' politics.

With love and gratitude to my life partner Elelwani and our daughter Masana Nelly. Individually and together they allow me to see more clearly what causes are worth fighting for.

Lots of thanks to students and colleagues worldwide, particularly at the University of the Western Cape in South Africa, Hogeschool Zuyd in the Netherlands and the European Network of Occupational Therapy in Higher Education (ENOTHE). I value you all as 'compañeros de viaje' on the journey of learning together about the 'big picture(s)' of the ways of the world.

Last but not least, I wish to thank 'partners in crime' Nick Pollard and Dikaios Sakellariou for their ongoing (moral) support with the transition process and family life events that we underwent during the genesis of this publication. And a special thank you to Linda, Emma, Sally, Molly, Joshua and Daisy for allowing us to meet, work and PLAY in your home away from home.

The three of us would like to thank Dinah Thom and Catherine Jackson of Elsevier for their valuable support.

Introduction

Occupational therapy regarded itself, until recently, as an apolitical profession. However, during the first years of this century occupational therapists began to become concerned with a range of political questions as they expressed dissatisfaction with the way in which the practice of occupational therapy was constrained by events outside their control. In the UK, many of the changes were a product of health service restructuring, itself the result of government intervention. Although governments of both hues had intervened in the regulation of state health and social care, the end of the 1990s saw an increasing momentum in change and reform, which has been maintained. Occupational therapists appear to have had little voice in this change. Many of the measures concerning risk taking and efficiency do not seem to take account of the client-centred and needs-led approaches that have been developed within the profession.

Although occupational therapists often perceive themselves as advocates for the patients' interests through their client-centred focus, they do not have the monopoly of this position; this is shared with other professions. Nor does this put occupational therapists at loggerheads with an organization demanding efficiency at all costs, and risk assessment over positive risk taking. Occupational therapists in the UK have also seen themselves as apolitical because they are part of a state structure, the National Health Service, which has historically been respected by all political parties. Occupational therapists have professional associations whose aim is to protect their interests as a profession from other people practising similar professions without the same degree of qualification, or simply posing as occupational therapists. Whether working for business or for the state they are part of the social apparatus that determines the health status of other individuals. Occupational therapists can assess with other team members whether a patient is well enough to return to their own home, or else the steps that should be taken so that they can. They can give a second opinion about the state of health of other individuals. They can advise whether a person is complying with aspects of their treatment programme. They are therefore part of the apparatus of social control, among the soft police officers operating in the health and social care services. In this capacity it is difficult to see occupational therapists as genuinely apolitical.

This book explores the features of a political practice of occupational therapy. How is it possible to introduce the political into a profession that is linked to health and social care? What form could a political practice take, and how could the political components of practice be analysed and evaluated?

Clearly in most countries the provision of health and social care is determined by government policy along with other central concerns such as education, law, defence and transport infrastructures. Decisions made by government and as a consequence of political pressure have an impact on the provision of facilities and implementation of practice to individuals and communities. These political pressures result not only from the influence of politicians, their constituencies and their need to retain power but also from cultural forces (e.g. pressure from religious groups, or as a consequence of gender dominance), corporate pressures (e.g. in the pharmaceutical industry) and structural forces (e.g. economic risks and legal considerations about the effects of policy changes).

A political practice of occupational therapy pertains to the understanding of the interaction between these decision-making forces and the political actors involved. The authors argue that the political context that underpins health and social care policy, for example the evidence of health disparities created by economic disadvantage, the differences of life quality across the globe, suggest very strongly that occupational therapy, indeed all health and social care, is inescapably political. Furthermore as occupational therapists, whether employed in state apparatuses to provide health and social care or operating privately, professionals are applying criteria that determine the right of individuals to have access to meaningful occupation or to be enabled to participate in their communities. Occupational therapists are social activists in opening up occupational opportunities, and they are also agents of social control in that they are also concerned with operating limits on access, for example, since they have to work within a budget defined by their employers that means that, irrespective of need, no more resources are available within the financial year.

Occupational therapists therefore have to face ethical choices – to comply with the needs of clients, or with the needs of the system that employs them. The choice is never clear, even though the clients' needs may seem starkly defined: an individual requirement sometimes has to be balanced against wider values and conditions. These demands may be complex, depending on a combination of cultural, social, economic, environmental and political factors that may either form a significant component of professional responsibilities or act as a restraint on therapeutic autonomy. While there are various apparatuses available to practitioners, such as processes of clinical reasoning, reflection and supervision that offer some means of understanding and making these issues explicit, they rarely offer a means for political analysis – the politics of these problems are often not framed clearly.

What would such political analysis achieve and how could it be used? Is it possible to distinguish a concept of 'political competence' in occupational therapy? Political competence is the product of political reasoning, which can be developed through the use of pADL and 3P archaeological processes. While it cannot be specific to the occupational therapy profession, every new set of circumstances requires forms of political competence that are particular to that situation. Political competence arises from the combination of experience and the use of analytical tools to assess the information available in order to determine the best course of action. However, the use of the term competence does not imply that the strategy chosen will always prove to be the right one, instead that it must always be adjusted to suit developing and changing needs. A political competency, therefore, is a kind of pilot's licence, enabling the therapist to navigate waters in which currents, sandbars and weather conditions are always in flux.

Political activities of daily living (pADL) takes a view of the broader situation, attempting to encompass a synthesis of all the factors known to the user of the tool, while 3P archaeology enables users to investigate their personal resources and motivations. They do not apply solely to occupational therapists but can be used by any group. They were developed in response to the needs of occupational therapists and the people they work with as a means for rethinking objectives, priorities and occupational goals.

Occupational therapists are defined as a professional group. Like all other individuals, the circumstances in which they do, are, become and belong give a particular set of elements to the experience of being an occupational therapist. The position is akin to that of a chess piece for which certain manoeuvres are possible but others are not. Perhaps this is most clear when the occupational therapist is considered as a component of a multidisciplinary team, where each member has both overlapping and discrete functions. However, since we are not dealing with a rigid set of rules, such moves are not so much disallowed as perhaps more difficult to achieve or regarded as unorthodox. Using 3P archaeology and pADL tools enables the people involved to rethink the rules by which they play and establish tactical approaches that work towards their needs. It is possible, for example, for internal rules to be developed (as in fact often happens in team cultures) that offer a means of resolving conflict and cooperation issues within a group of people. Internal rules may operate quite differently from the way in which a group has to conduct itself in a wider environment. For example, minority cultures often maintain a set of practices when they are 'at home' that differ from those when they are 'abroad' in the dominant culture.

Thus the political dimension of interaction is potentially open-ended. Competence is limited only by the ability to reason, but other factors such as resources, the availability of information, luck and environmental elements may all combine to produce outcomes. Competence may give a tactical advantage in developing a project but, to continue with a game analogy, the object of the game itself may change, the game may suddenly develop new rules, or rules may emerge that have been hidden to some of the players. Competence is not a constant, neither is it finite, and it therefore requires an openness to new situations. The pADL and 3P archaeological reasoning tools aim to produce that openness in each situation to which they are applied.

An individual or an organization may be very politically competent in local community negotiations but unable to exercise the same influence on a larger scale. A person who has acquired good managerial expertise in a commercial organization may find difficulty in operating the outcomes of this experience in state- or community-based organizations, which run on different principles. Different cultures also operate different business and social rules. It is therefore important to reconsider, in all new situations, rather than to attempt to make initiatives and achieve an impact from the beginning. Progress may be set on a course from which it is difficult to return to the starting position if it turns out that elements of groundwork are missing. As with a chess game, the wrong opening move may determine the rest of the match.

Of course, many occupational therapy interactions are not a contest. Rather, the therapist is seeking to work with the client. However, it may be necessary to persuade the client of certain goals that may be helpful to them. The client may need to advise the therapist. There are goals to be realized with other team members and there may be objectives for which the therapist has to form a team with the client or the carers. There are many possible conflicts and cooperation opportunities. This can be defined as achieving a good rapport with the client, but whether this always occurs can be questioned. The occupational therapist, it appears, sometimes makes choices about whether to serve the client or to serve the employing organization. These choices can be difficult to resolve and may not always be apparent, since the assessment of performance generally occurs within the context of appraisals conducted by the employing organization rather than the user of a service. The occupational therapist is therefore operating in a multiperspective environment – which we describe as a heteroglossic context – and needs to be able to develop the skills to navigate the conflict and cooperation situations it presents for both their own practice and the occupational choices open to their clients. In this context holistic practice does not arise from a static or fixed competence but depends on the ability continually to negotiate meanings, purposes, choices and processes.

The pADL and 3P archaeology tools are intended to enable therapists, perhaps in combination with their clients, to look at their political contexts independently. The actions taken on the basis of such analytical tools have to be carefully considered too. They offer a snapshot, not a long-term view. Political reasoning does not depend just on reviewing immediate information but on interpreting how that information may translate into future actions over time. For example, it may seem in the short term that it is appropriate to take immediate action, for example to stop interventions that are inadequately resourced, but this approach may make it difficult to maintain a rapport with other actors. A longer-term view may suggest that other actors can gradually be persuaded of an argument for more resources, even though this appears to compromise interventions that are currently being carried out.

This interpretative approach is described as occupational literacy, an ability to read the processes in which the individual or community is engaged. Successful navigation depends on a capacity to map the terrain with reasonable accuracy, but also to understand where the map is inaccurate. Occupational therapists often possess power by virtue of their professional status, but this is in turn compromised by the gendered nature of the profession in the patriarchal hegemonies in which they work and the consequences this has for being able to influence practice and the policies that determine practice. Consequently the occupational therapist has to navigate interests with clients, employers, colleagues and other professionals and professional bodies in order to maintain a position in which he or she can act at all. There is a line along which the professional walks between personal interest and altruism, between professional responsibilities and personal responsibilities, between the needs of the client and the needs of the institution, between what is needed and what can be allocated, and between what the rules allow and what can be wangled.

Unless we are able to maintain these balances, using the skills we have acquired both as professionals and as ordinary people, we will be unable to practise or engage with our clients. Our role as agents of social control is perhaps an inevitable consequence of this balance; therefore the path along this line has to be negotiated with conscientiousness, integrity and modesty. Above all, as occupational therapists, despite the enormous responsibilities posed by the concept of a holistic sense of human occupation, we have to remember that we are also merely human and occupational beings.

Theory

THEORY

This section of the book contains theoretical discussions to set out some of the foreground for a political practice of occupational therapy. The first chapter explores political aspects of human occupation. It sets out an examination of why political considerations apply to the contexts of occupational therapy practice and development, and considers ways in which they can be actively pursued through occupational therapy practice. The authors argue that while occupational science concepts such as occupational justice and concerns with issues such as occupational deprivation and apartheid are useful, some further development has to take place if they are to be applied in working situations. One of the principal difficulties is finding a way by which occupational therapists can incorporate the rhetoric of these terms into the constraints and realities of practice. If they are to be agents of social change, occupational therapists have to reconceptualize the basis from which they work. If occupational rights, i.e. the right to meaningful and purposeful occupation, is a goal for the profession, there has to be a critical examination of the alliances it makes. Occupational therapists have to consider whether they are the unquestioning implementers of policy as salaried employees of health and social care systems, or whether they can challenge the perpetuation of occupational injustices that result from the divide between government and experience.

The second chapter proposes a concept of political competence that may enable the navigation of these contexts. The tools offered here are not intended to be complicated but to offer the basis by which occupational therapists and the individuals and communities with whom they work can explore political aspects of the programmes they are developing together. An important part of these considerations is the location of personal motivation; a theme that follows through these chapters is a perspective that individual action is not disconnected from the whole and that responsibility is shared.

The final chapter in this section explores the concept of occupational literacy. This ability to read and interpret occupation as a process may serve to underpin a competency by enabling people to be aware of the political implications of what they do. Providing a means to make these issues explicit could become a means for empowerment and the negotiation of change. This term, first coined in the context of understanding work practices in industrial environments, is taken beyond its industrial birthplace and considered in the wider context of human occupations as having the potential to facilitate the interpretation of individual and collective action.

A political practice of occupational therapy

1

Nick Pollard, Frank Kronenberg,
Dikaios Sakellariou

Abstract

Occupational therapy is said to be based on the belief that there exists a universal and funda-mental relationship between people's dignified and meaningful participation in daily life and their experience of health, well-being and quality of life. However, who decides what occupa-tions are dignified and meaningful is not only culturally informed but is also probably politi-cally negotiated. This describes a practice of strategic engagement in conflict and cooperation situations that concern people's capacity and power to construct their destiny. It requires occupational therapists to view enabling access to meaningful occupation as a right, not just 'treatment' but a political endeavour. The purpose of this chapter is to explore meanings of politics in relation to occupational therapy and explain how this might be applied to activities of daily living. A set of key questions provides a framework for developing political reasoning within occupational therapy.

3

pADL

pADL is an acronym that stands for (small 'p') political activities of daily living. It emphasizes the need to develop and integrate political literacy and political engagement within occupational therapy education, practice and research. Strategic involvement in conflict and cooperation are the concern of pADL. The small 'p' in pADL distinguishes this *aspect* from the *domain* approach, which views 'Politics' (with a capital 'P') merely as a particular, defined sphere of human relationships, indicated by terms such as 'the state', 'government', 'public administration', or a political party. Our use of the small 'p' in this discussion refers to a politics that is not determined by party ideologies but by local conditions, the intricacies of accountability, interprofessional relationships, user and carer needs and individual motivations, issues that are often managerial concerns.

3P archaeology

3P archaeology describes an in-depth exploration of *p*ersonal, *p*rofessional and *p*olitical values (3Ps), which are seen as interrelated since each impacts on the others. Archaeology is concerned with finding and investigating cues from the past. A better understanding of one's occupational narrative in terms of these 3Ps enhances one's positioning to make informed decisions about objectives in the present. Engaging in 3P archaeology can allow one to come to terms with the conflict and cooperation situations that one is strategically to engage in. It is necessary to do this to put into practice what one stands for as a citizen and as a professional.

Introduction

Increasingly, occupational therapists are recognizing that there is a political component in the work that they do. For a long time, as allied health professionals, occupational therapists have perhaps tended to work towards a treatment process that has been defined by medicine (Pollard & Walsh 2000, Wilcock 2002; see Ch. 7), but this has often been difficult to reconcile with the knowledge that the causes and experience of disability are linked to social, economic and geopolitical conditions (Wilcock 2002). During the 2004 World Federation of Occupational Therapists (WFOT) Council meeting in Cape Town, occupational therapists agreed a position paper on community-based rehabilitation that recognized the systematic exclusions that prevent disabled people from realizing their right to meaningful occupation (see Ch. 5). The use of the term 'occupational apartheid' (World Federation of Occupational Therapists 2004, Kronenberg & Pollard 2005a; see Ch. 4) for these forms of exclusion derives from both the former South African political regime and the experiences of one of the authors in working with street children in Central America (Kronenberg 2005).

Enabling access to meaningful occupation as a right is not just treatment but a political endeavour. The purpose of this book is to explore the meaning of politics in relation to occupational therapy and explain how this might be applied to activities of daily living. It draws on the contemporary experience of occupational therapy practitioners and educators as well as political and historical literature to consider how a political understanding may be of value to the profession and its clients.

Occupational therapists have been concerned with problems arising from the social conditions of the people they have been working with, their families and communities throughout the history of the profession (Townsend 1993, Wilcock 2002). Many of the ideas that have informed current perspectives of the profession derive from an understanding of occupation that has its origins in socialist and utopian political philosophies of the 18th and 19th centuries (Wilcock 2001). The legacy of these philosophies has been powerful and includes tyrannies and revolutionary movements that continue to raise strong antipathies (Latey 1972). When using words that have become value-laden, such as 'social' and 'political', it is important to be clear that this is not a new reductionism (Galheigo 2005). Although occupational therapy may have, over much of its history, considered itself to be 'apolitical', politics is something that occurs everywhere, in all aspects of life (Vaneigem 1983, Tansey 2000, Van der Eijk 2001, Kronenberg & Pollard 2005b).

There is a worldwide change in occupational therapists' perception of their professional objectives. Two examples are the position statements of the World Federation of Occupational Therapists on community-based rehabilitation (2004) and human rights (2006), which gave prominence to the experiences of occupational apartheid, occupational injustice and occupational deprivation. In these, occupational therapists are urged to acknowledge meaningful occupation as a right and critically to explore occupations and disabling situations in their context.

This political consciousness has arisen at a time when many occupational therapists have become concerned about the political nature of the challenges they face in meeting the occupational needs of the people they work with. Occupational therapists have been recognizing extremes of poverty, occupational injustice (Townsend & Wilcock 2004) and occupational apartheid (Cage 2007), even in relatively wealthy states of Europe and North America. Occupational therapists are beginning to recognize the relationship between human occupation, global poverty and disabling conditions, and their professional organizations are attempting to facilitate their members in taking up this new direction (Wilcock 2002, Pollard et al 2005, Sanz Victoria & Garcia Rezio 2005, Kronenberg & Pollard 2006, Lawson Porter & Pollard 2006a,b). If occupational therapy is to live up to the holism that is often claimed for it, this entails the development and maintenance of a broad view of human complexity and a living interest in the diversity of cultures (see Chs 6, 7, 21).

Occupational therapists have a responsibility towards the enactment of occupation as a human right (World Federation of Occupational Therapists 2006). Community membership or citizenship is enabled through occupational justice. This doesn't just stop at the hospital exit but extends into the heart and soul of the communities we belong to ourselves.

The linking of occupation to citizenship and community participation requires an awareness of the political nature of occupational therapy. Many important political issues have their origins at the community level (Ward 1985, Tansey 2000), in the very issues and among the very strategies addressed by and through community-based rehabilitation (Kay & Dunleavy 1996, Edmonds & Peat 1997) and other approaches linked to health outcomes, such as community development (Pollard et al in press). These issues are often symptomatic of the systematic oppressions that create occupational apartheid and prompt occupational therapists to consider the relationship between rehabilitation and social change.

Knowledge and domination in occupational therapy

English-speaking discourses of knowledge have dominated the field of occupational therapy from its very outset (see Ch. 7). The Western or northern hemisphere domination of the dissemination of theory and practice may present some barriers to the exchange of knowledge in the profession and also to the development of an understanding of the complex contexts in which people live and occupy themselves (Kondo 2004, Iwama 2005, Odawara 2005).

The 2005 World Federation of Occupational Therapists survey of occupational therapists engaged in community-based rehabilitation, for example (Sakellariou et al 2006), revealed that therapists from southern hemisphere countries such as Colombia and South Africa tend to have longer community-based rehabilitation engagement than those from wealthier Western countries, often with established interventions supported by many local structures (Sakellariou & Pollard 2006, Sakellariou et al 2006, Pollard & Sakellariou 2007, 2008). The short-term involvement of expatriate therapists precludes an understanding of the cultural construction of occupation and disability in ways that could inform occupational therapy theory and practice.

Language presents a significant difficulty. Occupational therapy represents a small part of the international health science textbook market. The publishers of this book have informed us that a good target sales figure might be 4 500 copies worldwide. Breaking into this market from other languages, given the dominance of English as a teaching medium even where it is a second language, is difficult. There are relatively few occupational therapy texts available even in other major languages, such as Spanish, and certainly many fewer examples of articles or books originating in other languages being translated into English. Many therapists who speak English as a first language do not have good foreign language skills and come from countries where, as in the UK, there is a long established problem of a lack of facilities or emphasis on foreign language education (see Ch. 7). Occupational therapy education in many countries often requires students to access material in English, yet developments in professional practice, particularly in relation to approaches that recognize the issues associated with poverty alleviation, community-based rehabilitation or social approaches produced by these programmes are often set out in other languages. Despite initiatives such as the social occupational therapy developed in Brazil (Galheigo 2005) being well established, with a history dating back to the 1970s, these experiences have not until recently been available to the English language-dominated professional literature.

Understanding the political context of occupational therapy requires an open exchange of knowledge or a facility of curiosity that enables therapists and those they work with to acquire a functional awareness synthesis of the diverse perspectives they encounter in their practice (see Chs 3, 6, 7, 21). The current dominance of Western epistemologies in occupational therapy inhibits the development of culturally appropriate models of practice responding to local needs, or else restricts the exchange of knowledge. However, we do not suggest that one cultural perspective should be valued over the other.

'Community focused?'

'Community' is often perceived as a benign concept (Williams 1976) but it masks a range of differences drawn up on the lines of class, ethnicity, regionality and gender (Woodin 2005). Occupational therapists frequently belong to a different culture, class and sex (see Chs 5, 8–13, 15–20) from the one in which projects are being carried out, and terms such as 'social change' have to be used with caution. Social change is a phenomenon that operates at many levels within a society, traversing concepts such as cultural groups, class, generations and professional groups. The processes are not all completed simultaneously and many natural, geographical, economic and cultural as well as political factors may affect the outcomes (Skocpol 1980, Landman 2000).

In a profession concerned with human occupational activity, and therefore facilitating people in virtually all aspects of human life in which they want to participate, occupational therapists are at risk of taking on a greater range of knowledge than they (or anyone else) can really hope to assimilate. Even dominant occupational therapy perspectives have been made only partially available across language and cultural barriers, with consequent differences and confusions about the implementation of ideas in other localities (Kondo 2004, Iwama 2005, Odawara 2005).

Given these circumstances the dissemination of ideas is partial and generally one way. The distribution of knowledge and the accessibility of research and literature searching procedures favour a market in which the English language prevails. This produces exclusions, because people either cannot access knowledge or cannot share or distribute it. If the approach being implemented cannot address the needs of the person the therapist is working with, there is a danger that the therapist is actually operating a mechanism for exclusion rather than a technology for treatment. Resolution often requires an adaptation, based in local needs (Kondo 2004). Therefore the term 'rehabilitation' is not always useful where it applies to communities if it is associated with the acceptance of values or compliance with a 'normality' that may not actually be shared.

Occupational apartheid is about systematic exclusion. Confronting situations and approaches that perpetuate it are, we suggest, at the heart and soul of occupational therapy practice. Every society contains invisible voices, whether street children or psychiatric survivors, voices of people who are marginalized through race, culture, disability, sex, economics or educational level, and often, through their concern with human activity, occupational therapists and other health and social care professionals are concerned with eliciting these narratives in order to work out solutions to their problems. Invisibility can occur whether or not facilities exist to address a particular issue. Workers attached to services may not be sufficiently empowered to obtain the resources they need, or problems may be ignored simply because they are not heard at all and no agency exists to address them.

It is inevitable that those who have wealth seek to isolate themselves from the poor. They protect their lifestyles through security measures and high prices, which insulate them from the daily awareness of deprivation, even though their wealth is generally obtained at the expense of others' impoverishment. Thus people may physically live in close proximity with each other but be unaware of the occupational nature of each other's lives (Putnam 2000, Galvaan 2005). The opportunities for exploring each other's narratives may be there but require active mediation to evolve into a conscientious consciousness.

The development of political skills and awareness: politics as a human occupation

In the opening chapter of our previous book (Kronenberg & Pollard 2005b), we set out a series of principles. One of these is that 'everybody is responsible for everything'. This does not mean that occupational therapy should include every dimension of every occupational problem. Instead what it suggests is a principle of contiguity, of interconnectivity between all people, something that is entirely compatible with the feminine origins of the profession and with the best of its practice (Pollard & Walsh 2000). This contiguity is something that cannot be insular but of its nature must reach out and connect, just as individuals must recognize the connection they have with the community and society around them.

This process of making connections is something that begins very early on in human life. In early infancy a child is entirely focused on its own needs, perceiving its mother almost as an extension of itself (Winnicott 1992). Later it begins to recognize that its mother is absent at times but returns at others, and that it can survive and continue independently in the gaps in her presence (Winnicott 1990, Bowlby 1992). The child becomes aware of its separate existence, becomes increasingly self-reliant, sustaining an understanding of its continuous existence by symbolizing the presence of its mother through a transitional object, such as a blanket or comforter.

Children soon acquire attachments to other aspects of their environment, regular routines and preferences (Bowlby 1992). They seek to maintain the security that these routines give them, demanding that Mummy, not Daddy, reads the bedtime story but on occasion, because it is a novelty, that Daddy, not Mummy, reads the bedtime story. These are early experiments with power and influence. 'I want Mummy' is a statement of need but it can also be a political statement if, for example, Daddy has just reprimanded the child and it hopes that Mummy will contradict Daddy's admonishment. Mummy and Daddy inevitably differ, no matter how much they may try to cooperate to offer consistent parenting, and from this the child will learn about situations where it can try and produce conflicts – for example to get the sweets that the other parent has said should wait till after mealtime, 'But Mummy said I could have them'.

If we reflect, we can all remember employing childhood experiments like this to obtain the things we wanted. Often we found that, by observing certain rules, adopting pieces of etiquette like saying 'please' or performing some household chore without being asked, we could ensure favourable conditions for some requests through cooperation. In other situations making a fuss might obtain a concession to keep us quiet. Learning which methods were best and when they might be most effective formed part of the acquisition of social skills and also entailed the germ of a political ability. This ability has perhaps been described by Berne (1968, 1975) as complementary transaction in human relationships, the ability to use a script or a plan successfully to negotiate the satisfaction and exchange of needs with others.

Everyone, therefore, acquires the ability to operate within their local sphere as a 'politician', motivated by interests that relate to their particular needs but are shaped by their particular experience. This use of the term 'politics' is rather wider than the limited sense that applies to issues of government or the definition of ideas about policy. In Berne's theory of transactional analysis (1968), the games people play are largely at an unconscious level, although some motivations may be clear. Players of political games are generally more explicit in identifying, at least to themselves, their strategic goals. As we shall explore, political ideas extend from personal interests to having a global, as well as a local, impact and are realized in the means we have as individuals to pursue our daily occupations (Wicks & Whiteford 2005). Just as Berne used the idea of games to explore human relationships, it is sometimes possible to analyse larger political movements in terms of games. Landman (2000) explores the late 20th century transitions to democracy in Poland, Russia and Portugal in which actors in political factions employed clear tactics to develop their desired outcomes through strategic moves, as in a game of chess.

Politics is thus a human occupation and the skills and components from which it is composed are developed over time, both through the rites of passage that make up personal development and through the historical process through which societies develop (Wilcock 1998, 2001, Fernández-Armesto 2000). The nature of society is itself determined by the way in which people occupy raw territory and the tasks that are necessary for people to maintain themselves in the environments in which they settle, including conflict and cooperation with neighbouring societies (Fernández-Armesto 2000, Landman 2000; see Chs 10, 20). The interrelationship between human occupation and the fundamental basis of politics is therefore a very significant one, which is realized through the ability of individuals to participate in community activities at every level of society. Political activities therefore can range from highly localized individual or community issues through to matters of global significance (Ward 1985, Landman 2000, Wicks & Whiteford 2005). Sometimes individual issues can have a powerful enough effect, as a popular symbol for particular causes, to exert a global influence. Similarly, wider events, the fallout from decisions made at the domain level, impact on the occupations of individuals – for example where they find themselves living near nuclear radiation or pollution hazards and are consequently shunned as a potential source of contamination (Kasperson et al 2001).

Tools for political reasoning

To address this kind of complexity we have derived a framework for political reasoning from the work of Van der Eijk (2001). Van der Eijk describes 'politics' as being classifiable into two main types, the *aspect* approach and the *domain* approach. The aspect approach acknowledges the presence of politics in every facet of life and human interaction. It implies that politics is present in the tensions between conflict and cooperation in almost every human occupation and human relationship. Van der Eijk (2001) explains that conflict and cooperation provide the motor for all political engagement and, since this provides the motivating principle for action, neither should be regarded as necessarily good or bad. Conflict and cooperation are the concern of political activities of daily living (pADL) (Kronenberg & Pollard 2005a). The lower-case 'p' in pADL distinguishes this *aspect* from the *domain* approach which views 'Politics' (with a capital 'P') merely as a particular, defined sphere of human relationships, indicated by terms such as 'the state', 'government', 'public administration' or a political party.

In participating in domain politics, politicians, political functionaries and the apparatus of government and administration are also practising aspect politics, or pADL. This may frequently be observed in political diaries, where individuals record their personal relationships with their professional colleagues. Clearly in the behaviours that arise from the interaction of political figures at a personal and aspect level there is an interaction that both affects and is affected by larger domain issues such as international conflict, cabinet changes or the development of new policies (e.g. Luthuli 1963, Clark 1994, Howe 1994, Mandela 1995, Thatcher 1995a, Gorbachev 1997, Major 1999, Guevara 2001, Currie 2002, Mowlam 2002, Blumenthal 2004). Similarly, the behavioural styles and actions of politicians are frequently linked to experiences in their early lives, for example the relationships that Iain Macleod (Shepherd 1994), Edward Heath (Campbell 1993), Harold Macmillan (Davenport-Hines 1992) and Fidel Castro (Thomas 1986, Szulc 1989) had with their parents, as they occasionally admit themselves (Thatcher 1995a,b). The conduct of politics is not something removed from personal behavioural styles.

Earlier political theories have discussed the conflicts or cooperation of political forces as being engineered or motivated by classes but more recently theorists have argued that this analysis does not take account of the evidence of complexity, of the action of groups within classes, of factions and even individuals (Skocpol 1980). In other words, conflict and cooperation arise from the occupational histories of the various individuals involved (Beagan 2007; see Ch. 5). Political processes are a human occupation, the rich product of occupational behaviours and performances in particular environments. Although often not specifically mentioned in the theoretical models of occupational therapy, they are an important element of the social and cultural aspects that are incorporated in them, particularly where they concern issues around justice. There is a need to lobby for better resources and further developments in health and social care policy (Barbara & Whiteford 2005). To do this, and get the resources to meet the needs of the people they're working with, occupational therapists need to embrace a deeper political awareness and the facility to employ political argument. In her account of the management of peace negotiations in Northern Ireland, Mowlam (2002) describes the personal and reflective approach she used, stressing values such as honesty and clarity but, above all, using her person as a means to gain rapport with those on differing sides. Irrespective of political stance or professional standing, individual personality is a vital element in the way objectives are attained.

If the characteristics of individuals are key to the way they employ their abilities in political occupations, then it follows that political ideology cannot be fixed. Its interpretation often depends on individual factors, just as again we might see in the history of the Russian Revolution and the differences between the key protagonists both before and after (Latey 1972, Lenin 1976, 1988, Trotsky 1977) or the conservative governments of the later part of the last century (Campbell 1993, Thatcher 1995a, Major 1999). As the pADL reasoning tool identifies, other political variations can occur according to the aims, motives, interests and contextual factors involving the actors. These can range from limitations to means in terms of physical resources as well as limitations in perception and ability on the part of those carrying out actions (Pugh 1994) or the perception that mistakes are being made, as revealed by the marked policy shifts in some socialist dictatorships (Skocpol 1980, Thomas 1986).

These shifts in ideology and the aims, motives and interests, or even the perceptions, are not always admitted or, conversely, are admitted when in fact there hasn't been a shift, or a clear ideology may not actually exist, as was claimed of the UK Conservative Party during the 1980s (Honderich 1991). There had been a 'one nation' consensus policy in the late 1960s and early 1970s based on a mixed economy (i.e. a combination of private and state-run businesses) under Ted Heath but an ideological shift led to the emergence of a tougher, market-determined approach under Margaret Thatcher. It was later acknowledged that Heath was the architect of Thatcherism – but could not put it into effect. The perception that remains is that Thatcher commanded the determination to carry this policy out and is associated with it, whereas Heath lacked the opportunity and the power to do so (Campbell 1993). Such phenomena may not be fully apparent until a historical process has taken place. The cause and effect of political events is not always apparent to participants at the time, even when these actors are driving the strategy. Truth is relative and history a matter of debate.

The search for evidence in evidence-based practice suffers a similar limitation if it is to be used in constructing models. Models have a limited usefulness and, if too rigid, cannot be adapted to meet the inevitable shifts in circumstances that occur between conception and the experience of application. Practice that is client-centred and negotiated locally is going to vary widely in definition, as is clear in explanations of multidisciplinary practices in mental health (Lloyd et al 2004) or community-based rehabilitation (Fransen 2005). When people work in different teams there may be a tension between the core values they hold in one team and the ability to practise in the same way in another (Lloyd et al 2004).

Models offer a framework for analysis but the therapist is a political actor and has to develop a flexible critical awareness. Despite hierarchies of evidence and the weight of precedence, therapists need to maintain their individual critical judgement based on their own experience if they are to be an effective tool, and must be able to argue for this approach, based on their own reflective practice and in consultation with the others with whom they are working. This is part of the negotiating environment in which therapists work, whether implementing programmes with clients or discussing strategies with other team members. Change is not driven by evidence unless it matches local experience. If they are to be useful, models are not static and have to be adapted to fit local needs as well as matching global considerations.

Professional knowledge and experience and a further set of lay knowledge and experience are built up in the process of treatment. Occupational therapists, like all other people delivering specialized services, have to negotiate the border between professional and lay expertise, the community knowledge base and the expertise that disabled people and their carers have about their own conditions and needs. Often, through professional standards, the means of evaluating evidence are supplied from sources external to a local situation, and the evaluation, the perceptions and the solutions will not accommodate local needs unless local people themselves are engaged in their interpretation.

The authors describe this kind of relationship as the 3P dialectic triangle, one of the tools for developing a competence in political reasoning. The 3P archaeology process explores political values (and even the absence of political values is 'political') as a consequence of personal motivation and their professional enactment. It is termed 'archaeology' because unravelling the links between these components requires an in-depth self-questioning investigation of one's values and actions to put these into practice (Fig. 1.1).

The three corners of the triangle represent the Political, Professional and Personal components of the perception that actors take of themselves and events around them. Again, each of the three Ps is interdependent, as the shape of the perception depends on all three elements being present. However actors consider the circumstances of which they are part, each takes a different personal perspective, according to their different political and professional experiences and interests. This means that people have to perform a process of 'personal archaeology' and explore how these perceptions have developed. We suggest that the interaction of these dimensions colours the way we see the world, as if through 3P glasses (Fig. 1.1). We have to know how our 3P glasses affect our perception of both the events around us and the behaviours we adopt to pursue our goals.

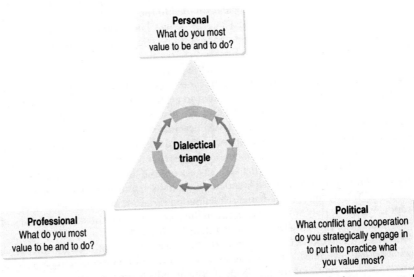

Figure 1.1 ● The process of 3P archaeology. In-depth exploration of who we are and what we stand (up) for at three interrelated levels.

Personal, professional and political

The dialectical triangle depicts the personal, professional and political elements of a developmental process. Just as the self is a therapeutic tool for the therapy professional (Hagedorn 2000), personal resources often determine the individual basis for community engagement. For many people it is difficult to acknowledge the political aspect of this and there are legitimate concerns about politicizing the profession through activism.

This problem extends into the issue of recognizing not only the political nature of the occupational therapy profession but also the political issues within the profession, for example the tensions that affect the relationship between qualified and unqualified staff or the function of the occupational therapist's role as an agent of social control (Pollard & Walsh 2000, Hammell 2007, Mackey 2007). It is, more fundamentally, an aspect of being a predominantly female profession, concerned with daily activities but leaving them behind in favour of those interventions that are more overtly science-based since the route to power and influence lies in being allied to the male dominant mode of medicine (see Chs 5, 7). Deeper still, it is an aspect of being feminine in that women are not expected to express themselves politically, or, if they do, are dismissed or belittled (Thatcher 1995a, Mowlam 2002). Finally, politics have not traditionally been regarded as a subject of polite conversation due to the potential to offend, or bore, others (Sproule 1981). Despite the popularity of political issues as a media topic, any expression of in-depth interest is often perceived as hectoring and frequently descends to be so.

This book is not a blunt instrument of the Popular Front for Occupational Therapy. Our use of the small 'p' in this discussion refers to a politics that is not determined by party ideologies but local conditions, the intricacies of accountability, interprofessional relationships, user and carer needs and individual motivations, issues that are often managerial concerns (Owen 2002, Stewart 2007). This small p also occurs in *partnership* and in the local focus of *practice*. It is a small p that reflects the *personal rapport* on which partnership and practice at this level depend. The small p offers just one key to open up some of the important mystery boxes in the context of occupational therapy as a complex intervention.

The dialectical triangle, therefore, involves the personal in the political and vice versa. In other words, the dialectical triangle enables therapists and others to see, think and act critically with awareness from these three interrelated perspectives.

Political activities of daily living

In order to achieve goals, actors have to determine how they can cooperate with other actors to obtain them. In the pursuit of these goals, for example the right of occupational therapists to occupational justice, it is quite possible that the territorial occupation of certain aspects of professional status may result in occupational injustices for others. Professional peers and clients may find the rights they previously enjoyed are now compromised by changes.

Politics is concerned with the development of conflicts between groups of people, cooperative strategies to influence the outcome in one or another group's desired direction, and the resolution of conflict (Kronenberg & Pollard 2005a). To determine the political nature of a situation one can ask a set of specific questions, set out in the 'pADL reasoning tool' box. The answer to any pADL question will have implications for the other interrelated and interdependent questions. The pADL framework therefore recognizes the dynamic impact of gains in knowledge and information in the shaping of human occupation and activities of daily living. It is intended to raise awareness of the context in which decisions are made, whether by individuals or through negotiations between groups of actors.

pADL (political activities of daily living) reasoning tool

1. What are the characteristics of the conflict and cooperation situation?
2. Who are the actors?
3. How do the actors conduct themselves? What are their aims, interests, motives, perceptions and attitudes?
4. What are their means?
5. What does the political landscape look like?
6. What is the broader context for conflict and cooperation?

What are the characteristics of the conflict and cooperation situation?

Often very different situations appear to share characteristics: aspects of conflict and cooperation at local level are to be found at domain level in national and international issues, conflicts at a local level such as personal conflicts between individuals and the departments they run within political administrations can also affect the enactment of policy, as has frequently been asserted in accounts of government (e.g. Brogan 1990, Healey 1990, Honderich 1991, Davenport-Hines 1992, Cole 1995, Gorbachev 1997, Blumenthal 2004). They can provide models for explaining the origin and interrelationships of different factors and develop a general understanding of political situations. This enables us to make sensible predictions and set realistic outcomes.

Who are the actors?

Situations of conflict are often based in exclusion yet they can sometimes be met through cooperation with actors, who are often part of the excluding and marginalizing apparatus (Mandela 1995, Landman 2000, Mowlam 2002). One reason for this is that the excluded can eventually become part of the threat to the stability of the interests that those in power and operating the exclusions wish to preserve (Skocpol 1980, Mandela 1995, Landman 2000). Because they are institutions, whether publicly or privately funded, health care services are often unintentionally part of this process because of the part they play in providing for the needs and rights of citizens. Health care services and the people they work with can be described as actors, but when we ask the question, 'Who are the actors?', pADL reasoning is concerned not so much with actors but with the conflicts and cooperations that develop between them, between one occupational situation and the next. This question could be reworded as, 'Who is whose ally, partner or opponent?'. Actors cooperate in some areas and conflict in others according to their interests and the particular occupational goals they are trying to realize. Since each actor's goals are specific to them, it follows that allies or partners do not agree on everything but will provide a source of power and influence for each other through cooperation in conflict situations with other actors if their interests coincide, as can be explored through the next pADL question (Kronenberg & Pollard 2005a).

Actors may be people within the institutions or other agencies with a relationship to a project. Such a relationship may concern the allocation of funding or enabling of access to resources. The actors may include all the people involved: service users, an occupational therapist, adult educator, support workers, volunteers and additional others including, for example, people like the readers of this book. As part of their continuing need for leverage with local managers, and as dictated by the ethics of a continuing research process, these actors may have discussion of their activities regularly disseminated to an audience in the form of articles, papers or book chapters. All these individuals and the agencies to which they belong are interlinked through a complex nexus of occupational goals and motivations. An inter-meshing of purposes makes it difficult to extricate one aspect of this without considering how it is dependent on others: 'Everybody is responsible for everything.'

How do the actors conduct themselves? What are their aims, interests, motives, perceptions and attitudes?

There can be many aims, motives and interests not only for each actor but also shared between actors, producing a complex interplay of conflict and cooperation. *Aims* refers to the objec-tives for which the actors are consciously striving, *motives* refers to desires the actors may have but do not outwardly express and *interests* refers to what actors strive for consciously in a way that is clear to others (Kronenberg & Pollard 2005a). We need to recognize the aims, interests and motives of the actors in any situation in order to get an idea of what they are trying to achieve.

Each of the groups involved in a project will have their own aims, motives and interests, thus increasing the likelihood of conflict but also different opportunities for cooperation. Actors have to learn from each other to find new ways of defining their roles, for example as practitioners or patients. Where actors are able to cooperate they may work to recognize and reduce barriers, such as traditional or even professional practices, that inhibit their human interaction. They may realize new possibilities and exercise these both for themselves and for the development of the groups to which they belong through working together (Werner 1998). Many of the 'occupational spin-offs' (Rebeiro & Cook 1999) that arise from this kind of activity are derived from the range of aims, motives and interests that can be met through a project.

In order to understand the actors' political behaviour, besides investigating their aims, interests and motives one must also take note of their perceptions and attitudes. This includes the 'logic' that the actors employ with their goal-oriented behaviour. And it doesn't matter if this logic is fact or fantasy, complete or incomplete. It is simply based on how one thinks that the world functions and it can include one's preferred political and economic ideologies and religious beliefs. This subjective logic forms the basis for each actor's assessment of situ-ations in terms of risk and the possibilities for the realization, costs and benefits of goals, just as therapists must account for risk and benefit in making use of occupations. It is particularly important to consider the actors' attitudes towards themselves, towards others, towards power and authority, etc. (Van der Eijk 2001) when attempting to understand their political con-duct. All these estimations and expectations form the basis for an actor's decisions and actions (Kronenberg & Pollard 2005a).

What are their means?

This key question is concerned with influence, power and related notions. *Influence* is the capacity of actors to determine or change the availability to other actors of a range of behav-iours or choices. *Power* is often viewed as the capacity of actors to determine or change the behaviours or choices of others.

The capacity indicated by the term *power* is based on:

- the means of power, including force and coercion; *means* refers to everything that actors can use to realize their political aims in conflict and cooperation situations
- the resources of power, such as connections, money, information or means of communication (Van der Eijk 2001).

Asking the question 'What are their means?' facilitates an understanding of where actors' power comes from and what kind of power results from their means. 'Means' refers to any-thing that may be turned to the actors' advantage, including other actors, as well as resources and opportunities (Werner 1998).

Where does occupational therapists' power come from? What are occupational therapists' means? Often when working with disabled people, for example in community-based rehabilitation situations, practitioners can be led to suppose that there are no means other than the skills the therapist has brought with them. Similarly, disabled people can be persuaded that they have no means other than the solutions being offered by others. This is why it is often important to tap into the power of human occupation that everyone possesses (Kronenberg & Pollard 2006), through the exchange of narratives and experience (Werner 1998, Galvaan 2005, Simó Algado & Cardona 2005). What emerges from this is an occupational literacy (see Ch. 3), a reading of the stories that individuals share about themselves, their communities and what has happened to them in a way that begins to offer solutions around which cooperation can be built, or conflicts can be resolved (Werner 1998). Determining whether these solutions will work needs a more in-depth exploration of the systems through which they will have to be enacted (Landman 2000). All the actors, whether practitioners or other participants in projects, need to develop an understanding of these political landscapes and what is possible in them.

What does the political landscape look like?

Conflict and cooperation take place within political systems. How they arise and develop is partly dependent on the organization of the system, which includes, among other things, institutions and rules. Political institutions are more or less established forms for the organization of behaviour. They include:

* concrete institutions, such as the British House of Commons, professional occupational therapy associations such as the American Occupational Therapy Association or the British College of Occupational Therapists
* procedural institutions, such as regular and free democratic elections, annual general meetings.

Rules are codes for the political methods that are permitted or appropriate in conflict and cooperation. In the arena of politics rules are not laws but are often vague; there is no external referee. Rules thus present an important source of conflict and cooperation. They are a significant area of political interest, as just a few examples from the history of UK and US governments show. The disputes over questions of loyalty that produced cabinet shuffles during Thatcher's administration (Clark 1994, Howe 1994, Thatcher 1995a, Major 1999), the rapid transition to independence of African states in the British Empire driven by economic considerations over ideas of colonial responsibility (Healey 1990, Davenport-Hines 1992, Shepherd 1994), the conduct of the peace process in Northern Ireland (Mowlam 2002) and attempts to suborn legal processes to political power in the USA during the Nixon and Clinton administrations (Brogan 1990, Blumenthal 2004) were all critical issues in which 'rules' were breached. In each of these situations factional groups of individuals attempted to work around other groups in order to satisfy particular objectives in which they had an interest. Where rules were operated by one group to consolidate power or obstruct objectives, other groups used differing interpretations of them or developed internal rules to bind members of their own faction into protecting their interests. Knowledge of how rules are continuously subject to change and reinterpretation enables participants better to understand and deal with situations of conflict and cooperation (Kronenberg & Pollard 2005a).

These nuances of domain politics also occur in the political circumstances of local environments. The degree of professional autonomy held by occupational therapists varies across the world's different health systems. Simmond (2005) found that, simply because she was a Westerner in Vietnam, she was expected by local people to find solutions to issues that were beyond her professional remit as an occupational therapist. This demand was the product of different cultural perceptions of the roles of health professionals. Although Simmond could not accept these responsibilities, her being unable to do so was at first perceived as undermining her professional ability. This made it difficult to set boundaries about how much she was capable of doing or what could reasonably be expected of her. In such situations thwarting some of these expectations (e.g. by arguing that one's own professional rules allow you to practise in certain ways but not others) may create temporary difficulties and appear to transgress local rules but leads to a further point of negotiation in asking the question: What is the broader context for conflict and cooperation?

What is the broader context for conflict and cooperation?

Politics is not a spare-time or academic occupation. If, as the feminist adage has it, the personal is the political, individuals have to pay attention to this question in order to see how their individual perspectives fit into the wider social and occupational environment (Wilcock 1998). As Chapparo and Ranka (1997) suggest, this environment contains many interlocking and also conflicting elements. Although apparently simple, this question is one that is never completely answered. Instead, actors develop an experiential picture over time.

Community-based rehabilitation projects are often dependent on many factors, not the least of which may be having to work across different languages and cultures and different social practices while maintaining efficiency and negotiating needs and solutions. A local embarrassment might have significant implications for the future development of projects and the people they are intended to reach.

In the development of psychiatric services occupational therapists may find that there are clients who have complex needs arising from their culture, condition and personal circumstances. New arrangements have to be worked out to meet the requirements of each individual, often against the background of changes in service definitions, social benefits and facilities.

Conclusion

Occupational therapists work in diverse and multivariate arenas, some of which, such as those in community-based rehabilitation projects, are themselves subject to many interpretations (Fransen 2005) or to the rapid development of new specialisms, as in several Western health environments (Lloyd et al 2004, Whiteford 2005). In the broader context in which we live there are many challenges, which have multiple causes and effects. In recent years we have become acutely aware of disasters that appear to be linked to environmental changes, such as the increase in tropical storms in the Gulf of Mexico and the Caribbean and the extensive famines of central Africa. In their turn they are indicative, if only in the difference in the levels of aid given to American storm victims and those on the other side of the Atlantic in Africa, of the rising global divergence between wealth and poverty. Poverty is recognized as one of the key issues in determining life quality and opportunities to reduce the impact of disability, but an applied and lasting solution is difficult to achieve. The sheer number and different mechanisms of the agencies involved both suggest and present numerous challenges in themselves. Obtaining efficacy is difficult in the resulting confusion.

For example in the wake of hurricane Katrina in 2005, some occupational therapist colleagues in the USA were told that because they were not 'certified mental health professionals' they were legally unable to offer assistance to some of the displaced and very distressed people with whom services had not yet engaged. These occupational therapists were local to that situation and so were directly available. On the other hand it is arguable that the occupational therapist role is more usefully applied as a secondary resource – in community-based rehabilitation and other strategies of follow-up – rather than in acute disaster intervention.

The experience of hurricane Katrina in 2005 refocused attention on the differences in quality of life and opportunities within the USA, but conflict and disaster have displaced communities all over the globe and it is anticipated that, through population growth, increased demands on the environment and failure to manage ecological damage these problems will increase (Voss & Hidajat 2002, De Souza 2004). Even in the wealthiest communities there are well established intergenerational pockets of extreme poverty. For example, life expectancy in the UK varies by as much as 10 years in neighbouring communities (Shaw et al 2005).

The application of a pADL reasoning tool and the recognition of the political in everyday life will not by itself address these complex problems. Finding community solutions through negotiation with all the actors involved, working with conflict and cooperation requires an approach that takes account of the impact of political factors on human occupation as one element in a diverse context. If occupational therapists are to take on an understanding of a right to meaningful occupation through such terms as occupational justice, occupational deprivation and occupational apartheid as the basis for the negotiation of community-based rehabilitation projects (World Federation of Occupational Therapists 2004), then occupational therapy will not only be 'one of the Great Ideas of the Twentieth Century' (Reilly 1962, p. 1) but may perhaps offer some strategies for the uncertainties of this millennium.

It is important to make clear that we are not suggesting an ideological approach through our concern with the political, but a means for reading political complexity. It is when attempts are made to translate an ideology from one context to another without concession to historical, social, cultural and other local differences that problems and even catastrophes arise (Latey 1972, Skocpol 1980), just as we have explored the difficulties that arise through the translation of occupational therapy models and approaches (Kondo 2004, Iwama 2005, Odawara 2005). The last century was replete with these, whether the export of political revolution or economic policy. The Cuban revolution did not provide a model that could be easily exported, as Guevara found in Congo and Bolivia (Guevara 1975, 2001, Thomas 1986). For example, the history of Cuba and that of the UK under Thatcher have both been depicted as dangerous adventurism and oversimplification, in which adherence to ideology created severe problems (Thomas 1986, Campbell 1993, Pugh 1994). A political literacy can at best enable only a partial reading of any situation, because of the simple problem that it is never possible to know what everyone else is thinking, even with historical hindsight.

References

Barbara A, Whiteford G 2005 The legislative and policy context of practice. In: Whiteford G, Wright-St Clair V (eds) Occupation & practice in context. Elsevier Churchill Livingstone, Marrickville, New South Wales: p 332–348

Beagan B L 2007 Experiences of social class: learning from occupational therapy students. Canadian Journal of Occupational Therapy 74: 125–133

Berne E 1968 Games people play. Penguin, Harmondsworth

Berne E 1975 What do you say after you say hello? Corgi Books, London

Blumenthal S 2004 The Clinton wars. Penguin, Harmondsworth

Bowlby J 1992 The making and breaking of affectional bonds. Routledge, London

Brogan H 1990 The Penguin history of the United States of America. Penguin, Harmondsworth

Cage A 2007 Occupational therapy with women and children survivors of domestic violence: are we fulfilling our activist heritage? A review of the literature. British Journal of Occupational Therapy 70: 192–198

Campbell J 1993 Edward Heath. Jonathan Cape, London

Chapparo C, Ranka J 1997 Occupational performance model (Australia), monograph 1. Total Print Control, Sydney. Available online at: http://www.occupationalperformance.com/index.php/au/home/structure: accessed 19 October 2007

Clark A 1994 Diaries. Phoenix, London

Cole J 1995 As it seemed to me. Weidenfeld & Nicholson, London

Currie E 2002 Diaries 1987–1992. Little, Brown, London

Davenport-Hines R 1992 The Macmillans. Heinemann, London

De Souza R M (2004) In harm's way: hurricanes, population trends, and environmental change. Population Reference Bureau. Available online at: http://www.prb.org/articles/2004/InHarmsWayHurricanesPopulationTrendsandEnvironmentalChange.aspx: accessed 19 October 2007

Edmonds L J, Peat M 1997 Community based rehabilitation (CBR) and health reform: a timely strategy. Canadian Journal of Rehabilitation 10: 273–283

Fernández-Armesto F 2000 Civilizations. Macmillan, London

Fransen H 2005 Challenges for occupational therapy in community based rehabilitation. In: Kronenberg F, Simó Algado S, Pollard N (eds) Occupational therapy without borders. Elsevier Churchill Livingstone, Oxford: p 166–182

Galheigo S 2005 Occupational therapy and the social field: clarifying concepts and ideas. In: Kronenberg F, Simó Algado S, Pollard N (eds) Occupational therapy without borders. Elsevier Churchill Livingstone, Oxford: p 87–98

Galvaan R 2005 Domestic workers' narratives: transforming occupational therapy practice. In: Kronenberg F, Simó Algado S, Pollard N (eds) Occupational therapy without borders. Elsevier Churchill Livingstone, Oxford: p 443–454

Gorbachev M 1997 Memoirs. Bantam, London

Guevara E 1975 The secret papers of a revolutionary: the diary of Che Guevara. American Reprint Company, New York

Guevara E 2001 The African dream: the diaries of the revolutionary war in the Congo. Grove Press, New York

Hagedorn R 2000 Tools for practice in occupational therapy. Churchill Livingstone, Edinburgh

Hammell K W 2007 Client-centred practice: ethical obligation or professional obfuscation? British Journal of Occupational Therapy 70: 264–266

Healey D 1990 The time of my life. Penguin, Harmondsworth

Honderich T 1991 Conservatism. Penguin, Harmondsworth

Howe G 1994 Conflict of loyalty. Macmillan, London

Iwama M K 2005 Situated meaning, an issue of culture, inclusion, and occupational therapy. In: Kronenberg F, Simó Algado S, Pollard N (eds) Occupational therapy without borders. Elsevier Churchill Livingstone, Oxford: p 127–139

Kasperson R E, Jhaveri N, Kasperson J X 2001 Stigma and the social amplification of risk: toward a framework of analysis. In: Flynn J, Slovic P, Kunreuther H (eds) Risk, media and stigma. Earthscan, London: p 9–27

Kay E, Dunleavy K 1996 Community-based rehabilitation: an international model. Pediatric Physical Therapy 8: 117–121

Kondo T 2004 Cultural tensions in occupational therapy practice: considerations from a Japanese view-point. American Journal of Occupational Therapy 58: 174–184

Kronenberg F 2005 Occupational therapy with street children. In: Kronenberg F, Simó Algado S, Pollard N (eds) Occupational therapy without borders. Elsevier Churchill Livingstone, Oxford: p 269–284

Kronenberg F, Pollard N 2005a Overcoming occupational apartheid, a preliminary exploration of the political nature of occupational therapy. In: Kronenberg F, Simó Algado S, Pollard N (eds) Occupational therapy without borders. Elsevier Churchill Livingstone, Oxford: p 58–86

Kronenberg F, Pollard N 2005b Introduction, a beginning… In: Kronenberg F, Simó Algado S, Pollard N (eds) Occupational therapy without borders. Elsevier Churchill Livingstone, Oxford: p 1–13

Kronenberg F, Pollard N 2006 Political dimensions of occupation and the roles of occupational therapy (AOTA Plenary Presentation, 2006). American Journal of Occupational Therapy 60: 617–625

Landman T 2000 Issues and methods in comparative politics. Routledge, London

Latey M 1972 Tyranny: a study in the abuse of power. Pelican, Harmondsworth

Lawson Porter A, Pollard N 2006a Think, consider and convey. Part I. Occupational Therapy News 14(1): 20

Lawson Porter A, Pollard N 2006b Think, consider and convey. Part II. Occupational Therapy News 14(2): 28

Lenin V I 1976 One step forward, two steps back. Foreign Languages Press, Beijing

Lenin V I 1988 What is to be done? Penguin, Harmondsworth

Lloyd C, King R, McKenna K 2004 Actual and preferred work activities of mental health occupational therapists: congruence or discrepancy? British Journal of Occupational Therapy 67: 167–175

Luthuli A 1963 Let my people go. Fontana, London

Mackey H 2007 'Do not ask me to remain the same': Foucault and the professional identities of occupational therapists. Australian Occupational Therapy Journal 54: 95–102

Major J 1999 The autobiography. Harper Collins, London

Mandela N 1995 Long walk to freedom. Abacus, London

Mowlam M 2002 Momentum. Hodder & Stoughton, London

Odawara E 2005 Cultural competency in occupational therapy: beyond a cross-cultural view of practice. American Journal of Occupational Therapy 59: 325–334

Owen J 2002 Management stripped bare. Kogan Page, London

Pollard N, Sakellariou D 2007 Occupation, education and community-based rehabilitation. British Journal of Occupational Therapy 70: 171–174

Pollard N, Sakellariou D 2008 Operationalizing community participation in community-based rehabilitation: exploring the factors. Disability and Rehabilitation 30: 62–70

Pollard N, Walsh S 2000 Occupational therapy, gender and mental health: an inclusive perspective? British Journal of Occupational Therapy 63: 425–431

Pollard N, Alsop A, Kronenberg F 2005 Reconceptualising occupational therapy. British Journal of Occupational Therapy 68: 524–526

Pollard N, Sakellariou D, Kronenberg F (in press) Community development. In: Molineux M, Curtin M, Supyk J (eds) Occupational therapy and physical dysfunction, 6th edn. Elsevier Science, Oxford

Pugh M 1994 State and society: British political and social history 1870–1992. Arnold, London

Putnam R 2000 Bowling alone, the collapse and revival of American community. Simon & Schuster, New York

Rebeiro K L, Cook J V 1999 Opportunity, not prescription: an exploratory study of the experience of occupational engagement. Canadian Journal of Occupational Therapy 66: 176–187

Reilly M 1962 Occupational therapy can be one of the great ideas of the twentieth century. American Journal of Occupational Therapy 16: 1–9

Sakellariou D, Pollard N 2006 Rehabilitation: in the community or with the community. British Journal of Occupational Therapy 69: 562–567

Sakellariou D, Pollard N, Fransen H, Kronenberg F, Sinclair K 2006 Reporting on the WFOT-CBR master project plan: the data collection subproject. WFOT Bulletin 54: 37–45

Sanz Victoria S, Garcia Rezio E (eds) 2005 Trascendiendo fronteras. Monográfico 38. Terapia Ocupacional. Asociación Profesional Española de Terapeutas Ocupacionales, Madruid

Shaw M, Davey Smith G, Dorling D 2005 Health inequalities and New Labour: how the promises compare with real progress. British Medical Journal 330: 1016–1021

Shepherd R 1994 Iain Macleod, a biography. Hutchinson, London

Simmond M 2005 Practising to learn: occupational therapy with the children of Vietnam. In: Kronenberg F, Simó Algado S, Pollard N (eds) Occupational therapy without borders. Elsevier Churchill Livingstone, Oxford: p 285–294

Simó Algado S, Cardona C E 2005 The return of the corn men: an intervention project with a Mayan community of Guatemalan retornos. In: Kronenberg F, Simó Algado S, Pollard N (eds) Occupational therapy without borders. Elsevier Churchill Livingstone, Oxford: p 347–362

Skocpol T 1980 States and social revolutions. Cambridge University Press, Cambridge

Sproule A 1981 Table manners. In: Burch D E (ed) Debrett's etiquette and modern manners. Pan, London: p 87–120

Stewart L S P 2007 Pressure to lead: what can we learn from the theory? British Journal of Occupational Therapy 70: 228–234

Szulc T 1989 Fidel Castro: a critical biography. Coronet, London

Tansey S 2000 Politics: the basics, 2nd edn. Routledge, London

Thatcher M 1995a The Downing Street years. Harper Collins, London

Thatcher M 1995b The path to power. Harper Collins, London

Thomas H 1986 The history of the Cuban revolution. Weidenfeld & Nicholson, London

Townsend E 1993 Occupational therapy's social vision. Canadian Journal of Occupational Therapy 60: 174–183

Townsend E, Wilcock A A 2004 Occupational justice. In: Christiansen C, Townsend E (eds) Introduction to occupation: the art and science of living. Prentice Hall, Thorofare, NJ: p 243–273

Trotsky L 1977 The history of the Russian revolution (trans Eastman M). Pluto, London

Van der Eijk C 2001 De kern van politiek. Het Spinhuis, Amsterdam

Vaneigem R 1983 The revolution of everyday life (trans Smith DN). Left Bank Books/Rebel Press, London

Voss H, Hidajat R 2002 International symposium on disaster reduction and global environmental change. German Committee for Disaster Reduction/German National Committee on Global Change Research, Bonn. Available online at: http://www.dkkv.org/DE/publications/ressource.asp?ID=82; accessed 19 October 2007

Ward S 1985 Organising things. Pluto, London

Watson R, Swartz L (eds) Transformation through occupation. Whurr, London

Werner D 1998 Nothing about us without us: developing innovative technologies for, by and with disabled persons. HealthWrights, Palo Alto, CA. Available online at: http://www.dinf.ne.jp/doc/english/global/david/dwe001/dwe00101.htm; accessed 19 October 2007

Whiteford G 2005 Knowledge, power, evidence, a critical analysis of key issues in evidence based practice. In: Whiteford G, Wright-St Clair V (eds) Occupation & practice in context. Elsevier Churchill Livingstone, Sydney: p 34–50

Wicks A, Whiteford G 2005 Gender, occupation and participation. In: Whiteford G, Wright-St Clair V (eds) Occupation & practice in context. Elsevier Churchill Livingstone, Sydney: p 197–212

Wilcock A A 1998 An occupational perspective of health. Slack, Thorofare, NJ

Wilcock A A 2001 A journey from self health to prescription. Occupation for Health, vol. 1.

British Association and College of Occupational Therapy, London

Wilcock A A 2002 A journey from prescription to self health. Occupation for Health, vol. 2. British Association and College of Occupational Therapy, London

Williams R 1976 Keywords. Fontana, London

Winnicott D W 1990 The maturational process and the facilitating environment. Karnac, London

Winnicott D W 1992 Through paediatrics to psychoanalysis. Karnac, London

Woodin T 2005 Muddying the waters: changes in class and identity in a working class cultural organization. Sociology 39: 1001–1018

World Federation of Occupational Therapists 2004 Position paper on community based rehabilitation (CBR). Available online at: http://www.wfot.org.au/officefiles/CBRposition %20Final.pdf; accessed 19 October 2007

World Federation of Occupational Therapists 2006 Position paper on human rights. Available online at: http://www.wfot.org/office_files/ Human%20Rights%20Position%20Statement% 20Final.pdf; accessed 19 October 2007

Political competence in occupational therapy

2

Nick Pollard, Dikaios Sakellariou,
Frank Kronenberg

Abstract

In order to practise effectively, occupational therapists need to have sufficient power to be a credible force in their negotiations and to inspire confidence in those with whom and for whom they are negotiating. Political skills are essential to demonstrate the relevance of the profession to others with whom they are working. However, lack of focus, dilution, isolation and erosion are political factors that combine to make the political representation of the profession both a local and a global problem. It is due to these problems that professional associations themselves are recognizing the need to develop political competence in individual members to enable them to represent and assert core values.

Ultimately if occupational therapists do not listen to the voices of the people they are working with and take them into account in the development and delivery of practice, the profession will cease to be relevant. The concern of the profession to work with people towards autonomous goals or toward community participation is connected with enabling active citizenship and achieving a reciprocated sense of value. This is an occupational goal but it cannot be realized without political initiatives.

Political competence

Political competence refers to a dynamic set of critical knowledge, skills and attitudes that enables one to engage effectively in situations of conflict and cooperation that are about responding to people's needs and demonstrating the relevance of the profession. Examples of components of political competence are: political reasoning (pADL), strategic planning and decision-making, networking, lobbying, debating.

Introduction

In order to practise effectively, occupational therapists need to have sufficient power to be a credible force in their negotiations and to inspire confidence in those with whom and for whom they are negotiating (Wilcock 1998; see Ch. 7). The central issue is that political skills are essential to demonstrating the relevance of the profession to others with whom therapists are working.

This concern is not just about evidence-based practice or pedigrees in client-centred practice. The 'allied' health professional status of occupational therapy presents it with problems (see Chs 5 & 6). Allied to the medical profession in which the male order predominates, occupational therapists are mostly women and so both 'not-men' and 'not-doctors' (Pollard & Walsh 2000). Occupational therapy is often not well understood by other professionals (Craik et al 1999, Lloyd et al 1999a,b, Peck & Norman 1999, Munoz et al 2000) and does not have the profile in popular awareness that many of their professional colleagues possess, partly as a consequence of this. The power occupational therapists have as agents of social control in the negotiation of treatment depends upon their professional status, but this is precarious. They can act in ways that are professional-centred rather than client-centred because they are not directly employed by the client but by a state health and social care system or private health system with its own agenda, to which they may feel more obligated (Hammell 2007).

As Hammell (2007, p. 266) argues, occupational therapists are 'not victims of oppressive institutional practices. We are often complicit' in their perpetuation. Occupational therapists may chafe about the secondary nature of their 'allied' health professional status and its erosion of the position that occupational therapists occupy. But occupational therapists can only take on this issue when they have amassed sufficient evidence to win the contest and demonstrate a capacity to accept the liabilities of clinical consultancy. In the carnivorous world of legal-fee-chasing litigation, these may be dangerous waters.

Accepting the limitations has enabled therapists to remain engaged with clients, propose activities, share knowledge and maintain value as team members (Peck & Norman 1999). Many changes have been driven by policy, such as, in the UK, the introduction of general management under the Thatcher government in 1990 with the introduction of the internal market in the National Health Service (Wilcock 2002) and the introduction of a series of National Service Frameworks or guidelines from the National Institute for Clinical Excellence (Morley et al 2007, Stewart 2007). These have altered the structure and delivery of health services, often translated into a need for cost containment, reduced therapist–client contact, involved the loss of occupational therapy positions in senior management and increased the importance of the multidisciplinary team. These issues can have an adverse effect on the alliances that occupational therapists can establish and ultimately on the power occupational therapists have to negotiate solutions for the benefit of their clients.

Sometimes the multidisciplinary relations in which occupational therapy has been involved are presented as an uneven conflict. Practitioners feel themselves to be a minority, whose identity is threatened by generic pressures (Hughes 2001, Parker 2001, Cook 2003), especially when their managers come from other professions. There has been much discussion concerning the implications of change and service redesign for occupational therapists; these mostly offer a series of apparently contradictory vignettes and suggest a negative process that therapists have to combat.

Lack of focus

The profession has difficulties in promoting itself because its identity and purpose are often unclear. Rebeiro (1998) points to a confused tradition of separating functions out from a view of the whole person, which has prevented focus on occupation as a core component of mental health and has detrimentally affected public awareness of occupational therapy. Craik et al

(1999) indicate concerns about the increasing pressure towards genericism contrasted with lack of resources to research core values.

Occupational therapists have been perceived as unskilled, unfocused and filling gaps (Fortune 2000, Munoz et al 2000), with a limited knowledge of medication and crisis intervention that renders them less useful in generic team frameworks (Trysenaar et al 1997). In finding a high degree of convergence between the roles of community occupational therapists and psychiatric nurses, Filson and Kendrick (1997) found that the assessment of activities of daily living was the only area where a significant occupational therapy specialism could be evidenced. Their solution to this was further training for psychiatric nurses, rather than development of occupational therapy. On the other hand, an over-specialization that focuses on one particular area may also be detrimental to the value of professional input, as Fitzpatrick and Presnell (2004) attest in their discussion on the compatibility of occupational therapy with hand therapy. Occupational therapy appears to find itself caught in a paradox: between being too specialized to be regarded as *occupational* therapy and being insufficiently specialized to be of value. This suggests a further issue of dilution.

Dilution

Hughes (2001) suggests that the generic nature of community mental health teams both produces the effect of not having the space in which to practise occupational therapy effectively and also puts the activities of daily living skills of the professional worker in potential conflict with the hands-on role of the generic support workers in the team. These dilutions are potentially increased by the need for community teams to work on shift rotas. Therapists may be able to meet a wider range of client needs by working more flexibly (Wigham & Supyk 2001); however, their time may be prioritized for more generic areas of practice when team strength is reduced to offer an out-of-hours service.

Isolation

In the move from institution to community, occupational therapists are more and more finding themselves working in multidisciplinary teams as the sole representative of their profession (Lloyd et al 1999a). The break-up of unidisciplinary departments has resulted in occupational therapists being managed and supervised by people from other professions with limited managerial knowledge of occupational therapy (Craik et al 1999, Lloyd et al 1999a,b, Munoz et al 2000). Peck and Norman (1999) have also highlighted the shorter working experience of most occupational therapists compared to that of workers in other disciplines in mental health settings such as social work and nursing, leading to professional isolation and misunderstandings in community teams. These issues may encourage occupational therapists to avoid conflict and seek consensus in teams, to fit in and be flexible rather than to assert their professional identity. Isolation, loss of career structure and lack of role clarity contribute to increased levels of stress and burn-out amongst therapists (Bassett & Lloyd 2001).

Erosion

The loss of higher professional staff grades during the 1990s in the UK left the occupational therapist vulnerable to team structures led by managers from other disciplines. Working relationships often depend on the attitudes of line managers and others; for example, in mental health the team psychiatrists play a significant role. Since the latter years of the last century interventions based in medication and psychotherapy have predominated in many areas of practice, because of improvements in medication and continued research (Shorter 1997,

Pringle 1998, Burns & Firn 2002). Although the development of consultant therapy posts in the UK and master's level entry to professional registration may have begun to address this issue, occupational therapy has not been enabled to evidence itself effectively because it has rarely been able to access adequate research and educational development opportunities (Bannigan 2001, Bannigan & Duncan 2001, Illot & White 2001, Wilcock 2002).

For many years there have been insufficient therapists to fill the posts available. Rather than budget for vacancies that cannot be filled, managers under pressure to maximize their use of resources have often responded to a lack of therapists by asking people from other professions to carry out specialist interventions (Stalker et al 1996, Wilcock 2002). If an unqualified 'activity therapist' position can be created for a support worker that appears to answer the diversional needs of clients, the need for a scarcely obtainable occupational therapist becomes unclear. Senior staff have been less available to work alongside newly qualified staff, particularly in mental health environments, to the detriment of the experience accessible to their junior colleagues (Morley et al 2007). Occupational therapists continue to be challenged in disseminating a robust and clear understanding of the profession to many of their peers. For example, occupational therapists often find their concerns about the discharge of clients over-ridden by the decisions of others because their opinion is discounted or because they have been unable to argue their case effectively (e.g. Lymbery 2002, Atwal & Caldwell 2003).

These same confusions may feed into the cause and result of deficiencies in education. Mental health in particular has experienced a historic lack of community placements (Trysenaar et al 1997, Lloyd et al 1999a) and good occupational therapy role models for students (Craik & Austin 2000, Morley et al 2007). Unsurprisingly Peck and Norman (1999) suggest that a high turnover of occupational therapists in mental health has contributed to the erosion of posts when specific vacancies have been left unfilled.

Changes and opportunities?

Greaves et al (2002, p. 385) point to the 'consumer-focused value base' of the profession as a source of occupational therapists' adaptability and competence. In the medically dominated field of hand therapy it has been suggested that occupational therapists adapt to change and find ways to responding to new challenges, without losing sight of the need to be holistic (Dale et al 2002). Peck and Norman (1999, p. 240) found that occupational therapists were valued by adult community mental health team members for their 'ambition for service users (e.g. employment)', 'therapeutic optimism' and 'long-term perspective', issues that in turn are highlighted as key parts of the practice of occupational therapists in assertive community treatment (Orford 1999, Auerbach 2001, Krupa et al 2002), along with their 'therapeutic use of self' (Burns & Firn 2002, p. 60).

These attributes have led occupational therapists to work in new fields, such as community-based rehabilitation, despite their occasional concerns about the relevance and adequacy of their education (Sakellariou et al 2006, Stewart 2007; see Chs 11, 15–18). While some have found it hard to retain their specialist function as multidisciplinary team approaches have demanded more generic working in mental health (Brown et al 2000, Cook 2003), others have found new specialisms emerging in the process of service development, as has been the case for occupational therapy in the expanding economies and social reform contexts of eastern Europe (see Chs 7, 11).

However, most of these attributes can also be claimed by other professionals, volunteers, carers and clients with whom therapists work. If traditional activities such as woodwork, gardening and socializing show the motivating power of occupation (Mee & Sumsion 2001), these and many of the interventions carried out with clients in community services do not specifically require occupational therapists to ensure they happen. Nor are therapists' attributes evidence that objectives are being realized, as Greaves et al (2002, p. 385) remark, 'caution is needed ... in presuming that self-efficacy implies task competence'.

Even competence may be misplaced. Therapeutic optimism, long-term perspectives and ambition for service users may not be appropriate if, as Corrigan suggests (2001), the profession is unable objectively to question the basis for its practice. There have been increasing questions about the dominant paradigm of occupation that informs the theoretical base of the profession, a particular view of social responsibility through individual productivity. It has been suggested that occupational therapy has as a consequence encountered difficulties of application in non-Western cultures (Iwama 2005a,b, Odawara 2005). The self-efficacy of therapists may be harnessed to competence in tasks that are geared to forms of social control and a limited sense of client-centred benefit in which individual clients make progress. However, outside these conditions of compliance the status quo is unchallenged, or else unresolved cultural issues may produce confusion and even detrimental outcomes (Kronenberg & Pollard 2005a, Hammell 2007).

This problem of ideology and ethics is a product of the professionalization of the facilitation of occupation. The simplicity of doing is the perennial stumbling block in the case for occupational therapy (Perrin 2001). Occupational therapists themselves have not always placed a high value on domestic activities, while other professionals have consequently been ambivalent about the value of occupational therapy (Hamlin et al 1992, Pollard & Walsh 2000, Wilcock 2002, Hammell 2004, Clark 2007). It is not merely that 'work lacks scientific kudos' (Perrin 2001, p. 134) but that, despite all the concerns with the development of occupational therapy's theoretical models, what a service really needs are people who will encourage clients to take part in activity and can facilitate them in doing so (Burns & Firn 2002).

One answer has been to review generic pressures on professional experiences in the light of an occupation-focused model of practice (Reeves & Summerfield-Mann 2004) but, as Fish (1998) remarks, the theoretical models into which occupational therapists often retreat have little to say about the *art* of practice, which is evident in many professional transactions concerning the management of clients and clinical interventions (Detweiler & Peyton 1999, Peloquin 2005). Fish and Coles (1998) place the revelation of artistry in practice as a critical process essential to insider practitioner research. They make the point that, despite all the evidence that may be amassed to support intervention, it is the practitioner's understanding of the process of treatment that is essential to its effectiveness. The practitioner is an inside researcher, embedded in practice, and thus has an advantage over the outside researcher in unpicking the nuances of practice narratives. This applies not only to interventions in clinical settings but also where occupational therapists become involved in community development. To answer the common problems in this field of much official rhetoric but little sustainable involvement (Kapasi 2006, Lowndes et al 2006, O'Brien & Penna 2007), those involved have to interpret and critically review their experiences in a systematic way (see Chs 7, 10, 15–17).

These are just two sides of the 3P triangle (see Ch. 1). The problem described here in terms of professional and personal attributes cannot be resolved by these means alone. Lack of focus, dilution, isolation and erosion are political factors that combine to present both a local and a global problem (since these sources are from many different occupational therapy practices) of the political representation of the profession. It is because of these problems that professional associations themselves (e.g. Pollard et al 2005, Alsop 2006, College of Occupational Therapists 2006, Lawson-Porter & Pollard 2006a,b) are recognizing the need to develop political competences in enabling individual members to be able to represent and assert core values.

However, representing occupational therapy effectively does not just concern well articulated professional narratives of practice or examples of advocacy. The stories of practitioners involve others whose voices do not always emerge except as recounted by the professional – disabled people, their carers and the communities they belong to often do not possess the methodologies required to present evidence in ways that will be understood and exert influence in professional hierarchies (Fine 1998, Hammell 2007). If occupational therapists are to concern themselves with describing their artistry, there is a need to explore and facilitate the articulation of other perspectives as part of the process of empowerment. These, in turn, need to be valued for themselves, not as quaint and curious points of view that, having been accorded a patriarchal (or, perhaps with occupational therapy, maternal and nurturing) smile of encouragement, can be dismissed when the professionals get down to the *real* business of determining interventions.

The production of professional discourses leads to the imposition of cultural values, to what our colleague Elelwani Ramugondo has called occupational colonization (E L Ramugondo, personal communication, 2007). She explains that occupational colonization refers to the valuing of occupations only when those who represent a dominant group begin to engage in them. This can even lead to some occupations from indigenous people being commodified without benefiting the people from whom these originated. An example is the song 'The lion sleeps tonight' in the musical the *Lion King*. Had it not been for his family pointing out the copyright issues involved, the song would not have rightfully been credited to Solomon Linda. The underlying dynamics in these copyright issues are historical and political, arising from differences in power and the development of one group's dominance over others. These are political processes. A profession espousing client-centred practice has to listen to the voices of its clients as well as the evidence of professional colleagues. Occupational therapy appears to be caught up in understandings of health and social care that inhibit its full development and the recognition of its interests (see Ch. 1). On one hand it has to accommodate a medical agenda rather than deliver occupation-centred objectives. On the other, the profession sometimes appears reluctant to address gaps in understanding between therapists and clients (Abberley 1995, Maitra & Erway 2006, Hammell 2007) and ways in which it might be failing to engage with clients' occupational needs (Stagnitti 2005, Hammell 2007).

Since participation in occupational therapy depends on people feeling that it will meet their needs and that they have a reason to take part in the activities offered, there will always be challenges. Clients do not always want what is in their best interests, cannot always be realistic, articulate, rational (Carr 2001). Cultural and class differences may stand in the way of them being empowered to identify their needs appropriately (Kronenberg 2005; see Chs 16–19). There may be significant problems, perhaps due to official doctrines and cultural differences, in identifying ways in which needy groups can be accommodated as clients (Kronenberg 2005; see Chs 10, 16–19). Ultimately, however, if occupational therapists do not listen to the voices of the people they are working with and take them into account in the delivery of practice, the profession will cease to be relevant.

Recognizing political situations

The complex and multidisciplinary environments of the institutions and communities in which occupational therapists work evoke tactical questions about picking the right battles and only taking part in conflicts that can be won (Sun Tzu 1998). If occupational therapists take part in conflicts without adequate resources and sufficient evidence, and without the assent of others – for example clients – they can find themselves wasting their energies and, in the long term, damaging their chances of mounting a credible position in subsequent and possibly more significant contests.

Identifying a 'conflict and cooperation situation' can in itself be a political issue. The actors who define a problem generally have a stake in determining how it is to be addressed. For example occupational therapists have the power to guide assessment and intervention processes through their choice of practice framework and assessment batteries.

Conflict and cooperation situations can be identified through a narrative strategy. Each situation arises from a particular context. This uniqueness may not fit a systematic formula but depends on lived experiences (Clouston 2003). Such accounts can be termed 'occupational narratives' (Kielhofner et al 2002, p. 127), which combine a description of identity with an account of making sense of and interacting in the environment, which includes exchanging stories with other people (see Chs 3, 14, 20). The therapist might ask 'What is the story?' and thereby combine narrative and political reasoning:

- What story am I telling, and what stories are the other actors telling? An incident recounted by different witnesses is described according to each person's perspective. To get an overview it is necessary to ask each person what they saw in their own words (Clouston 2003)
- Where do they agree or disagree? What features do they share and which are different?
- Why do the agreements and differences occur?
- What is the core of the story, and which of the differences threaten its integrity? Can ways be found to incorporate them into the outcome?

It should be noted that, in the analysis of the story, the questions employed here are concerned with revealing the critical qualities of experiences and perceptions and can be worked alongside the '3P archaeology' and 'pADL' processes identified in Ch. 1. There is no linguistic ascent into technical terms for, as Fish (1998) points out, discussion has to be open and enabling, rather than elevated to a theoretical and exclusive discourse to which some of the participants do not have access (see Ch. 6).

The points of conflict and cooperation that emerge can be ranged on a scale. At the cooperation end of the axis there is no conflict but it is unlikely that this point will be achieved. At the other end of the axis there is full conflict but, even where this is so, the possibility of cooperation is not fully excluded; as a rule war is expensive and exhausts the combatants to the point where eventually they have to seek peace (Sun Tzu 1998).

What we usually observe is not conflict *or* cooperation but conflict *and* cooperation. Actors can cooperate in some areas and conflict in others (Kronenberg & Pollard 2005a). Separating out individual elements carries a danger that they are not seen as a whole process. An effective politician manages both conflict and cooperation strategies in simultaneous fields with the same actors, like foreign policy. A foreign minister can rattle sabres against another country but still act to maintain a trading relationship and joint interests in a federation with other actors. The same applies to individuals and the groups to which they belong. For example, occupational therapists working in different departments within a hospital have alliances with occupational therapists and also with the departments in which they work relating to different fields of health and social care. This can be overlaid with their patterns of social relationships with colleagues, particular interests in areas of practice and other possible affiliations such as membership of professional groups within their main professional body or different health unions, membership of course cohorts, peer supervision groups, and so on. This is of course in addition to other aspects of their social and family life that may not involve work. All answer particular needs in the individual, and in the heavily gendered context of occupational therapy are incorporated into strategies that Wicks and Whiteford (2005, p. 210) have referred to as 'women's ways of doing', because social restrictions acting on these complexities generally affect women differently from men. They may also affect men who work in occupational therapy environments in similar ways to their female colleagues because the surrounding conditions impacting on the profession arise in part from the gendered nature of the allied health professional career structure (Pollard & Walsh 2000, Meade et al 2005).

A wider role for occupational therapy

Throughout its history occupational therapy has responded to changing demands in health and social care systems with many new ideas and innovative practices. This book is part of a recent re-examination and reconceptualization of occupational therapy to recognize a broader, global and social responsibility and acknowledge a need for the profession to realize the goals of occupational justice by addressing inequality and poverty (Pollard et al 2005; see Introduction, Chs 1, 7).

This re-examination is at the forefront of the strategies of many occupational therapy professional associations. It is recognized that for occupational therapists to meet the challenges of poverty and inequality they need to build on their abilities in working cooperatively and in partnership with communities. Effective occupational therapy depends on gaining acceptance and permission to practise and to offer responses to the needs of local populations. This is a problem of aspect politics in that it requires skills in negotiation and the ability to work with actors across social and political power structures. 'Politics' and 'political' in this discussion are not about party politics, although an awareness and recognition of party differences is often important (see Ch. 1). Occupational therapists require political competencies to work with problems arising from the social, political, economic and environmental contexts in which they work. An effective occupational therapy needs to:

- upon invitation build the future with people, rather than for them (Kronenberg & Pollard 2005a,b)
- offer strong political commitment to equity in meeting all people's basic needs (Fransen 2005).

Historically, occupational therapists in some countries have had periods of political engagement (Thibeault 2002, Wilcock 2002, Barros et al 2005; see Ch. 7) but this has not often been sustained. Perhaps as a consequence many practitioners have not appeared to appreciate the political nature or importance of occupational therapy (Kronenberg & Pollard 2005a; see Chs 5, 7). However, its engagement with enablement, advocacy and social reform underpins the development of occupational therapy as an agency for social change and as a form of intervention that has the capability to address complexity (Creek 2003, Whiteford et al 2005). It has been argued that occupational therapy could be more valued in the community base, and to realize this practitioners need to increase activity and networking in the community to find and engage with their clients (Wilcock 1998, Whiteford 2000, Creek 2003, Scriven & Atwal 2004).

Occupational therapists have been lamenting their position for many years, bemoaning the lack of research and evidence, the poverty of resources allocated to smaller professions (Wilcock 2002). The authors of these articles, including ourselves (Pollard 2002a), have seen the way forward as calling for more research, but this is not the only way of raising awareness (Kronenberg & Pollard 2006). One of the difficulties the profession has also had to confront is the relatively low profile of occupational therapy as a career. Compared to physiotherapy and nursing, for example, it is not as widely known to school children or their career advisors (Craik et al 2001, Royeen et al 2001, Greenwood et al 2005; see Ch. 5). Popular culture has been important in this; television dramas in hospital settings and a subgenre of romantic fiction, for example the Sue Barton novels of Helen Doyle Boylston (Philips 1999), emphasize nursing and medicine (Hockenberry 2006).

Human occupation is such a ubiquitous aspect of society that it is perhaps taken for granted and becomes a matter of common sense that is difficult to objectify from a lay perspective (Hockenberry 2006). It lacks the tension of life-and-death drama, of traumatic events that enable people to make neat narrative resolutions in time for the news programme. Assessment and treatment approaches have not, in the main, lent themselves to more than bit parts in fiction.

Occupational therapists often use their own stories to negotiate and work out with people what their needs are and how they can be met. This facility, enshrined in a professional versatility, produces problems in the professional context of demands for generic working. Occupational therapists are often managed by other professionals or are allocated referrals by other professionals and work for opportunities to develop their role rather than their role being clearly understood. This can have the effect that work with a client develops along occupational therapy lines, or has an occupational therapy flavour, rather than the client having been given a specific occupational therapy referral. Therapists may sometimes find themselves taking on referrals in order to have a role and through it to demonstrate the value of occupational therapy (Cook 2003).

This can be a positive strategy that provides opportunities to discover the occupational potential of people who perhaps have not responded to other approaches, or to find new ways of developing a rapport from which to negotiate intervention. There are both problems and advantages in this issue. Some occupational therapists have argued for a long time that they cannot engage in every aspect of human occupation, such as, for example, many of the issues connected with sex, politics and religion (Kielhofner 1993, Couldrick 2005, Pollard & Sakellariou 2007; see

Chs 5, 6, 21). Occupational therapists have to concentrate their energies or dissipate their effectiveness and even risk burnout, or missing priorities, for being concerned with tangential issues (Brown et al 2000, Fortune 2000, Morley et al 2007, Stewart 2007).

However, in being adaptable, occupational therapists are in touch with the creative and catalytic aspect of the profession. Therapists should ensure the strategic use of their successes to give publicity to the services they work with. Generating good news stories and positive public relations through a well presented media profile enhances the value of the profession to the people who manage the service, but it also provides evidence of efficacy (Kronenberg & Pollard 2006). Good public relations provide a source of power that enables occupational therapists to do more of what they are good at. Occupational therapists are often working creatively on the margins (Lloyd et al 2004). The clients that occupational therapists work with are their source of power; mutually, they are the means for enabling each other.

An alliance with clients

One example we can draw upon is our participation in the Federation of Worker Writers and Community Publishers. This network, which includes a large number of people who belong to Survivors' Poetry groups, has given us the opportunity to discuss disability issues, for example experiences as mental health survivors, outside a health context (Pollard & Smart 2005, Pollard 2008; see Ch. 14). Through friendships and cooperation based in a shared interest in community publishing (e.g. Smart 2005), rather than that of patient and therapist, it has been possible to combine efforts and resources to develop interventions for work with other people with mental health problems (Pollard 2002b, Pollard & Steel 2002, Ryan & Pollard 2002). One outcome was that the therapists, the service users and the survivor poets developed several published results: articles, a video, a newspaper article and a conference presentation. These in turn led the continuing collaboration and discussion that has contributed to this book and other publications (Kronenberg & Pollard 2005a,b, Pollard & Kronenberg, in press). Ch. 14 is another example of this experience. We strongly feel that the collaboration with 'survivors' is core to the future development of the profession, as we attempted to indicate through the foregrounding of survivor stories in *Occupational Therapy Without Borders* (Kronenberg 2005, Kronenberg et al 2005a). Relevant examples are given in Chs 11, 12, 13 and 15.

This kind of activity is linked to a form of literacy that is at the core of a political consciousness, because it operates at the level of community, the local events that are immediate to people, or social actors. As a vehicle for this, community publishing has long been viewed as a form of social action, a grassroots political activity that is outside party politics but operates at the level of neighbourhoods or localities (Morley & Worpole 1982, O'Rourke 2005, Smart 2005, Woodin 2005a,b). Occupational therapy has a very similar potential by reason of its sphere of engagement with communities, as a vehicle for social engagement (Kronenberg et al 2005b, Pollard & Kronenberg 2005, Simó Algado et al 2005). Often, although it has been rarely written up as 'community publishing', occupational therapists have used the activities of creative writing as part of the interventions toward occupational justice and expressing the needs of disabled people (Pollard 2004, Pollard & Smart 2005, Simó Algado & Burgman 2005).

People Relying On People (PROP) is a group of people who have early-onset dementia and their carers (Jubb et al 2003, Chaston et al 2004), discussions with whom also contributed to the development of the pADL framework (Kronenberg & Pollard 2005a; see Ch. 1). Using their networking skills and basing their work around a social programme with a young people with dementia nursing team, this group has demonstrated a positive approach to their condition through the development of conference presentations and other events that have the goal of raising a local and national profile. A recent DVD, *Out of Sight, Out of Mind* (People Relying on People 2005), aimed at educating service users, carers and others about early-onset dementia, has used comedy sketches acted by group members to illustrate the typical fears and difficulties they have experienced (Webster & Kendrew 2005). These communication-centred activities are especially important where groups like those with early-onset dementia are liable to experience marginalization and stigmatization (Reidpath et al 2005; see Ch. 3).

While there are many strategies and legislative arrangements in place to produce and enforce 'equalities' in treatment and social opportunity, these often have the limited and even negative effect of making those who manage community resources 'go through the motions' without enabling local people to sustain developments for themselves (Kapasi 2006, Lowndes et al 2006, O'Brien & Penna 2007; see Ch. 10). Adherence to the letter of the law is not the same as a belief in the appropriateness of the justice that the law provides. Approaches like the PROP group's DVD cut across this barrier of recognition, using comedy sketches to deal with a subject that many people find difficult and perhaps even feel they should not be laughing about, persuading their audience to laugh *with* them. However, it is not only at this level that an exchange of value, through humour, takes place. The DVD and the other community activities in which the group is engaged demonstrate that dementia is not a condition that suddenly makes the individual unable to deal with the social world, and that people with dementia can continue to educate and enrich others (Jubb et al 2003, Chaston et al 2004).

Recognizing and analysing engagement in 'conflict and cooperation' situations

The pADL questions set out in Ch. 1 can be applied as a filter to assist the analysis of the story of the relationship with the client (see Chs 8, 10). This enables both the therapist and the client to set their present situation in the historical context of the intervention process. In long-term interventions this can be an important factor in determining what is going on in the present – a therapist might involve the client in looking back over the course of their work together to see if there had been issues similar to the one of current concern. For the practitioner this might well also occur during peer supervision, or through team processes that draw on the experiences of other health professionals who have been working with the same client. It would not be unusual to contact individuals in other teams who had previously seen a person, in order to find out whether they had had similar experiences with the client, what strategies had been employed, and what the outcome had been.

It is inevitable that, while some of this discussion will involve clients directly, much of it will occur when the client is absent. Even where a therapist is working in community-based interventions it is inevitable that at times there will be discussions among professionals that do not include representatives of the community. It must be recognized that there will be similarly exclusive discussions taking place in family groups or in community meetings. Although good working relationships may continue it is essential to ensure trust by finding a way to communicate the import of these discussions. The audience of this recounted narrative will be quick to notice discrepancies and inconsistencies (Fish 1998) and this can be potentially detrimental to communication, especially across cultures (see Chs 10, 17).

Similar issues operate in service settings. In many aspects of the provision of care situations can arise that lead to emotional tensions and communication failure. For example, a distressed client may use inappropriate means to gain attention from staff. Although the client needs care and assistance in identifying the kind of help or reassurance needed, they may express this need by making threats. This could result in the client being labelled dangerous (and, perhaps, there may be a point where the client may become dangerous if this is not addressed). Such decisions are based on risk criteria operated by practitioners (Blank 2001). The facilities to assess communication issues that stem from institutional processes are often lacking or inadequate (O'Connell & Farnworth 2007). What is then recorded is the client's threat but not the reason for the threat, e.g. 'You're not listening to me', which may after all be due to the circumstances of compulsory detention.

While contributory factors such as the use of drink or drugs may be recorded, other social indicators that may affect the ability to negotiate with professionals – such as lack of educational opportunity linked to poverty (Warner 1994, Blank 2001) – may be less evident in assessments, compromising human rights (Carr 2001). Of course the effective presentation of more information, and better information, is not the only answer to this problem but it would make it more difficult to evade responsibilities. Occupational therapists routinely gather social information about the people they work with but if they are unable to present this clearly at the time when risk is being assessed then it cannot contribute to decision-making processes (O'Connell & Farnworth 2007). Occupational therapists need to find ways of researching and effectively disseminating such information, not only in the day to day practice of team meetings and case conferences but where it will be read by their fellow health professionals, managers and the lay public, who are often carers and clients capable of lobbying hospital management or local councillors and parliament members.

This information is needed to develop a wider and nuanced understanding of many of the issues concerning experiences of disability, and to encouraging a public responsibility in living with them. Generally, innovations in health practices are positively reported, while mental health issues frequently receive negative coverage (Byrne 2003, Huang & Priebe 2003). These matters need to be understood in ways that do not offload a medicalized and professionalized responsibility on to health and social care services for complex social factors that are partly due to patterns of consumption and other behaviours. A further danger arising from the popular awareness of mental health issues is the degeneration of information into psychobabble or, for example, stimulating the harmful emulation of suicide methods in adolescents (Byrne 2003). Collaboration in dissemination between services users and professionals may be one means to address this (Thomas 1997).

Byrne (2003) suggests that professionals need to be aware of popular media, both news and entertainment, and their significance in the marginalization and construction of negative images of all people who are perceived as being 'different' (Murphy 1987; see Ch. 5) This is especially so in community settings, where stigma is very much associated with fear.

Occupational therapists as political actors

Political power can be strengthened through making allies, for example with service user organizations (Lawrence 2004). An example of this might be encouraging the awareness of fluctuations in mental health as an everyday occupational issue. Many mental health users' organizations, such as MIND or Survivors' Poetry, are already engaged in this work, but the recovery journey of mental health survivors finding their way back to employment in health services is not always facilitated by the attitudes of colleagues (Lawrence 2004).

Health and social care interventions often have the effect of depriving people of power and responsibility, of depriving them of opportunities for meaningful occupation, for example because the resources required are not available or are restricted (Hammell 2007), or because treatment requires them to be detained involuntarily (O'Connell & Farnworth 2007). Preventive health strategies could include effective personal and social education, for example to enable people, whether as school students or perhaps as new citizens, to learn to avoid inappropriate behavioural strategies to resolve their problems based on a critical concern for others (Clarke 1996; see Ch. 3) and reduce their risk of being exposed to health risks or deprivation through the promotion of occupational justice values. However, such educational strategies have been in place for many years and have made little impact on systems that are either run by powerful corporations or institutions running on corporate lines.

Consequently, encouraging people to be responsible for themselves is a stance that is hedged with reasonable caution. It does not suppose that everyone is to blame for everything, or that everyone else can be blamed for everything (see, for example, Abberley 1995). What it does suggest (see Ch. 1) is that people do the best that may reasonably be expected of them. This might be more complicated than it appears, as research suggests health professionals often do less than they believe they should do (Smith et al 1991). To ensure congruence between a sense of personal consistency and ethical practice, occupational therapists who are aware of poor practice should take steps to do something about it, and this includes weighing up the issue of ethical practice, for example to provide adequate resources or complete interventions, against employer obligation. However, to meet the obligations of responsibility requires a critical awareness based in evidence (Hammell 2007; see Ch. 3).

Occupational therapists continue to disseminate models of occupational justice based in occupational science approaches. While the frameworks proposed in this book (see Chs 1, 3, 7, 10) and others (Kronenberg et al 2005a, Whiteford & Wright-St Clair 2005) provide processes for describing politically aware practice and form a basis for political competencies, they are interdependent with other competencies such as the ability to assemble evidence, communication and leadership skills, the capacity to adapt, concede, resist, attack, defend and negotiate effectively, and cultural competence. These abilities are themselves dependent on personality and experience (see Ch. 1).

Both conflict and cooperation provide insights

Van der Eijk (2001) explained that 'conflict and cooperation' are the motor of all political engagement. It is important to remember that it does not follow that conflict is 'bad' or that cooperation is 'good'. As Binmore (2006) argues, individuals, or groups, cooperate for many reasons, including the development of conflicts among themselves. The Norwegian island of Givaer, in the Arctic Circle, has 15 permanent inhabitants. In winter strong snow-storms restrict the living space on the island to $1\,km^2$. People there appear to embody perfect cooperation; they meet every evening for knitting or smoking, go out fishing together and organize a summer celebration, a sort of homecoming event for Givaer-born people who have left the island. As one woman points out, while they are not all friends, open conflict between individuals would threaten the sustainability of the community (Schulz 2007).

The terms 'conflict' and 'cooperation' merely refer to the aims and objectives of individuals and groups (see Ch. 1; Kronenberg & Pollard 2005a). Conflict occurs when individuals or groups work against each other to realize their own goals and interests while these are mutually incompatible. Conflicts are inevitable and often cannot be fully resolved, but to reach a solution for a community or society as a whole requires cooperation. Cooperation can be viewed as the other side or reverse of conflict, and it can also be understood as inevitable. In both conflict and cooperation one can distinguish two different aspects: one with respect to content and another with a behavioural or occupational aspect. The content aspect suggests that 'it's about *something*', objectives usually indicated by the terms aims and interests. The occupational aspect indicates that conflict or cooperation can be perceived in behaviour. If occupational therapists assume that there is a right to human occupation and a potential in all for meaningful occupation, we actually need to engage in conflict and cooperation situations in order to facilitate the realization of this potential. Traditionally, occupational therapists have favoured cooperation over conflict (see Ch. 5) but this has given them limited negotiation power and an impression that occupational therapy can be accommodative without being demanding (e.g. Hammell 2007).

Politics is everywhere in everyday life

Mundane interactions are ripe with unnoticed, unintended, taken-for-granted politics that simmer away in the historical process and develop or die out over time. These everyday, unexamined small-'p' politics (see Ch. 1) can be more dangerous or may even be masked by open political discussion and events in the domain field of big-'P' politics. A premature exploration of them may provoke unnecessary conflicts, yet 'If it works, why fix it?' is an excuse sometimes for not examining how things work, especially if the way they work is unequal – both sides appear to benefit but the exchange is loaded more on one side than the other.

A small cog has to turn many more times than a big cog to drive the same shaft. It may seem preferable just to accept that the gears work. However, the bearings for the small cog may wear

32

down faster and over a long period need to be more frequently replaced. This may be acceptable but only in inanimate objects. A social mechanism consumes health, not bearings. The settlement of industrial injury claims is full of these problems. Tort law was developed to deal with the tendency of capitalist enterprises to regard workers and the public as expendable items in the pursuit of profit (Abel 1981).

However, in many communities the law may be an inappropriate tool that takes the power of negotiation away from the people most directly affected in conflict and cooperation. It may not be as useful as simple conversation, persuasion and understanding, particularly if the issues are nuanced, based in daily details of existence. Many forms of oppression are buried in the activities of daily living to the point that people living under them are able to accept them and even cooperate with them enough to get by. As discussed in Ch. 1, a consciousness can even develop that these conditions are acceptable.

Working towards political competence

Rehabilitation is more than just adaptation and recovery. When disabled people remain socially excluded, relieved of social responsibility and denied facilities for social participation, they have also been denied citizenship, for citizenship is inextricably connected with access to political involvement (Arendt 1998). If an occupational therapy process that claims to be concerned with *all* human occupation thereby signs up to holism it is, or needs to be, in tension with social forces that restrict occupational potential – perhaps, as we have explored, through constraints on resources. The hole in some occupational therapy perspectives of holism is that they avoid the bits that are difficult to deal with (see Chs 5, 6). The authors see 'occupation' as a liberating principle where it encompasses a sense of access for all to human occupation. However, it is also fraught with potential for misuse that arises as much from a limited perspective of holism that perhaps overlooks occupational injustices (Hammell 2007) as from overstretching the professional focus. There is always going to be somewhere out of the profession's gaze in the field of human occupation.

A political role for occupational therapy

Issues of access to occupation are essentially rights-based issues, issues about affirming citizenship. Occupational therapists and occupational scientists, in employing terms like 'occupational deprivation', 'injustice' and 'apartheid', are recognizing the need to incorporate a political vision as a missing part of the holistic jigsaw. People are often uncomfortable with the 'political' word. It is often taken to imply a left-wing perspective, something that only people committed to social revolution would be interested in. Just as occupational therapists sometimes argue that they are constrained by the medical model that dominates many services, a political model and even a social model can be just as reductionist.

In eschewing the arts, craft and domestic origins and practice of the profession for a more scientific and treatment-based approach during the 1970s and 1980s (Wilcock 2002), occupational therapy may have temporarily shifted its focus from something that had, since hippocratic times, been held essential to good health: a concern with lifestyle and the activities of life (Porter 1997). It is, after all, negotiation and control of the right to access to these fundamentals that is often the focus of stigmatization, and occupational injustice or occupational apartheid.

Despite its concern with social transformation (see Ch. 7), occupational therapy has itself occasionally sought to exclude the political, religious and sexual from a model of human occupation. Kielhofner (e.g. 1993, and cited in Couldrick 2005) has asserted that these areas are not occupations. The consequence of this exclusion is that it offers occupational therapy only a partially holistic vision and as a result only a partial basis for empowering the people therapists work with. The concern of the profession to work with people towards autonomous goals or toward community participation is connected with enabling an active citizenship and achieving a reciprocated sense of value. This is an occupational goal but it cannot be realized without political initiatives.

References

Abberley P 1995 Disabling ideology in health and welfare – the case of occupational therapy. Disability and Society 10: 221–232

Abel R L 1981 A critique of American tort law. British Journal of Law and Society 8: 199–231

Alsop A 2006 Think, consider and convey. Part III. Occupational Therapy News 14(3): 31

Arendt H 1998 The human condition, 2nd edn. University of Chicago Press, Chicago, IL

Atwal A, Caldwell K 2003 Ethics, occupational therapy and discharge planning: four broken principles. Australian Occupational Therapy Journal 50: 244–251

Auerbach E S 2001 The individual placement and support model versus the menu approach to supported employment: where does occupational therapy fit in? Occupational Therapy in Mental Health 17(2): 1–19

Bannigan K 2001 Annual AOTMH lecture 2001: sharing the evidence for mental health occupational therapy practice. Mental Health Occupational Therapy 6(2): 4–9

Bannigan K, Duncan E 2001 A survey of post registration research students in occupational therapy. British Journal of Occupational Therapy 64: 278–284

Barros D, Ghirardi M, Lopes R 2005. Social occupational therapy: a socio-historical perspective. In: Kronenberg F, Simó Algado S, Pollard N (eds) Occupational therapy without borders: learning from the spirit of survivors. Elsevier Churchill Livingstone, Edinburgh: p 140–151

Bassett H, Lloyd C 2001 Occupational therapy in mental health: managing stress and burn-out. British Journal of Occupational Therapy 64: 406–411

Binmore K 2006 Why do people cooperate? Politics, Philosophy and Economics 5: 81–96

Blank A 2001 Patient violence in community mental health: a review of the literature. British Journal of Occupational Therapy 64: 584–589

Brown B, Crawford P, Darongkamas J 2000 Blurred roles and permeable boundaries: the experience of multidisciplinary working in community mental health. Health and Social Care in the Community 8: 425–435

Burns T, Firn M 2002 Assertive outreach in mental health: a handbook for practitioners. Oxford University Press, Oxford

Byrne P 2003 Psychiatry and the media. Advances in Psychiatric Treatment 9:135–143

Carr J 2001 Reform of the Mental Health Act 1983: implications of safety, capacity and compulsion. British Journal of Occupational Therapy 64: 590–594

Chaston D, Pollard N, Jubb D 2004 Young onset of dementia: a case for real empowerment. Journal of Dementia Care 12(6): 24–26

Clark D H 2007 The story of a mental hospital: Fulbourn 1858–1983. Available online at: http://www.human-nature.com/free-associations/clark/index.html; accessed 4 July 2007

Clarke P B 1996 Deep citizenship. Pluto, London

Clouston T 2003 Narrative methods: talk, listening and representation. British Journal of Occupational Therapy 66: 136–142

College of Occupational Therapists 2006 Recovering ordinary lives: the strategy for occupational therapists in mental health services 2007–2017. College of Occupational Therapists, London

Cook S 2003 Generic and specialist intervention for people with severe mental health problems: can interventions be categorised? British Journal of Occupational Therapy 66: 17–24

Corrigan K 2001 Doing time in mental health: discipline at the edge of medicine. British Journal of Occupational Therapy 64: 203–205

Couldrick L 2005 Sexual expression and occupational therapy. British Journal of Occupational Therapy 68: 315–318

Craik C, Austin C 2000 Educating occupational therapists for mental health practice. British Journal of Occupational Therapy 63: 335–339

Craik C, Austin C, Schell D 1999 A national survey of occupational therapy managers in mental health. British Journal of Occupational Therapy 62: 220–228

Craik C, Gissane C, Douthwaite J, Philp E 2001 Factors influencing the career choice of first-year occupational therapy students. British Journal of Occupational Therapy 64: 114–120

Creek J 2003 Occupational therapy defined as a complex intervention. College of Occupational Therapists, London

Dale L, Fabrizio A, Adhlakha P et al 2002 Occupational therapists working in hand therapy: the practice of holism in a cost containment environment. Work 19: 35–45

Detweiler J, Peyton C 1999 Defining occupations: a chronotypic study of narrative genres in a health discipline's emergence. Written Communication 16: 412–468

Filson P, Kendrick T 1997 Survey of roles of community psychiatric nurses and occupational therapists. Psychiatric Bulletin 21: 70–73

Fine M 1998 Working the hyphens: reinventing self and other in qualitative research. In: Denzin N K, Lincoln Y S (eds) The landscape of qualitative research: theories and issues. Sage, Thousand Oaks, CA: p 130–155

Fish D 1998 Appreciating practice in the caring professions. Butterworth Heinemann, Oxford

Fish D, Coles C 1998 Developing professional judgement in health care. Butterworth Heinemann, Oxford

Fitzpatrick N, Presnell S 2004 Can occupational therapists be hand therapists? British Journal of Occupational Therapy 67: 508–510

Fortune T 2000 Occupational therapists: is our therapy truly occupational or are we merely filling gaps? British Journal of Occupational Therapy 63: 225–230

Fransen H 2005 Challenges for occupational therapy in community-based rehabilitation: occupation in a community approach to handicap in development. In: Kronenberg F, Simó Algado S, Pollard N (eds) Occupational therapy without borders: learning from the spirit of survivors. Elsevier Churchill Livingstone, Edinburgh: p 166–182

Greaves A J, King R, Yellowlees P, Spence S, Lloyd C 2002 The competence of mental health occupational therapists. British Journal of Occupational Therapy 65: 381–386

Greenwood W, Lim K H, Bithell C 2005 Perceptions of occupational therapy compared with physiotherapy and nursing among minority ethnic and white United Kingdom school and college students: implications for recruitment. British Journal of Occupational Therapy 68: 75–84

Hamlin R, Black L, Kathryn M, Froelich J, MacRae N 1992 Feminism: an inclusive perspective. American Journal of Occupational Therapy 46: 967–970

Hammell K W 2004 Dimensions in meaning in the occupations of everyday life. Canadian Journal of Occupational Therapy 71: 296–305

Hammell K W 2007 Client-centred practice: ethical obligation or professional obfuscation? British Journal of Occupational Therapy 70: 264–266

Hockenberry J 2006 Keynote address. AOTA Congress, Charlotte, NC

Huang B, Priebe S 2003 Media coverage of mental health care in the UK, USA and Australia. Psychiatric Bulletin 27: 331–333

Hughes J 2001 Occupational therapy in community mental health teams: a continuing dilemma? Role theory offers an explanation. British Journal of Occupational Therapy 64: 34–40

Illot I, White E 2001 College of Occupational Therapists' research and development strategic vision and action plan. British Journal of Occupational Therapy 64: 270–277

Iwama M 2005a Situated meaning: an issue of culture, inclusion, and occupational therapy. In: Kronenberg F, Simó Algado S, Pollard N (eds) Occupational therapy without borders: learning from the spirit of survivors. Elsevier Churchill Livingstone, Edinburgh: p 127–139

Iwama M 2005b Occupation as a cross cultural construct. In: Whiteford G, Wright-St Clair V (eds) Occupation & practice in context. Elsevier Churchill Livingstone, Sydney: p 242–253

Jubb D, Pollard N, Chaston D 2003 Developing services for younger people with dementia. Nursing Times 99(22): 34–35

Kapasi H 2006 Neighbourhood play and community action. Joseph Rowntree Foundation, York

Kielhofner G 1993 Occupation as the major activity of humans. In: Hopkins H, Smith H (eds) Willard and Spackman's occupational therapy, 8th edn. J B Lippincott, Philadelphia, PA: p 137–144

Kielhofner G, Borrell L Friedheim L 2002 Crafting occupational life. In: Kielhofner G (ed) A model of human occupation: theory and application, 3rd edn. Lippincott, Williams & Wilkins, Baltimore, MD: p 124–144

Kronenberg F 2005 Occupational therapy with street children. In: Kronenberg F, Simó Algado S, Pollard N (eds) Occupational therapy without borders: learning from the spirit of survivors. Elsevier Churchill Livingstone, Edinburgh: p 261–276

Kronenberg F, Pollard N 2005a Overcoming occupational apartheid: a preliminary exploration of the political nature of occupational therapy. In: Kronenberg F, Simó Algado S, Pollard N (eds) Occupational therapy without borders: learning from the spirit of survivors. Elsevier Churchill Livingstone, Edinburgh: p 58–86

Kronenberg F, Pollard N 2005b A beginning. In: Kronenberg F, Simó Algado S, Pollard N (eds) Occupational therapy without borders: learning from the spirit of survivors. Elsevier Churchill Livingstone, Edinburgh: p 1–13

Kronenberg F, Pollard N 2006 Political dimensions of occupation and the roles of occupational therapy. American Journal of Occupational Therapy 60: 617–625

Kronenberg F, Simó Algado S, Pollard N (eds) 2005a Occupational therapy without borders: learning from the spirit of survivors. Elsevier Churchill Livingstone, Edinburgh

Kronenberg F, Fransen H, Pollard N 2005b The
WFOT position paper on community based
rehabilitation: a call upon the profession to
engage with people affected by occupational
apartheid. WFOT Bulletin 51: 5–13

Krupa T, Radloff-Gabriel D, Whippey E, Kirsh B
2002 Reflections on occupational therapy and
assertive community treatment. Canadian
Journal of Occupational Therapy 69:
153–157

Lawrence J 2004 Mental health survivors: your
colleagues. International Journal of Mental
Health Nursing 13: 185–190

Lawson-Porter A, Pollard N 2006a Think,
consider and convey. OT News 14(1): 20

Lawson-Porter A, Pollard N 2006b Think, consider
and convey. Part II. Occupational Therapy News
14(2): 28

Lloyd C, Kanowski H, Maas F 1999a Occupational
therapy in mental health: challenges and
opportunities. Occupational Therapy
International 6: 110–125

Lloyd C, King R, Maas F 1999b The impact
of restructuring mental health services on
occupational therapy. British Journal of
Occupational Therapy 62: 507–513

Lloyd C, King R, McKenna K 2004 Actual and
preferred work activities of mental health
occupational therapists: congruence or
discrepancy? British Journal of Occupational
Therapy 67: 167–175

Lowndes V, Pratchett L, Stoker G 2006 Locality
matters: making participation count in local
politics. Institute for Public Policy Research,
London

Lymbery M 2002 Transitional residential
rehabilitation: what helps to make it work?
Building Knowledge for Integrated Care 10: 42–48

Maitra K, Erway F 2006 Perception of client-
centred practice in occupational therapists and
their clients. American Journal of Occupational
Therapy 60(3): 298–310

Meade I, Brown G T, Trevan-Hawke J 2005 Female
and male occupational therapists: a comparison
of their job satisfaction level. Australian
Occupational Therapy Journal 52: 136–148

Mee J, Sumsion T 2001 Mental health clients
confirm the motivating power of occupation.
British Journal of Occupational Therapy 64:
121–128

Morley D, Worpole K 1982 The republic of letters.
Comedia, London

Morley M, Rugg S, Drew J 2007 Before
preceptorship: new occupational therapists'
expectations of practice and experience of
supervision. British Journal of Occupational
Therapy 70: 243–253

Munoz J P, Sciulli J, Thomas D L, Wissner R S 2000
Utilization of occupational therapy in mental
health facilities in Western Pennsylvania.
Occupational Therapy in Mental Health 16:
33–51

Murphy R 1987 The body silent. W W Norton,
New York

O'Brien M, Penna S 2007 Social exclusion in
Europe: some conceptual issues. International
Journal of Social Welfare 17: 84–92

O'Connell M, Farnworth L 2007 Occupational
therapy in forensic psychiatry: a review of
the literature and a call for a united and
international response. British Journal of
Occupational Therapy 70: 184–191

Odawara E 2005 Cultural competence in
occupational therapy: beyond a cross cultural
view of practice. American Journal of
Occupational Therapy 59: 325–334

Orford J E 1999 From asylums to assertive
community treatment: a personal reflection.
Mental Health Occupational Therapy 4(4): 11

O'Rourke R 2005 Creative writing, education,
culture and community. NIACE, Leicester

Parker H 2001 The role of occupational therapists
in community mental health teams: generic
or specialist? British Journal of Occupational
Therapy 64: 609–611

Peck E, Norman I J 1999 Working together in
adult community mental health services:
exploring inter-professional role relations.
Journal of Mental Health 8: 231–242

Peloquin S M 2005 The art of occupational
therapy: engaging hearts in practice. In:
Kronenberg F, Simó Algado S, Pollard N (eds)
Occupational therapy without borders: learning
from the spirit of survivors. Elsevier Churchill
Livingstone, Edinburgh: p 99–109

People Relying on People 2005 Out of sight,
out of mind (DVD). People Relying on People,
Doncaster

Perrin T 2001 Don't despise the fluffy bunny:
a reflection from practice. British Journal of
Occupational Therapy 64: 129–134

Philips D 1999 Healthy heroines: Sue Barton,
Lillian Wald, Lavinia Lloyd Dock and the Henry
Street Settlement. Journal of American Studies
33: 65–82

Pollard N 2002a On the line: continuing
professional development between research
and practice. British Journal of Occupational
Therapy 65: 242–244

Pollard N 2002b Doncaster-Dumfries Part 1.
Federation 24: 13–15

Pollard N 2004 Notes towards an approach
for the therapeutic use of creative writing in
occupational therapy. In: Sampson F, Kingsley J
(eds) Creative writing in health and social care.
Jessica Kingsley, London: p 189–206

Pollard N 2008 Voices talk, hands write:
sustaining community publishing with people
with learning difficulties. Groupwork 17(2):
36–56

Pollard N, Kronenberg F 2005 El marco
conceptual de las actividades de la vida diara,
la rehabilitación basada en la comunidad y la

terapía ocupacional. Terapia Ocupacional 38: 16–24

Pollard N, Kronenberg F (in press) Working with people on the margins. In: Creek J, Ormston C (eds) Occupational therapy in mental health, 4th edn. Elsevier, Oxford

Pollard N, Sakellariou D 2007 Sex and occupational therapy: contradictions or contraindications? British Journal of Occupational Therapy 70: 361–365

Pollard N, Smart P 2005 Voices talk and hands write. In: Kronenberg F, Simó Algado S, Pollard N (eds) Occupational therapy without borders: learning from the spirit of survivors. Elsevier Churchill Livingstone, Edinburgh: p 287–301

Pollard N, Steele A 2002 From Doncaster to Dumfries. OT News 10(11): 31

Pollard N, Walsh S 2000 Occupational therapy, gender and mental health: an inclusive perspective? British Journal of Occupational Therapy 63: 425–431

Pollard N, Alsop A, Kronenberg F 2005 Reconceptualising occupational therapy. British Journal of Occupational Therapy 68: 524–526

Porter R 1997 The greatest benefit to mankind: a medical history of humanity from antiquity to the present. Harper Collins, London

Pringle R 1998 Sex and medicine. Cambridge University Press, Cambridge

Rebeiro K L 1998 Occupational-as-means to mental health: a review of the literature and a call for research. Canadian Journal of Occupational Therapy 65: 12–19

Reeves S, Summerfield-Mann L 2004 Overcoming problems with generic working for occupational therapists based in community mental health settings. British Journal of Occupational Therapy 67: 265–268

Reidpath D, Chan K Y, Gifford S M, Allotey P 2005 'He hath the French pox': stigma, social value and social exclusion. Sociology of Health and Illness 27: 468–489

Royeen C B, Zardetto-Smith A M, Duncan M, Mu K 2001 What do school-age children know about occupational therapy? An evaluation study. Occupational Therapy International 8: 263–272

Ryan H, Pollard N 2002 Poetry on the agenda for Scottish weekend. Adults Learning January: 10–11

Sakellariou D, Pollard N, Fransen H et al 2006 Reporting on the WFOT-CBR master project plan: the data collection subproject. WFOT Bulletin 54: 37–45

Schulz S 2007 Wir Kinder von Givaer. Der Spiegel. Available online at: http://www.spiegel.de/reise/europa/0,1518,497859,00.html; accessed 19 October 2007

Scriven A, Atwal A 2004 Occupational therapists as primary health promoters: opportunities and barriers. British Journal of Occupational Therapy 67: 424–429

Shorter E 1997 A history of psychiatry. John Wiley, New York

Simó Algado S, Burgman I 2005 Occupational therapy intervention with children survivors of war. In: Kronenberg F, Simó Algado S, Pollard N (eds) Occupational therapy without borders: learning from the spirit of survivors. Elsevier Churchill Livingstone, Edinburgh: p 245–260

Simó Algado S, Sakellarious D, Datsira M et al 2005 Terapia ocupacional al Sur del Alma. Terapia Ocupacional 38: 25–35

Smart P 2005 A beginner writer is not a beginner thinker. In: Kronenberg F, Simó Algado S, Pollard N (eds) Occupational therapy without borders: learning from the spirit of survivors. Elsevier Churchill Livingstone, Edinburgh: p 46–53

Smith T, McGuire J, Abbott D, Blau B 1991 Clinical ethical decision making: an investigation of the rationales used to justify doing less than one believes one should. Professional Psychology 22: 235–239

Stagnitti K 2005 The family as a unit in post-modern society: considerations for practice. In: Whiteford G, Wright-St Clair V (eds) Occupation & practice in context. Elsevier Churchill Livingstone, Sydney: p 213–229

Stalker K, Jones C, Ritchie P 1996 All change? The role and tasks of community occupational therapists in Scotland. British Journal of Occupational Therapy 59: 104–108

Stewart L S P 2007 Pressure to lead: what can we learn from the theory? British Journal of Occupational Therapy 70: 228–234

Sun Tzu 1998 The art of war (trans Yuan Shibing). In: The art of war/The book of Lord Shang. Wordsworth Editions, Ware

Thibeault R 2002 Muriel Driver memorial lecture: in praise of dissidence: Anne Lang-Etienne (1932–1991). Canadian Journal of Occupational Therapy 69: 197–204

Thomas P 1997 The dialectics of schizophrenia. Free Association Books, London

Trysenaar J, Ball J, Klassen K 1997 Employers' perceptions of occupational therapy in community mental health. Occupational Therapy in Mental Health 13: 63–79

Van der Eijk C 2001 De kern van de politiek. Het Spinhuis, Amsterdam

Warner R 1994 Recovery from schizophrenia: psychiatry and political economy. Routledge, London

Webster A, Kendrew C 2005 Working with younger people with dementia. Design and Print Services, Doncaster

Whiteford G 2000 Occupational deprivation: global challenge in the new millennium.

British Journal of Occupational Therapy 63: 200–204

Whiteford G, Wright-St Clair V (eds) 2005 Occupation & practice in context. Elsevier Churchill Livingstone, Marrickville, New South Wales

Whiteford G, Klomp N, Wright-St Clair V 2005 Complexity theory: understanding occupation, practice and context. In: Whiteford G, Wright-St Clair V (eds) Occupation & practice in context. Elsevier Churchill Livingstone, Marrickville, New South Wales: p 3–15

Wicks A, Whiteford G 2005 Gender, occupation and participation. In: Whiteford G, Wright-St Clair V (eds) Occupation & practice in context. Elsevier Churchill Livingstone, Marrickville, New South Wales: p 197–212

Wigham S, Supyk J 2001 Should occupational therapists work shifts? British Journal of Occupational Therapy 64: 151–152

Wilcock A 1998 An occupational perspective of health. Slack, Thorofare, NJ

Wilcock A A 2002 A journey from prescription to self health. Occupation for Health, vol. 2. British Association and College of Occupational Therapy, London

Woodin T 2005a Building culture from the bottom up: the educational origins of the Federation of Worker Writers and Community Publishers. History of Education 34: 345–363

Woodin T 2005b 'More welding than writing': learning in worker writer groups. History of Education 34: 561–578

When Adam dalf and Eve span:
occupational literacy and democracy

3

Nick Pollard

Abstract

Occupational literacy is a term that is used to describe the acquisition of new skills in response to developments in work processes. This article explores the term occupational literacy and discusses how it might address a wider set of issues – needs and rights. Commencing with a discussion of some examples of the relationship between literacy and power, it addresses the implications of reinterpreting occupational literacy through the lenses of occupational therapy, occupational science and critical literacy. The article concludes with the position that an ability critically to read and interpret occupation offers a way to democratic civic participation.

Occupational literacy refers to the capacity to make sense of, i.e. read or interpret, human occupations. As a literacy it provides a set of navigation skills which enable the user to explore and make use of contextual factors in order to access occupations of need and choice.

Delving into power, games and literacy

If the mark of civilization is an interest in the political values of citizenship (Aristotle 1962, Arendt 1998), then education and literacy must be a prerequisite for democracy (Friere 1972, Mill 1991) as they form the basis for access to political discourses and thus the enactment or pursuit of full citizenship rights. This is especially so if democracy is to enable social change through opportunities for civil participation (Friere 1972). That this social change should come from the grass roots of society is a long established discourse against privilege and the exclusions it creates. In 1381 the rebel priest John Ball, a leader in the Peasants' Revolt, is reputed to have made the point that all people were naturally equal but inequalities were imposed through social structures. This was the tenor of his provocative 'When Adam dalf and Eve span, who was thanne a gentilman?' (Dobson 1970, p. 374). With this rereading of the Bible Ball challenged the most widely distributed text underpinning the authority of the church and king, and the key passage illustrating God's moral authority over men. At the same time access to this knowledge was restricted to those who knew Latin in a society where most people were illiterate in their own tongue. This simple couplet cut through all that to give a short education in the politics of both equality and, since a 'gentilman' by definition did no work, the occupational nature of humans.

Another lesson in the practice of moral authority can today be derived from *The Sims* (Electronic Arts 2002), a computer game in which players create and manipulate families of individuals in an environment that is also designed by the player. If the player fails to endow the characters he or she creates with life skills, they have accidents, fail to eat or drink, and die. Their ability to participate and respond to events in their virtual environment depends on their ability to interpret the phenomena around them. Without being able to understand how what they do affects their world, their behaviour quickly becomes chaotic.

An antecedent to *The Sims* occurs in Philip K. Dick's dystopian novel *The Three Stigmata of Palmer Eldritch* (Dick 1973). Here the players are linked to each other through taking a drug that enables them to assimilate the roles of the figurines that are used to play the Perky Pat game in a simulated environment. The Perky Pat layout provides an exciting and absorbing alternative reality to the occupationally deprived conditions of the protagonists, whose main motivation in life becomes the pursuit of the game and the accessories linked to it. This dystopia explores a recurrent theme of Dick's novels, a view of social participation being largely centred on the pursuit of trivia to the extent that it becomes hard for the characters to distinguish what is significant and meaningful in their lives from the fantasies in which they are enmeshed. Essentially they are faced with the problems of literacy and interpretation that confined the lives of the serfs whom John Ball addressed. The unequal distribution or restriction of knowledge to prevent the realization of natural rights is a concern of the Declaration of Persepolis (International Symposium for Literacy 1975), a call for the development of literacy for human political enablement. That access to power should begin with commonplace activities (such as digging and delving) is reflected in Heath's (1983) study of the relationship of language use to daily occupations. She found that the most frequent uses of writing, for example, were in the writing of personal correspondence and lists, such as shopping lists, which reflected immediate functional concerns. Perhaps through more recent technological advances these phenomena would be replaced by mobile phone texts (Ofcom 2003).

Occupational literacy – not just workplace literacy

The development of literacy to encompass not just reading and writing but a new range of skills to meet the requirements of industrial and socioeconomic change (Hull & Grubb 1999, Smith 1999) has led to new concepts such as 'workplace literacy' and 'occupational literacy'. Often, however, it is difficult to show that the changes brought about by these literacies have resulted in changes in the relations of power that govern occupations, because they have been developed with built-in limitations.

Occupational literacy has emerged out of workplace literacy, one definition of which is 'written and spoken language, math and thinking skills that workers and trainees use to perform specific job tasks' (Stein 2000, p. 3). The definitions of occupational literacy that are available so far also relate to a whole range of work-related skills such as a personal work ethic, business-like appearance and time management (Carvin 2000), but also to the competent reading of documents associated with work (Rush et al 1986).

For occupational therapists and occupational scientists, whose prime concern is with 'occupation' (Gray 1998) or 'the human as an occupational being' (Yerxa et al 1990, p. 6), the term has a much broader range of application than the narrow sense of work, 'including the promotion of health and wellbeing' (Rebeiro 1998, p. 13). In this wider scope the complementary ideas of occupational justice (Wilcock 1998) and social justice (Townsend

1993) consider the need for 'ethical, moral, and civic principles associated with fairness, empowerment, an equitable access to resources, and sharing of rights and responsibilities' (Wilcock & Townsend 2000, p. 84). Occupation is not merely related to work but to a political notion of having choice, participation and sharing in the community, making changes and requiring 'social revolution' (Wilcock & Townsend 2000, p. 85) to address issues of disadvantage, from individual through to political and organizational expression. Wilcock and Townsend apply 'meaningful occupation' as a 'practical means' for 'personal and community transformation' (2000, p. 85). This theme is further explored throughout the practice section of this book. In their discussions on empowerment through occupation, Kronenberg and Pollard (2005a, p. 5; see Chs 1, 2) derived from Molinas Maldonaldo and Monroy Peralta (1999) the following principles:

Everybody is responsible for everything
Think locally, act globally
Nothing changes if nothing is done to change
The aim is not to attain the goals proposed, but the process above all
There is no public ethic without a personal ethic.

Occupational literacy in this context then refers to a set of navigation skills (see Chs 6, 9) to explore and make use of contextual factors in order to access occupation of need and choice.

A critical tool – for whom?

We argued earlier that civil participation depends on literacy and education. If so, there is a need for a wider view of 'occupational literacy' as a critical tool if people are to be enabled to make informed choices about their social participation. Furthermore, as both Mill (1991) and Friere (1985) make clear, this should not necessarily be entrusted to the state, the interest of which is more efficient control. The problem has been, however, as we shall discuss, that perceptions of a literacy skills gap have produced strategies for individual responsibility in meeting new demands (Jackson 2000, Sandlin 2000). Occupational literacy, workplace literacy and a plethora of similar literacy demands – even agricultural literacy (Frick et al 1995) – have produced methods and mechanisms for the internalization and self-administration of controlling behaviours and the dissemination and interpretation of knowledge in the interests of private enterprise, state organizations and governments (Jackson 2000, McLaren & Baltodano 2000, Iedema and Scheeres 2003, Sandlin 2004). The participation that is being urged results not from the critical consciousness anticipated by Friere (1972) but from demands of efficiency and the maintenance of the social and economic order (McLaren & Baltodano 2000), demands that are produced by social and technological change rather than a decline in literacy (Sandlin 2004). None the less, the literacy project on which Friere embarked is one that encompasses an awareness of human beings and human development, a critical exploration of being (Peters & Lankshear 1994), and therefore parallels the concerns of occupational science. Depending on its use, and mechanisms of control constructed around it, an occupational literacy could be a resource for social change towards a society that values difference and promotes the right to occupation.

Apprenticeship

A parallel illustration in health, albeit based in neither Friere nor occupational science, is provided by the work of Ville (2005). In a study on the use of biographical approaches in the reintegration of people with paraplegic conditions to work, she describes a process of 'apprenticeship' (p. 340). This is used to describe the process by which people come to terms with their own changed story at their own pace. Ville (2005) suggests that this period of reassessment of priorities and life objectives is often constricted by the pressure to return to employment or meet externally imposed goals. Her study includes interviews with rehabilitation professionals who admit that the effect of setting goals for integration can be to compress the 'biographical time' (Corbin & Strauss 1987, p. 253) the person needs to the detriment of their success in making adjustments. Cole (2004) uncovered similar experiences in his collection of narratives by people living with spinal cord injury. This might be interpreted as a conflict of interests between the rehabilitation process demanded by a cost-driven health care system and the need for people with paraplegic conditions to read and interpret their new situations, thus restricting the extent to which they can effect choice in determining their lives.

Earlier work by Sartain and colleagues (2000) with chronically ill children also drew on the importance of narrative in enabling young people to articulate and interpret the disruptions created by hospitalization and so emerge as active participants in the process of determining their needs. Galvin (2005) similarly explored the value of biographical approaches in addressing a richness and complexity in the 'disabled identity' (p. 393), which is produced through negative social attitudes and reductive approaches to health and social care (see also Chs 13, 14). As Corbin herself (2002, p. 259) says, 'When the body becomes severely disabled, there is often a body/mind split... People start saying "I am more than my body."' In her analysis of the limitations that impact on people through illness, she lists a set of dimensions in 'time, space, aesthetics, morality, technology, information, and interpersonal relationship' (Corbin 2002, p. 259).

We might interpret this list as a set of dimensions in which the membranes of two universes intersect, akin to the multidimensional view of the universe presented in M theory (Duff 2003). M theory proposes that there are multiple, intersecting universes. We might see one universe as that in which the healthy person perceives a certain set of principles and the other universe, occupying much the same space, as that of people with disabilities (this idea is implied in the title of David Hevey's (1993) The Creatures Time Forgot: Photography and Disability Imagery). In M theory it is possible that what is perceived as size in one universe is understood as density in an intersecting universe (Duff 2003). Here, in the colliding universes of occupational literacies, although social actors within them perceive slightly different sets of principles, conducting operations in the 'disabled' universe is dependent on the set of principles being operated in the dominant 'healthy' universe. Thus, although invisible much of the time to the prevailing level of occupational literacy in the 'healthy' universe, people with disabilities confound the 'healthy' universe's principles by popping up unexpectedly and presenting situations that do not fit with the normative principles operant there. These situations, e.g. problems arising from exclusion by the physical design of the environment, lack of hearing induction loops, unavailability of large print, might well be normative to the 'disabled' universe experience. The perception of two universes is maintained where people in the dominant universe do not have to read the phenomena of the disabled universe, but this is a situation that repeated contact would weaken (see Ch. 14). As Duff (2003) illustrates, the development of a multidimensional M theory has occurred through the need to explain and incorporate the understanding of increasingly complex phenomena.

The gaze of the other

However, the metaphor of colliding universes does not accommodate the complexity that the concept of 'reading the phenomena' raises. To begin with, the two universes are not distinct but overlap – not everyone recognizes the same degree of disability or health and people with disabilities and illnesses conceal or make explicit their circumstances to differing degrees. Added to this is the issue of contact. The intermeshing of the two universes operates at different strengths; in other words both the contact between them and the interpretation of that contact is managed by many individuals according to their particular characteristics. One of the lenses through which that contact is managed is 'the gaze of the other' (Galvin 2005, p. 397). People with disabilities or chronic illness often experience feelings of rejection or being made to feel invisible and develop a 'diminished sense of self' (Galvin

2005, p. 398) in response to the disabling attitudes of others (Murphy 1990, Sontag 1991; see also Chs 5, 6, 14).

A precondition for an occupational therapy reconceptualization of 'occupational literacy' is the recognition of attitudinal barriers to enabling the development of an empowering literacy. Many of the social networks that operate in society work along lines of communication that are based in whether or not people share interests or like each other, usually on the basis of reciprocated values (Goffman 1968, 1971, Rogers & Kincaid 1981, Allan 1989, Putnam 2000). Therefore one of the problematic issues is that, although literacy may give access to knowledge, the ability to use that knowledge and express what has been synthesized from it still depends on access to social networks. Whether a person is liked or respected, or whether others feel that they will agree with the message, determines how they are able to communicate their needs.

The identification, admission and expression of interests or needs make them available for the information of and interpretation by others. For example, by telling their stories people with disabilities can challenge dominant and normative social and cultural forces (Galvin 2005; see Chs 13, 14). In view of this capacity to challenge cultural dominance, literacy has always been a political and economic issue, which has been both restricted and encouraged across many societies (Hoyles 1977a, Manguel 1996) and, as Friere and Macedo (1987) acknowledge, has been used both to empower and to disempower. Where the growth of literacy has been encouraged, those in power have sought to manage the range of cultural expression that has resulted (James 1963, Williams 1965, Hoyles 1977b). Capitalist society requires literacies for particular types of occupational functioning. Williams (1965, 1966) suggests that industry was (as with the new literacies) a driving force in their growth. However, this development, often in answer to new technological demands, has been accompanied by concerns about the kinds of culture, thought and understanding to which literacy gives access and the need to preserve power relations (Engels 1973, Smith 1993).

Under the guise of increasing participation through the closure of a mythical knowledge gap, industry and governments are using these new literacies for the purposes of surveillance and control. Rather than enabling openness, consistency and quality, they provide managers who fear loss of control with a data-driven governing apparatus (Jackson 2000, Iedema & Scheeres 2003), one that is in some fields, such as health and social care, actually called governance.

More power to those in power

Although there have been developments in the apparatus, the managerial culture has not changed. Workers are suspicious of management, managers fear loss of control and the very participation the new literacies are designed to produce (Jackson 2000, Scheeres 2002, Iedema & Scheeres 2003). The availability of so much data increases the identification of error and lower productivity, the voicing of dissent, while demanding more improvement in productivity, more evidence in behaviour and attitude of workers' adherence to corporate cultures and official ideologies, with a concomitant increase in lower-status workers' fear of job losses or other retaliatory measures for expressing criticism, failure or mistakes, and stress (Jackson 2000, Scheeres 2002, Iedema & Scheeres 2003). It is a climate for occupational injustices (Townsend & Wilcock 2004a), a new totalitarianism that echoes the dystopian experiences of Winston Smith (Orwell 1954) and D-503 (Zamyatin 1972), the internalization of the regime in which the workplace as a social community (Handy 1996) is one of many sites of social control. Workplace literacy has actually handed more 'power to those in power' (Darville 1995, p. 250), a psychological panopticon in which individuals focus the lens upon themselves. While it apparently offers a more open and blame-free social culture of individual self-reliance, it actually exposes and problematizes differences (Jackson 2000, Iedema & Scheeres 2003, Sandlin 2004).

Through concepts such as occupational justice (Townsend & Wilcock 2004b), occupational deprivation (Whiteford 2000) and occupational apartheid (Kronenberg & Pollard 2005b; see Ch. 4) occupational science offers a critical process for exploring and redirecting the scope of occupational literacy to recognize and decode conflict and cooperation situations, or everyday political situations, in order to address inequalities, enable empowerment and promote occupational justice through the recognition of shared social responsibility. In Chapters 1 and 2 (see also Kronenberg & Pollard 2005a,b) the authors suggest that occupational therapists can use these principles and the pADL framework tool to enable people to make active choices about their empowerment, a catalytic function of the practitioner in cooperation with others. An occupational literacy may be the result of this process, entailing a critical awareness of the occupational nature of being, one that enables the making of life choices and works for democracy.

If one of the problems resulting from the plethora of workplace literacies has been the 'textualization' of work into readable and recordable and standardizable data (Darville 1995, Jackson 2000, Iedema & Scheeres 2003), a wider occupational literacy limited to mere consumption of information without critical understanding would be pointless.

Widening literacies

Iedema and Scheeres (2003) point to the dangers in widening these limited literacies that reach beyond defined areas of practice such as work. One of the examples they use is medical practice. In remodelling their work practices clinicians begin to adopt altered identities and reshape themselves in line with the new interdependent relationships that are produced by the changes.

When people are asked to take ownership of new practices at work, they lose the distinction between their personal and their working lives; their working lives appear to them to be consequent upon personal decisions rather than structural ones. Being involved in the decision processes entails being implicated when problems arise (Jackson 2000). When workers are asked to collaborate on process improvements, it becomes harder to identify oneself as exploited by a process that is still, after all, dominated by capital (Sandlin 2004).

When these processes of conceptualizing the self are managed by an industrial or work-related literacy system, developing a critical occupational literacy becomes more urgent. The market and process demands of the new capitalism threaten to compromise and limit the expression of individual identity. It is not merely an issue of workplace literacy how we perform as an interdependent functionary in a productive process, but also as consumers of that process in other areas of our lives; for example, lifestyle choices that affect our health and may therefore impact on sickness rates are also connected to purchasing behaviours. On the one hand there are advocates of libertarianism, for example those who wish to lift restrictions on smoking, drinking, drug use, the sex industry and gambling, while on the other there are arguments for preventive legislation and health measures to limit the damage resulting from these activities (Laurance & Stevenson 2004). The debate is between those who maintain that there is a need to protect the vulnerable and reduce pressure on public services through legislation and education about health risks, as well as an economic argument based on the costs to both industry and the taxpayer. The opposing view maintains that these risks are overstated, that the occupations generate substantial tax revenues and that the consequences are a matter of individual responsibility (Laurance 2004, Luckhurst 2004).

The issues are complex: freedom for some means restriction for others. Current debate in the UK concerns on the one hand increasing anxiety about smoking, alcohol use, poor diet and the health risks, behaviours and loss of productivity associated with them (Department of Health 2004), while on the other hand large corporations are lobbying for more liberal licensing for casinos. The addictive behaviours related to either of these issues are of concern to health services and to occupational therapists, and most often impact on the more vulnerable and deprived groups. For example, although gambling behaviour is under-researched

(May-Chahal et al 2004), in my clinical experience there have been people who have had to agree to having restricted access to their social security benefits to prevent them from spending all their income on drink or gambling, while previously, as a betting shop employee, I witnessed at first hand the reckless betting and abusive behaviour associated with this form of occupation as entertainment. Whichever of the arguments is right, better education on the issues will enable people to make informed choices about the activities they participate in (May-Chahal et al 2004).

Similarly, a critical occupational literacy should be concerned with the full range and complexity of human doing, being, becoming and belonging (Wilcock 1999, Hammell 2004) and the enablement of occupational justice. Through occupational literacy people can make informed choices to exercise their freedom and their right to occupation, in diverse ways and diverse contexts.

An occupational literacy is not just about making a critical reading but also of developing critical modes of expression that enable reflection on experience. Consequently an occupational literacy encompasses the interpretation by the individual of internal and external events and the sharing of interpretations with others. As a mode of learning and reflection, the interpretations an occupational literacy offers may change through dialogue and with time. The significance of occupational events is not always immediately apparent but may be revealed through the course of life. According to Freeman (1993), this learning, reflection, interpretation and reinterpretation is an essential part of human functioning and has no objective standpoint. We are immersed in the process of doing and in multiple discourses of doing through reflection, interpretation and the development of our own narratives of experience (see Chs 2, 8, 10, 11, 13, 14, 19, 20).

Occupational therapy – literacy emerging from tension between discourse and practice

One such discourse is that concerning occupational therapy itself, which has been described as a narrative genre (Detweiler & Peyton 1999) but which, through a tendency to oral practices of narrative (Schwammle 1996), gives rise to the kind of distinction Smith (1993, p. 203) makes between 'discourse' and 'local practices'. Thus, although the profession of occupational therapy is managed through a discourse, it is not actually controlled by it, because at a local level individual practitioners continue to make individual choices. For example, according to Habermas (1987) it is this tension (we may assume that occupational therapists, like all people, experience multiple tensions of this nature; see Ch. 6) that generates the free consciousness through which knowledge, identity and culture are formed. None the less, the 'textually mediated'(Smith 1993, p. 209) progress of this discourse is intended to increase control and often, in the case of health and welfare, the systemization of equity in treatment, for example through the monitoring of ethnic, gender and cultural data. There are increasing pressures to conform to this discourse, for example through governance measures such as an evidence base for practice favouring quantitative approaches for a body of knowledge that is concerned with reading individual experience, despite assertions that for many areas of the profession the availability of evidence is undermined by a lack of research (Pollard 2002, Duncan et al 2007, O'Connell & Farnsworth 2007), and that combined perspectives offer the best research solutions (Duncan & Nicol 2004).

Occupational therapy has been described as a middle-class profession, with values that inhibit accessibility to would-be practitioners from lower-class backgrounds and minorities, and a discourse that carries a professional separation from a feminine domesticity in that its concerns with occupation frequently avoid the areas of domestic occupational needs that those who join the profession have left behind (Pollard & Walsh 2000; see Chs 5, 7). An occupational literacy is concerned with the interpretation or reading of occupation, the revelation of the meanings and a revaluing of occupation.

Cultural limitations

The meaning of occupational being has been little explored amongst the limitations of occupational therapy research and its tendency to respond to the demands of a biomedical scientific paradigm. Iwama (2005, 2006), for example, points to the cultural limitations of much of the supporting theory for a body of knowledge that purports to be concerned with the full range of human activity. An occupational literacy would enable occupational therapists, and perhaps occupational scientists, to map the holes in this holism, but a failure to engage in a critical process that enables practitioners and those they work with to read the complexities and multiple layers of meaning in occupation would risk the reproduction of a set of values that is advocated by therapists without sufficient question or reflection (Abberley 1995, Hammell 2007). In the management of care plans and the development and negotiation of interventions to enable the rehabilitation of people into societies and communities it is important to consider the political context in the process of doing so (as explored by many authors in this book).

Whereas one of the problems of increasing textualization or textual mediation has been a corresponding demand for sophistication in the literacies that deal with this phenomenon (Smith 1993, Jackson 2000), a critical occupational literacy should work for demystification and transparency. Through measures such as Kronenberg and Pollard's pADL tool and principles (2005a,b) in concert with the concepts of occupational justice (Townsend 1993, Wilcock 1998, Townsend & Wilcock 2004b) and Frank and Zemke's social transformation model (Ch. 7), a critical occupational literacy will not be yet another new technology for its own sake, producing another set of demands, but a tool for what Habermas (1987, p. 316) has called 'enlightened action'.

The enlightening reach of an occupational literacy is not confined to work practices but to the whole range of human occupation. Just as we enter training or education for work, we also undergo learning, both formal and informal, in the pursuit of domestic and leisure activities and social behaviours (Heath 1983). A wide range of popular and academic literature and other information is available to support this, while traditionally many activities, such as fishing, football or learning to ride a bicycle, are learned on an individual basis from peers, parents or relatives. The frequently oral and natural form of this learning none the less contains elements of a literacy. Fishing can entail learning to 'read' conditions in order to know when and where to find particular fish or the best places from which to fish (Toth 2000). Football requires the ability to interpret the movements and tactics of the members of the opposing team in order to defend or attack (Foers 2004). Riding a bicycle involves not only making the correct responses to road signs and signals from other road users, but also learning to anticipate the road ahead (Ballantine 1978).

For many people it may seem sufficient to leave it at that. But there are other potential components that an occupational literacy may choose to read. Fishing and football represent two major leisure industries in the UK. Extensive areas of rivers and lakes are maintained for coarse angling (Environment Agency 2005). Almost every community has access to a football pitch. Large numbers of boys, men and, increasingly, women and girls are involved in both activities. Cycling is also a popular activity, with national cycleways, a burgeoning demand for places for off-road cycling and political lobbies concerned with improving safety and the awareness of cyclists' needs (Sustrans 2005). All three are organized at many levels in UK society, from spontaneous 'kickabouts', fishing trips and bike rides to communal and work-centred clubs and local and national competitions, amateur and professional.

An activity analysis may reveal biomedical and kinesiological information about the effects of these occupations on those who take part in them. It may also determine the psychological, cognitive and social elements associated with them. There are, however, further occupational aspects to any activity that may impact on their value to the individual and the community. Some of these may be counted as occupational spin-offs (Rebeiro 2001) – for example through the occupations connected with the organization and membership of football teams, fishing trips or cycling clubs. Others, however, arise from the meaning, context and effect of these occupations in the community (see also Chs 12–14).

On the one hand areas may be maintained for people spontaneously to organize these activities as groups of individuals, simply because the activity answers their need for physical activity and maintaining social relations. At the community level it may be understood that it is beneficial to develop understanding and good social relationships through the activities associated with occupations such as these. Fishing, cycling and football are all potential vehicles for fostering appropriate relationships between peers and between generations. For example, all have been used in the rehabilitation of young offenders and the latter two in preventive police work to foster their relationships with the community they serve.

These occupations do not only serve the community for the purpose of developing good relationships, they also have an effect on environment and health. Aside from their health benefits as physical and social activities, each requires the maintenance of areas in which they may be safely practised, for example the upkeep of safe riverbanks and riverside paths, clean rivers for fish to breed in, and green communal spaces in urban and rural communities alike (Environment Agency 2005, Sustrans 2005). This not only provides employment, as does the manufacture and retail of equipment to support these activities, but also promotes interaction and respect for the green environment and education about environmental issues.

These occupations also, through the social relations connected with them and their dependence on the environment, and the availability and safety of equipment, require the learning of numerous practices. Each has a specialized technical vocabulary that may be the subject of conventional literacies; each requires participants to be considerate of the needs of other participants and others using the same environment. A person does not merely learn practice skills and the ability to assess risks connected with activities but ways of being a footballer, angler or cyclist in response to contexts of diverse relations. In the case of football it has been posited that the lessons learned may explain much else that happens in the world and ways of relating to it, and it is possible that this extrapolation might be applied elsewhere (Foers 2004). These are occupational choices, dependent on the acquisition and development of occupational literacy.

One way this might be realized is through the application of the principles Kronenberg and Pollard (2005a, p. 5) derived from Molinas Maldonaldo and Monroy Peralta (1999). Thus, if 'everybody is responsible for everything', 'the aim is not to attain the goals proposed, but the process above all' and if people are 'thinking locally, and acting globally' they might question whether, in the interpretation of football tactics, 'professional' fouls are permissible. When buying a football for the community psychiatric patient soccer team, should an occupational therapist be concerned about oppressive working practices operating in the country of its manufacture? If 'nothing changes if nothing is done to change', how should the team address other community members who allow their dogs to foul the pitch? If 'there is no public ethic without a personal ethic', how does an angler practise the sport in a way that minimizes risk to other people, wildlife and the environment, for example through the choice and use of tackle and bait? How can off-road cyclists reduce the damage caused by their machines on paths shared with walkers?

Politics with a small 'p' – literacy and justice

These concerns and practices are the issues of politics with a small 'p', issues around which the people involved in these occupations have to resolve the conflicts and possibilities of cooperation that arise from them with others sharing the same environments. Indeed bodies such as the UK's Environment Agency and the sustainable transport charity Sustrans are seeking to involve people engaged in popular activities such as cycling and angling in conservation and management issues (Environment Agency 2005, Sustrans 2005). Writers on politics and political action have indicated the importance of lobbying around these issues as the stuff of larger political debates (Ward 1985, Tansey 2000). The occupational literacy skills that are involved here (based on the principle that, since everyone shares the environment, everybody is responsible for everything) require the ability to cooperate with others. In many respects, they are similar to the workplace literacy skills required of industry. However, while optimizing production may be an outcome of occupational literacy, this would be secondary to the optimization of occupational justice.

As we have seen, workplace literacies do not address the fundamental issue of power but a critical occupational literacy can. One definition of 'occupation' (Irvine 1970, p. 327; Kirkpatrick 1983, p. 874) is 'possession'. Despite any claims of property law to the land and buildings in which we may live, everybody possesses the environment and the right to occupation within it. An occupationally literate person would be someone who is able to demonstrate appropriate skills and use them to achieve their occupational rights and the outcomes associated with these rights, or else are empowered to make choices about their participation. An occupationally literate society would not be one that optimizes occupational performances in limited sets of skills, or places emphasis on the high achievements of a few, but one where a critical consciousness enables people to respond in a facilitative way to the needs of others. The possibility of the construction of a society where occupational literacy is accessible to all requires overcoming power differentials that currently regulate access to resources. Access to facilities is directly connected with developing the skills and aptitudes that enable engagement in occupations of choice and need (see Ch. 5).

In each of the dystopias cited in this discussion the authors, Dick (1973), Orwell (1954) and Zamyatin (1972), are concerned with the management of information and the ability to interpret what is real and meaningful to individuals and wider communities. Their characters are struggling with a process of divining meaning amid the phenomena of the banal and everyday. After all, it is our immediate environment that concerns us most and where problems in occupational literacy first arise. Therefore, when occupational literacy questions power and status as the means by which occupational opportunity is obstructed, it has to work from a base in commonplace experience. Unless individuals and communities can resolve issues at this level they are unable to build higher levels of occupational capacity. The role of occupational therapists, therefore, is to facilitate occupational literacy through their practice and engagement with both individuals and communities.

In an earlier link between occupation, possession, interpretation and power, when John Ball said 'When Adam dalf and Eve span, who was thanne a gentilman?' he went on to advocate the complete destruction of the feudal social order (Dobson 1970). Over 600 years later, faced with a more complex social order, violent change is less possible, desirable or even necessary; however 'nothing changes, if nothing is done to change'. An occupational literacy process locates the questioning that supports and identifies the need for change. While a true occupational literacy process should perhaps serve the interests of those most disempowered, who may need to exercise their vision most, it may enable those with power to share responsibility through the facilitation of greater social participation.

Acknowledgements

Thanks to Dr Elizabeth Townsend, Dalhousie University, Canada, for her initial suggestion that this article be written and for her comments on earlier drafts.

References

Abberley P 1995 Disabling ideology in health and welfare – the case of occupational therapy. Disability and Society 10: 221–232

Allan G 1989 Friendship, developing a sociological perspective. Harvester Wheatsheaf, New York

Arendt H 1998 The human condition, 2nd edn. University of Chicago Press, Chicago, IL

Aristotle 1962 The politics. Penguin, Harmondsworth

Ballantine R 1978 Richard's bicycle book. Ballantine Books, New York

Carvin A 2000 More than just access: fitting literacy and content into the digital divide equation. Educause Review, November/

December, 38–47. Available online at: http://www.educause.edu/pub/er/erm00/articles006/erm0063.pdf; accessed 9 October 2007

Cole J 2004 Still lives. MIT Press, Cambridge, MA

Corbin J 2002 The body in health and illness. Qualitative Health Research 13: 256–267

Corbin J, Strauss A L 1987 Accompaniment of chronic illness: changes in body, self, biography, and biographical time. In: Roth J K, Conrad P (eds) Research in the sociology of health care, vol. 5. JAI Press, Greenwich, CT: p 249–281

Darville R 1995 Literacy, experience, power. In: Campbell M, Manicom A (eds) Knowledge, experience and ruling relations. University of Toronto, Toronto, Ontario: p 249–261

Department of Health 2004 Choosing health: making healthy choices easier. Available online at: http://www.dh.gov.uk/PublicationsAndStatistics/Publications/PublicationsPolicyAndGuidance/PublicationsPolicyAndGuidanceArticle/fs/en?CONTENT_ID=4094550&chk=aN5Cor; accessed 9 October 2007

Detweiler J, Peyton C 1999 Defining occupations: a chronotypic study of narrative genres in a health discipline's emergence. Written Communication 16: 412–468

Dick P K 1973 The three stigmata of Palmer Eldritch. Penguin, Harmondsworth

Dobson R B 1970 The Peasants Revolt of 1381. Pitman, Bath

Duff M J 2003 The theory formerly known as strings. Available online at: http://feynman.physics.lsa.umich.edu/~mduff/talks/1998%20-%20The%20Theory%20Formerly%20Known%20as%20Strings.pdf; accessed 30 September 2007

Duncan E A S, Nicol M M 2004 Subtle realism and occupational therapy: an alternative approach to knowledge generation and evaluation. British Journal of Occupational Therapy 67: 453–456

Duncan E A S, Paley J, Eva G 2007 Complex interventions and complex systems in occupational therapy: an alternative perspective. British Journal of Occupational Therapy 70: 199–206

Electronic Arts 2002 The Sims. Electronic Arts, Chertsey

Engels F 1973 The condition of the working-class in England. Progress Publishers, Moscow

Environment Agency 2005 Angling 2015 – getting more people into angling. Environment Agency, Bristol

Foers F 2004 How soccer explains the world: an unlikely theory of globalization. Harper Collins, New York

Freeman M 1993 Rewriting the self. Routledge, London

Frick M J, Birkenholz R J, Gardner H et al 1995 Rural and urban high school student knowledge and perception of agriculture. Journal of Agricultural Education 36(4): 7–8

Friere P 1972 Pedagogy of the oppressed. Penguin, Harmondsworth

Friere P 1985 The politics of education. Bergin & Garvey, New York

Friere P, Macedo D 1987 Literacy: reading the word and the world. Bergin & Garvey, South Hadley, MA

Galvin R D 2005 Researching the disabled identity: contextualising the identity transformations which accompany the onset of impairment. Sociology of Health and Illness 27: 393–413

Goffman E 1968 Stigma, notes on the management of spoiled identity. Pelican, Harmondsworth

Goffman E 1971 The presentation of self in everyday life. Pelican, Harmondsworth

Gray J M 1998 Putting occupation into practice: occupation as ends, occupation as means. American Journal of Occupational Therapy 52: 354–364

Habermas J 1987 Knowledge and human interests. Polity Press, Oxford

Hammell K W 2004 Dimensions in meaning in the occupations of everyday life. Canadian Journal of Occupational Therapy 71: 296–305

Hammell K W 2007 Client-centred practice: ethical obligation or professional obfuscation. British Journal of Occupational Therapy 70: 264–266

Handy C 1996 Beyond certainty: the changing world of organisations. Arrow Books, London

Heath S B 1983 Ways with words: language, life and work in communities and classrooms. Cambridge University Press, Cambridge

Hevey D 1993 The creatures time forgot: photography and disability imagery. Routledge, London

Hoyles M 1977a The history and politics of literacy. In: Hoyles M (ed) The politics of literacy. Writers and Readers, London: p 14–32

Hoyles M 1977b Cultural deprivation and compensatory education. In: Hoyles M (ed) The politics of literacy. Writers and Readers, London: p 172–181

Hull G, Grubb N 1999 Literacy skills and work. In: Wagner D, Venetsky R (eds) Literacy: an international handbook. Westview Press, Boulder, CO: p 311–317

Iedema R, Scheeres H 2003 From doing work to talking work: renegotiating knowing, doing and identity. Applied Linguistics 24: 316–337

International Symposium for Literacy 1975 Declaration of Persepolis. International Co-ordination Secretariat for Literacy, Paris

Irvine A H (ed) 1970 The Fontana English dictionary. Fontana, London

Iwama M 2005 Situated meaning: an issue of culture, inclusion, and occupational therapy. In: Kronenberg F, Simó Algado S, Pollard N (eds) Occupational therapy without borders: learning from the spirit of survivors. Churchill Livingstone, Oxford: p 131–143

Iwama M 2006 The Kawa Model: culturally relevant occupational therapy. Churchill Livingstone, Edinburgh

Jackson N 2000 Writing-up people at work: investigations of workplace literacy. Literacy and Numeracy Studies 10: 5–22

James L 1963 Fiction for the working man. Penguin, Harmondsworth

Kirkpatrick E M (ed) 1983 Chambers 20th century dictionary. W & R Chambers, Edinburgh

Kronenberg F, Pollard N 2005a Introduction: a beginning. In: Kronenberg F, Simó Algado S, Pollard N (eds) Occupational therapy without borders: learning from the spirit of survivors. Churchill Livingstone, Oxford: p 1–13

Kronenberg F, Pollard N 2005b Overcoming occupational apartheid: a preliminary exploration of the political nature of occupational therapy. In: Kronenberg F, Simó Algado S, Pollard N (eds) Occupational therapy without borders: learning from the spirit of survivors. Churchill Livingstone, Oxford: p 59–87

Laurance J 2004 Portrait of a nation addicted to fatty food, alcohol and tobacco. The Independent. Available online at: http://news.independent.co.uk/low_res/story.jsp?story=583263&host=3&dir=59; accessed 16 November 2004

Laurance J, Stevenson R 2004 Reid's smoking ban attacked by both sides. The Independent. Available online at: http://news.independent.co.uk/uk/health_medical/story.jsp?story=583679; accessed 17 November 2004

Luckhurst T 2004 Smoke screen. The Independent Review 16 November, p 8

McLaren P, Baltodano M P 2000 The future of teacher education and the politics of resistance. Teacher Education 11: 47–60

Manguel A 1996 A history of reading. Flamingo, London

May-Chahal C, Measham F, Brannock M et al 2004 Young people and gambling in Britain: a systematic and critical review of the research literature relating to gaming machine, lottery and pools coupons practice by children and young people under 18. Department of Culture, Media and Sport, DCMS Technical paper no. 8,

London. Available online at: http://www.culture.gov.uk/NR/rdonlyres/F4941636–7790–44B2-A994-F963853B6F77/0/YoungPeopleandGamblinginBritian.pdf; accessed 11 October 2007

Mill J S 1991 On liberty and other essays (ed J Gray). Oxford University Press, Oxford

Molinas Maldonaldo M M, Monroy Peralta J G 1999 Sistemización de experiencias: una invitación para la acción una propuesta para instituciones y/o programas que trabajan con el sector de la infancia. Childhope, Guatamela City

Murphy R 1990 The body silent. WW Norton, New York

O'Connell M, Farnworth L 2007 Occupational therapy in forensic psychiatry: a review of the literature and a call for a united and international response. British Journal of Occupational Therapy 70: 184–191

Ofcom 2003 Consumers' use of mobile telephony Q11 November 2002–27 January 2003. Available online at: http://www.ofcom.org.uk/static/archive/oftel/publications/research/2003/q11mobr0103.htm#chaptersix; accessed 11 October 2007

Orwell G 1954 Nineteen eighty-four. Penguin, Harmondsworth

Peters M, Lankshear C 1994 Education and hermeneutics, a Frierean interpretation. In: McLaren PL, Lankshear C (eds) Politics of liberation: paths from Friere. Routledge, London: p 171–192

Pollard N 2002 On the line: continuing professional development between research and practice. British Journal of Occupational Therapy 65: 242–243

Pollard N, Walsh S 2000 Occupational therapy, gender and mental health: an inclusive perspective. British Journal of Occupational Therapy 63: 425–431

Putnam R 2000 Bowling alone, the collapse and revival of American community. Simon & Schuster, New York

Rebeiro K 1998 Occupation-as-means to mental health: a review of the literature, and a call for research. Canadian Journal of Occupational Therapy 65: 12–19

Rebeiro K 2001 Occupational spin-off. Occupational terminology interactive dialogue. Journal of Occupational Science 8: 33–34

Rogers E M, Kincaid D L 1981 Communication networks: towards a new paradigm for research. Free Press, New York

Rush R T, Moe A, Storlie R 1986 Occupational literacy education. International Reading Association, Newark, DE

Sandlin J A 2000 Literacy for work: exploring everyday dominant discourses abut work and literacy in the everyday practice of adult literacy education. 2000 AERC Proceedings. Available online at: http://www.edst.educ.ubc.

ca/aerc/2000/sandlinj1-web.htm; accessed
11 October 2007

Sandlin J A 2004 'It's all up to you': how welfare-
to-work programmes construct workforce
success. Adult Education Quarterly 54:
89–104

Sartain S, Clarke C L, Heyman R 2000 Hearing the
voices of children with chronic illness. Journal
of Advanced Nursing 32: 913–921

Scheeres H 2002 Producing core values in the
workplace: learning new identities. Available
online at: nhttp://www.avetra.org.au/
abstracts_ and_papers_2002/scheeres.pdf;
accessed 11 October 2007

Schwammle D 1996 Are you listening? The oral
tradition of occupational therapy. Canadian
Journal of Occupational Therapy 63: 62–66

Smith D E 1993 Texts, facts and femininity.
Routledge, London

Smith D E 1999 Writing the social. University of
Toronto Press, Toronto, Ontario

Sontag S 1991 Illness as metaphor and AIDS and
its metaphors. Penguin Books, London

Stein S 2000 Equipped for the future content
standards: what adults need to know and be able
to do in the 21st century. National Institute for
Literacy, Washington, DC

Sustrans 2005 Charity information site. Available
online at: http://www.sustrans.org/default.
asp?sID=1090831665348&pID; accessed 23
January 2006

Tansey S 2000 Politics: the basics, 2nd edn.
Routledge, London

Toth M 2000 The complete idiot's guide to fishing
basics. Alpha Books, New York

Townsend E 1993 Occupational therapy's social
vision. Canadian Journal of Occupational
Therapy 60: 174–184

Townsend E Wilcock A 2004a Occupational
justice. In: Christiansen C, Townsend E (eds)
Introduction to occupation: the art and
science of living. Prentice Hall, Thorofare, NJ:
p 243–273

Townsend E, Wilcock A 2004b Occupational
justice and client centred practice: a dialogue.
Canadian Journal of Occupational Therapy
71: 75–87

Ville I 2005 Biographical work and returning
to employment following a spinal cord injury.
Sociology of Health and Illness 27: 324–350

Ward S 1985 Organising things. Pluto, London

Whiteford G 2000 Occupational deprivation:
global challenge in the new millennium.
British Journal of Occupational Therapy
63: 200–204

Wilcock A 1998 An occupational perspective of
health. Slack, Thorofare, NJ

Wilcock A 1999 Reflections on doing, being and
becoming. Australian Occupational Therapy
Journal 46: 1–11

Wilcock A, Townsend E 2000 Occupational
terminology interactive dialogue. Occupational
justice. Journal of Occupational Science 7:
84–86

Williams R 1965 The long revolution. Penguin,
Harmondsworth

Williams R 1966 Culture and society 1780–1950.
Penguin, Harmondsworth

Yerxa E J, Clark F, Frank G et al 1990 An
introduction to occupational science, a
foundation for occupational therapy in the
21st century. Occupational Therapy in Health
Care 6: 1–17

Zamyatin Y 1972 We (trans B Guilbert Guerney).
Penguin, Harmondsworth

Explorations of context

2

EXPLORATIONS OF CONTEXT

This group of chapters considers some of the contextual influences on occupation. The literature of occupational therapy sometimes has a tendency to focus on human occupations as if they were somehow disconnected from other elements of human behaviour or social influences. Although there are exceptions, much of the discussion of human occupation in the professional discourse has steered clear of gender, class, sexuality or political concepts. When these subjects arise they consequently stand out as if they were special cases rather than part of the general perspective of all human occupation.

In the first chapter the authors revise their earlier arguments for situations of occupational apartheid, acknowledging some of the challenges this term presents. The second chapter reviews a combination of dimensions of occupation that are also infrequently explored despite the strongly gendered professional membership and the importance of gender and class in occupational therapy's development. The reluctance to acknowledge or perhaps the lack of a perception of these issues has contributed to difficulties in navigating the profession through the different challenges it faces; the picture of occupational therapy as a holistic profession is blurred, difficult to capture and present in its complexity. The discussion of heteroglossia in the final part of this section suggests that a problem-based approach offers the means to relate both the wider environmental and contextual features of occupation and the application of interventions to the needs of communities and individuals.

Occupational apartheid

4

Nick Pollard, Frank Kronenberg,
Dikaios Sakellariou

Abstract

This chapter explores the concept of occupational apartheid as something that emerges through the uneven distribution of resources among different groups of people and a consequent imbalance of power. This imbalance arises through human occupation, which is often associated with forms of territorial occupation to the exclusion of other inhabitants (Ch. 20). Over time those groups with more power develop systematic measures to protect and maintain these inequalities from a fear that their privileges could be lost or taken away by force. Occupational apartheid is considered through a number of examples, and a concluding section appraises human occupation as a facet of being that contains both positive and negative aspects. While the term itself has to be applied to specific occupational circumstances arising from the oppression of one group by another, none the less much of human culture and development has depended on the experience of situations that may with hindsight be recognized as occupational apartheid.

Occupational apartheid is:

the segregation of groups of people through the restriction or denial of access to dignified and meaningful participation in occupations of daily life on the basis of race, colour, disability, national origin, age, gender, sexual preference, religion, political beliefs, status in society, or other characteristics. Occasioned by political forces, its systematic and pervasive social, cultural, and economic consequences jeopardize health and well being as experienced by individuals, communities, and societies.

Kronenberg & Pollard 2005, p. 67

An understanding of occupation as 'doing, being, becoming and belonging' (Wilcock 1999, p. 1, Hammell 2004, Iwama 2006) might seem inadequate where there are dominant and minority groups with distinct cultural experiences, for example in working with asylum seekers (Smith 2005; Chs 10, 15–20), and across classes and gender (Ch. 5). In any society it may become apparent from such differences that occupational therapists also need to

55

understand occupation in a territorial or possessive sense. Communities and the institutions that serve them are often conceived in geographical terms, or as occupying positions within social strata.

An extreme example of this could be found in South Africa under the previous apartheid system, where certain occupations were reserved for certain groups defined by their racial characteristics. These characteristics were determined by criteria set out by a powerful minority of white people. Our use of the term occupational apartheid refers to specific circumstances where the segregation of people is organized, systemic and intended to produce serious inequalities, or is operationally maintained by a dominant group despite the evidence of the harmful effects it produces in an oppressed group. There are many occupational situations that are determined by inequality: 'occupational apartheid' should not be used to describe minor inconveniences but reserved for the maintenance of restrictions by one group for the erosion or disregard for another's essential human rights.

In many instances the dominant group that determines the nature of the restriction does so to protect its interests and power. The restriction is based on the way the group in power defines itself; this becomes the qualification that determines occupational choice. In effect, the group in power takes steps to colonize aspects of occupation in order to define them as its territory – an example close to home might be the multidisciplinary conflicts that arise over professional boundaries, or in situations of domestic abuse (Cage 2007). Such restrictions are usually based on a fear of the excluded and an implicit recognition of the fact that power can be taken away, or laws and principles of exclusion can be subverted.

Forceful arguments may be made that a certain group defined by an arbitrary characteristic such as ethnic origin or class lacks the facility for certain occupations, but these are based on the implementation of restrictive measures to make the facility more difficult to obtain (Bush 2004). In other words the argument depends on crude manipulation of the evidence (Arendt 1986, Bush 2004). Eventually, as the history of South African apartheid demonstrates, such a restriction is morally unsupportable but it is also evident that the legacy of apartheid continues not only in the wide social and economic disparities but in the less visible, internalized self-perceptions of people and communities that hold themselves to be superior or inferior to their peers on the basis of race and culture (Bush 2004).

Aptly, perhaps, given apartheid's concern with gradations in skin colour, Card (2002, p. 6) describes such situations of continued oppressive contexts as 'grey zones'. This term, taken from Primo Levi's Holocaust experiences, refers to situations where people do what they have to do to survive and are even complicit in the perpetration of harm to others, without necessarily struggling against the oppression they experience. Card (2002) extends the concept of grey zones to allow them to refer to an accumulation of evil, which she defines as the product of wrongdoing and deliberate harm. These processes of accumulation may not be immediately clear, as discriminatory or disabling attitudes develop over time, for example through negligence or unscrupulousness. They manifest themselves in the abuses that human beings apply to each other, for example the development of racism as an associated cultural product of slavery, or the development of misogyny and its link to forms of domestic abuse (Bush 2004, Cage 2007).

Occupational apartheid is not an accident of human activity. It is either the result of laws and restrictions created to discriminate and exclude (as in the apartheid era in South Africa, Israel, and many other states that have operated regulations directed against, for example, indigenous minorities such as the Ainu People in northern Japan (Siddle 1999)), or else is recognized to be an effect of laws and restrictions, assumptions and attitudes. The conditions these produce may or may not be the result intended, but they are tolerated through expediency and complicity. These grey zones are an aspect of all human societies. While there may be conditional elements that clearly serve dominant interests or perceptions, whether locally (as in 20th century Northern Ireland (Bardon 1992) and the southern states of the USA (Brogan 1990))

56

or globally (as in the relationship between the 'developed' and 'developing' world), inhabiting them involves the assumption of 'grey' attitudes concerned with the preservation of self (Card 2002).

Consequently there is, as Card (2002) admits, a great deal of complexity and ambiguity. Consider, for example, a therapist who witnesses institutional bad practice and is obliged to report this. If the institution condones the practice, the practitioner risks being discriminated against (Harding 1991). Often, people who have attempted to report malpractice among their colleagues have themselves become victims of institutional bullying or discrimination. Consequently there can be a reluctance to do so. People may be aware of what they should do but are also fearful of the possible consequences for themselves.

Mattingly and Fleming (1994) found that occupational therapy values have often been at odds with dominant medical practices. This was principally because occupational or real-life issues did not fit the reductionist paradigm sometimes offered in treatment plans. However, in order to retain their value with colleagues of other disciplines therapists learned to record those of their interventions that concurred with biomedical issues while continuing their own interventions – which were not recorded. Consequently, some occupational therapists developed an 'underground practice' (Mattingly & Fleming 1994, p. 296).

This conflict of interests is an illustration of the difficulty of balancing everyday decisions, such as those therapists make in practice, in favour of right and wrong. Codes of practice can become opposed or may pose dilemmas in the face of client needs. Kazez (2007) argues that the maintenance of consistently good behaviour is a moral challenge because the more we explore the cause and effect of our occupations the more complex the issues become, 'there are no clear answers' (p. 157). We can take our complicity for granted since, in an interconnected society, 'everybody is responsible for everything'. This means that we are obliged to question our actions and probably to act on what we discover. *Probably*, because in that action we need both to be clear why we are acting in a certain way and to know that what we choose to do does not perpetrate some other negative effect. As Kazez (2007) frequently points out, this does not mean that we must do so without regard to our individual needs (Ch. 1).

This apparent political and moral complexity impacts on the occupational choices of daily functioning if, as human beings, we are to be concerned with making values of doing, being, becoming and belonging. Wilcock (1998) traces the evolution of occupation alongside human development, proposing that generally the separation of doing into categories of work and leisure emerged as societies grew in complexity, particularly with the development of agriculture and, later, industry. She argues that the development of capitalism created situations where the productive or occupational nature of humankind was turned against itself. Doing, being, becoming and belonging became subverted to mere subsistence in a wage economy and work became separated from leisure. Thus the political sense of occupation arises from a need for social justice, balance and equality in occupational opportunities. Whiteford (2005, p. 354–359) argues that to bring the political in a just and empowering way into everyday occupation requires a 'Third Way' perspective between the opposites of capitalism and socialism to bring about an 'enabling state'. Such a state mobilizes resources to address disabling experiences, restrictions and barriers to everyday occupational functioning through measures that devolve power to communities.

If this is to happen, political power cannot belong only to politicians, captains of industry or religious leaders. If everybody is to be responsible for everything, people and communities must insist on their rights. However, such a situation does not produce equality, only equality of the right to compete (Gomberg 2007). The 'enabling state' is consequently an illusory notion, since, as Gomberg says (2007, p. 19), 'the problems of competitive opportunity cannot be addressed by levelling the playing field'. Every state is unavoidably a disabling state (Graeber 2004). Every state will produce marginalizations and competition between different interest groups, or develop policies that cannot be applied equally to all its citizens. This is readily apparent when geographical location is considered with regard to access to health facilities (Ch. 10). In remote or sparsely populated areas it is difficult to provide the specialized facilities that may be available to city dwellers, even though there may be a right of access.

The uneven distribution of resources (whether health facilities, transport and communication infrastructure or opportunities for work) generates inequalities and the development of discriminatory attitudes (Fraser 1997). These become hardened into behaviours such as racism and can become intellectualized by professionals in order to justify policy decisions on the basis that to give people access to certain facilities would be a waste of resources (Gomberg 2007, e.g. Manning 1964)

Why 'occupational apartheid'?

The term occupational apartheid was first coined in relation to the designation of certain occupations for certain racial groups in US society and the promotion of affirmative action as a measure to counter the difficulties black people had in obtaining higher-status positions (Steinberg 1995, 2003). The use of the term apartheid has been controversial in the occupational therapy community. Some of the people with whom we have corresponded regard the term as counterproductive. They feel that apartheid is too strong, emotional and politically charged a word to describe this process, or else that it should specifically relate to the political and ethnic divides of the late 20th century South African government. Others agree that there is a real and systemic problem that the term 'occupational apartheid' recognizes but are not comfortable with its identification by liberal white males from privileged backgrounds in former colonizing powers, who, not having experienced direct oppression, may be considered part of the problem, as for example Biko (1987) has commented.

We respect such criticism. However, having raised this argument, we feel that there are valid issues to explore and that if marginalizing forces are in evidence we should not be complicit but seek to challenge them as best we can. These issues apply as much to the circumstances in which we live as anywhere else; no one lives very far from disparities in equality, so our work on occupational apartheid continues. Access to occupational therapy training is a privilege (Ch. 5); the global distribution of occupational therapists and educational opportunities is very uneven (Ch. 7). This book represents our current position but we are still developing these ideas as we receive welcome critique from our colleagues.

Occupational apartheid (Kronenberg 1999; Kronenberg & Pollard 2005, 2006) is a systematic and political process of marginalization and segregation leading to inequality and oppression. It is a relatively new term in occupational therapy but indicates an ancient phenomenon, evidenced in slavery and serfdom and the many situations where groups of people identify other groups which they deliberately and systematically subject to restricted occupations. Individuals can intentionally support conditions of occupational apartheid because it suits them, or they might think it is the right thing to do, or unintentionally through choosing not to know, or merely ignoring, how their choices and actions affect other groups of people. It is important to emphasize that occupational apartheid applies to the exclusion of groups, and conditions that affect individuals because they are members of excluded groups, rather than those exclusions applied between individuals, for example as a result of personal antipathy (Elelwani Ramugondo, personal communication, 2007). Occupational apartheid may set the systematic conditions for individual occupational circumstances but the extent to which these are operated between individuals depends on whether they observe them or not. For example, Wicks and Whiteford (2005) explore the history of barriers to occupational choice experienced by women. While they would not use the term occupational apartheid to describe these exclusions, it is arguable that it can be applied where overt restrictions are operated on the basis of sex or in situations of domestic violence in which the control of women by their partners is culturally sanctioned (Cage 2007).

In many countries street children are a social phenomenon whose existence and humanity is not only denied, but they are exploited by representatives of authority and even aid agencies, or else treated as vermin (Bonfim 2005, Kronenberg 2005). Disabled people have also struggled for many years to be allowed to articulate their own voices, to assert themselves and their right to be different (Mason 2000). Occupational apartheid is, consequently, not just a product of the relationships we make and the way we articulate them; it is evident in the failure to express critiques of injustices, to speak up and act for ourselves or with others. This in itself can be the result of oppression, being made to fear the consequences, being afraid of upsetting a situation so as to make conditions worse or preventing others from escaping by drawing attention to an issue (Arendt 1986), and should not necessarily be a criticism. Sometimes, in order to survive, it is tactically necessary to be silent until the opportunity to speak out effectively can be found.

An important aspect of occupational apartheid is that the process produces attitudes that become culturally embedded. Consequently it is difficult, to follow on from the points that Card (2002) makes about 'grey' behaviours, to avoid being complicit in its operation and the maintenance of the many structures that support it. Gomberg (2007) suggests that, whereas previous discussions of injustice have concentrated on the distribution of resources, work towards equity should instead centre on contributive justice. This is essentially an Aristotelian notion of transformation through valuing the social aspect of giving to others over material gain. It is through such an enabling stance that occupational apartheid may be challenged.

The emergence of occupational apartheid

Cultures of difference have evolved through the human occupational relationship with the environment and have themselves been instrumental in human evolution (Wilcock 1998). Human societies develop certain characteristics that reflect the need to maintain communities according to local conditions. Fernandez-Armesto (2000) describes how different civilizations emerged through the attempts of communities to live in various climates and topographies and the consequences of the effect the growing community had on the environment and resources around them. For example, living in a river delta facilitates cultivation on a replenishing supply of alluvial soil but requires a good deal of labour to maintain ditches and flood barriers to preserve crops. Increased need for labour increases the need for supplies to feed it and administrators to manage it but this increases the size of the community and makes bigger demands on the cultivators. Eventually an autocratic system emerges in which a clerical elite presides over the organization of agriculture and the engineering of flood management and repair.

The position of coastal communities, on the other hand, enables them to fish and to trade with inland and other coastal communities as goods find their way to the sea or to the interior. Trade creates opportunities for enterprise and cooperation, since in order to expand societies need to pool their resources. Through trade, complex societies emerged that were able to absorb influences, fables and knowledge from interactions with many others (Tacitus 1959, Herodotus 1972, Marcellinus 1986, Wilcock 1998, Fernandez-Armesto 2000). Although in the West some of the ancient societies that emerged may have had democratic features (Tacitus 1959, Aristotle 1962), many of these communities dealt in human captives and maintained strictly segregated societies (Thucydides 1972). For example the Greek warrior nobility saw themselves as above those who obtained their livelihoods by craft and trade (Aristotle 1962, Herodotus 1972).

The process of territorial occupation and exploitation is therefore associated with the development of individual occupations as components of social classes. As societies have developed these have necessarily become more diverse – the earliest literature in the British Isles from the warrior clans of the Celts describes a society primarily based on agriculture and feuding over land rights that clearly produced a nobility and a servant class (Taylor 2005). Through subsequent invasions and trade a wider range of occupations and roles gradually developed as different kinds of commodities were produced and new skills were required to supply them, market them and administer records of them. Sourcing goods also became increasingly important as societies became more complex. Because of their geographical position, however, sea-borne societies, such as the Greeks, Romans, Portuguese, Dutch and British, were able to spread their influence as their artefacts and ideas reached far beyond their borders and their increasing capacity for trade and exploitation brought wealth (Tacitus 1959, Thucydides 1972, Marcellinus 1986, Hobsbawm 1969, Boxer 1973a,b, Checkland & Checkland 1989, Fernandez-Armesto 2000).

The social, political and economic legacy of these empires remains in the imbalance of wealth between Western countries and much of the rest of the world and in many of the global economic and political structures, such as the British Commonwealth and patterns of trade (Ch. 7). They are also realized in many of our daily activities (Ch. 1). The British culture of tea drinking, with its combination of china, tea and sugar, would not have been possible without an empire. The wide dispersal of coffee, bananas, chillies, avocados, tomatoes and many other crops, which have become important elements of many national cuisines, is also due to the trading patterns of empire (David 1973, Ortiz 1977, 2002, Heal & Allsop 1986).

Inevitably the demand for labour in order to work in the mercantile ships that carried trade and the navies that protected them, to develop and maintain colonial administrations and to work in the great variety of supporting industries was very considerable. The process of territorial occupation, establishing land rights, conquest and the maintenance of the borders of empires and principalities has come, therefore, to require a plethora of supportive occupations, not only in military and administrative roles but also in supply of goods and services and even domestic settlement to further legitimize the colonies. These roles have further developed according to needs and opportunities created by changing social demands.

However, the same processes have also been destructive of roles and occupations. Just as through the successive invasions of Britain little is really known about pre-Roman society or pre-Saxon society, because these cultures were mostly obliterated (Whitelock 1972, Sowell 1994), the colonial enterprises of European and other cultures have been immensely destructive to those they have overwhelmed and consumed (Fanon 1986, 1990, Fernando 1991, Gomberg 2007). The Spanish and Portuguese incursions in South America (Boxer 1973a, Parry 1973, Hemming 1983) and of many European countries in Africa – in South Africa (Luthuli 1963, Arendt 1986, Biko 1987) and elsewhere such as the Congo (Ewans 2002), for example – were catastrophic events for the indigenous cultures and consequently whole ways of life were destroyed as people were subjugated, enslaved and killed through famine, disease and slaughter. Chapter 20 gives one account of the Native American experience. This list is far from exhaustive. So far, some of the most systematic development of human occupations connected with oppression in modern history has been under the regimes of Hitler and Stalin (Latey 1972, Arendt 1986). Arendt (1986) and Bettelheim (1970, 1992), among others, describe how the obliteration of people was turned into an industrial process in the Nazi period. The first to be thus murdered were the disabled.

Such events impact deeply on the way people understand themselves and perceive their abilities and needs, and as a result impact deeply on their occupational choices. Social destruction through colonization, even at times genocide, has often been accompanied by attempts at justification through the negation of indigenous cultures (Boxer 1973a, Hemming 1983, Arendt 1986, Biko 1987, Fernando 1991, Malik 1996). For example, Fanon (1990) illustrates how French colonial oppression in Algeria became internalized in the Algerian population to the extent that they accepted lower-status social roles and practised subservience to the colonial population.

Few peoples of the world have not experienced oppression by other people at some stage of their histories. The experience of being dominated or dominating others is an important aspect of many cultures (Arendt 1986, Biko 1987). Were it not for the vicissitudes of the Israelites and their neighbours described in the Old Testament, it is likely that many parts of the world would have a very different culture or society, although probable that some other story of conquest and conflict would feature prominently in whichever form it took.

Inevitably, also, an economic overdependence on wealth from imperial possessions led to economic decline as the vast territories became increasingly unsupportable and the expense of sustaining them became too much for weak home economies (Boxer 1973a,b, Parry 1973). Certainly in Britain the empire prevented progress in industry and agriculture, contributing to periods of unemployment and an increasingly unstable economy that, in turn, were combined with ideas of racial superiority to produce suspicion and hostility (expressed for example in fears of competition for work and the effects of inter-racial relationships) towards the people from subjugated countries who came to live there (Ramdin 1987, Fernando 1991, Malik 1996). As the balance of world power changes, perhaps to accommodate the demands of new super-economies, we suspect it is unlikely that these phenomena will cease to present problems. 'We know that no one ever seizes power with the intention of relinquishing it. Power is not a means, it is the end' (Orwell 1954, p. 211).

Discriminatory fictions

The term apartheid drew on a 'scientific' justification of biological differences, which were held to be evidence of the differences in ability and capacity between racial groups (Fernando 1991, Malik 1996). On this basis it was held appropriate that white people, who were presented as superior in development, should manage and govern people of other racial groups (Biko 1987). The corollary of this idea, however, was fear and exclusion of people who then might seek to destabilize this view, if not through active struggle, by the mere fact of their desire to live their chosen life.

Apartheid, then, was based on a discriminatory fiction that exploited and misrepresented differences. The false borders this created could be over-ridden even in a court trial for treason under the apartheid system to prosecute political activists who wanted to end that falsehood. Nelson Mandela (1994, p. 276) gives an interesting example from the South African Treason Trial where the ideology of apartheid was turned on its head. In an approving response to the medical achievements of one of the black defendants, Dr Wilson Conco, one of the white prosecution team, said, '*Sinjalo thina maZulu,*' which means, '*We* Zulus are like that' (emphasis added).

Law is less about what is in the public good, so much as what has been established through precedent. Many laws passed under many administrations, whether tyrannies such as those of Stalin or Hitler or more benign states, are frequently found to be unjust. A law that is initially just, perhaps protecting the rights of an oppressed minority, can eventually become unjust as the minority attains sufficient power to oppress others and upholds its ability to do so through principles once established for its protection. Although legal processes might eventually move in the direction of a concept of 'the public good', precedents have to be established through which the process of just law can move without compromising other aspects of the social apparatus that also operate for 'the public good' (Rawls 1973). As the influence of more powerful social elements has more force in determining the nature of 'what is good', legal processes prioritize some interests over others (Nussbaum 2003).

According to Sowell (1994), the importance of law is due to its provision of stable economic conditions in which industrial and agricultural developments can occur. The principle of stability is therefore recognized as good by those who benefit from it, and the development of law occurs to prevent the undermining of these conditions. In the Celtic society that existed in Britain before the arrival of the Romans, it is evident that the practice of cattle raiding and a culture of local conflict favoured a different pattern of social development from that which was enabled by imperial rule (Tacitus 1959, Taylor 2005). While pre-Roman Celtic society has a certain romantic appeal, it is clear that substantial areas of Britain quickly adapted to the practical advantages of living in cities and towns. The breakdown of this rule as the Roman Empire succumbed to external and internal conflicts led to the fragmentation that facilitated subsequent invasion (Whitelock 1972).

Although Roman law did not favour slaves, it did provide stability and conditions through which citizenship could be attained. Most Roman authors asserted that the underlying principles of their ordered society, even if based on slavery, were 'good'. They might use the Aristotelian argument that some people are born slaves, lack the capacity to be anything else and therefore need masters (Aristotle 1962). Civilian problems arise when the plebeians and slaves forget the lowly place ordained for them. Biko (1987) countered this by demonstrating that if the slave masters set the conditions for slavery then this perception is reinforced, not because it produces stability but because the value of the lives of the enslaved is so reduced that among them crime and other social problems are more common. The instability they experience is used to justify poorer occupational opportunities such as access to education, housing or land on the grounds of reduced ability and need.

Thus in South Africa the effect of the apartheid laws was increasingly to worsen and constrict the rights of the black majority of the population (Luthuli 1963, Mandela 1994, Sowell 1994). Ultimately this progressed to the extent that pressure mounted in other countries for the South African government to change, while the regime itself recognized the dangerous instability its policies had produced. The release of the Treason Trial prisoners was partly in response to the need to avert this crisis and its impact on the white population that the apartheid laws were intended to advantage (Mandela 1994).

Occupational apartheid is a term that recognizes the same category of false justice in which society is deliberately organized in order to benefit one group at the expense of negating another's occupational choices and human rights. At present, apartheid remains a politically emotive and sensational word, which demands that something is done.

Before we can take up the struggle against occupational apartheid, however, it is necessary to spend some time trying to understand how it has come about. Occupational apartheid manifests itself where individuals or groups experience limitations and segregations on spurious grounds, which deny them occupational opportunities such as being able to contribute to the community as a citizen. These denials constitute disabling conditions, or racial or gender segregation, the effects of which can be described as producing 'occupational apartheid'. It might be tempting to argue that the operation of rules such as preventing women from using some bars or participating in activities such as playing snooker, refusing entry to people on the basis of their skin colour or preventing people with physical disabilities from accessing facilities such theatres or cinemas on the grounds that they would block fire exits (as occurred in the UK during a large part of the last century) constitutes occupational apartheid. However, while these rules were oppressive and part of a systemic pattern of discrimination operated covertly and overtly, by and large they were not products of policy. They were locally applied rather than an instrument of control over sections of the population, so do not represent a form of occupational apartheid.

This nuance lies in the problem that, although equal rights legislation has addressed some of these issues, full equality cannot be established – there will always be groups of people who will remain disproportionately enabled in their access to facilities or opportunities. One person's occupational justice leads to another's occupational injustice. The concern anyone must have with this state of affairs is inevitably Sisyphean: we are obliged to attempt adjustments for the good of others rather than comply and accept inequity. We are also obliged to accept others' rights to the concrete terms of equity, not just the opportunity of access.

The restrictions in rights that emerge may be products of social, economic and political systems but in other instances may be unintentional, for example the result of geography or even personal choices. These we argue may be described as occupational deprivation. Opportunities are denied, but as a consequence of chance. They have the capacity to become elements of occupational apartheid where they become components of a system of oppression that operates to deny specific occupational choices. Thus occupational apartheid operates in larger terms. It could, for example, operate through a general law that restricted the rights of women from free association, a measure of which banned them from working men's social clubs, or if the partners of women prevented them from free association by systematic violence (Cage 2007). Occupational apartheid can also be the product of social expectation, for example strict social codes that operate to exclude specific groups from participating in activities (see Ch. 5). These are experienced by many disabled people in their right to work, access leisure or express their sexuality.

Recognizing instances of occupational apartheid

Where can we find occupational apartheid and how does it arise? These segregations do not suddenly and arbitrarily emerge but are the result of a complex historical process of human and social development (Arendt 1986, Fanon 1990, Sowell 1994, Card 2002). In other words, segregation is the product of human occupation and stems from the way people respond to and produce societies in relation to the environment. Our colleague Elelwani Ramugondo coined the term 'occupational colonization' in response to the difficulties of interpreting Western cultural conceptions of occupation in interventions with black South African clients (personal communication, 2007). This describes the domination of local discourses of occupation by powerful readings that are accepted as 'normal' because of their dominance. The result is that by a process of objectification people subject to occupational colonization are denied access to the natural expression of their own culture and identity. They come to understand themselves as inadequate or strange, take on the dominant cultural values and repudiate their former culture. For an approach to developing postcolonial affirmative understandings of culture with indigenous groups, see Chapter 20.

Apartheid developed from a process of colonization, by which a group of migrants occupied land in the southern part of the African continent and wanted to maintain their material gains. Like most colonial migrations the incoming people perceived themselves as more civilized than and technologically superior to the people already living in the country (Fanon 1986, 1990, Malik 1996, Fernandez-Armesto 2000). In time this translated itself into attempts to preserve the way of life experienced by the pioneers of what became a Boer tradition (Arendt 1986), or indeed, any colonial settler tradition experienced elsewhere (Fanon 1990).

Sowell (1994) argues that discrimination between groups of people need not necessarily be based on racial ideology. Notions of superiority or inferiority have often been based on perceptions of capability, in other words because of the access to opportunities one group has through a technical proficiency. For example the Roman Empire clearly operated restrictions on the basis of social status but for much of its development was successful through assimilating the people who were conquered and enabling them to become citizens. Romans recognized that the people they had defeated had the capacity to learn new ways of life. Giving them the opportunities to acquire the trappings of Roman culture was essential to maintaining the empire. Authors such as Tacitus are disparaging about those such as the tribes north of the Danube who refused to be annexed. Difference, and the fear of what that difference may mean to others, appears to be the main basis for discrimination (Kristeva 1991). This fear of others is also an acknowledgement of their capacity to effect changes and, by implication, their right to do so.

One of the antecedents of occupational therapy, moral treatment, was concerned with the use of work activities to regulate the behaviour of mentally ill people. Although the inference, as Wilcock (1998) points out, is that such methods were distinct from the humiliating and brutal treatment given to some patients, by the early 20th century occupational therapy was concerned with the development of appropriate life habits. Occupational therapy found its place within a medical hierarchy by the development of approaches that identified personal fulfilment with the compliance demanded of capitalism. Occupational therapy outcomes were connected with individual health, and this was realized through the adoption of good habits, but early occupational therapists concentrated on practical solutions over research. The result was that occupational therapy came to be seen in terms of a limited range of activities, often diversional rather than 'real work'. Instead of realizing the social and community focus of occupational interventions, many occupational therapists have since found themselves regarded more as instrumental in keeping patients quiet or facilitating discharge, in other words managing and containing difference. An increasing number of occupational therapists (e.g. Townsend 1993, Wilcock 1998, Creek 2003, Creek et al 2005, Whiteford 2005) have been arguing for a reappraisal of the core values of the profession and a political shift in direction towards public health, community-based approaches. They point to the need to address the underpinning social, economic and political factors that contribute to all forms of occupational injustice, with the facilitation of human occupation as a central focus. As occupational therapists work towards concepts such as the client-centred approach they have to reconcile themselves with new forms of cultural expression that have been developing in disability movements over several decades. Groups such as Mad Pride, Survivors' Poetry or the Disability Arts Movement are not concerned with compliance but with confronting stigmatization by demanding the acceptance and celebration of difference.

Occupation as oppression

Oppression and resistance are natural human occupations. It makes no sense to argue that there was an Arcadian time before the Fall when humans did not oppress each other. The Bible, as one example of the religious texts around which cultures have based themselves, contains many examples of people being shunned or exiled on the basis of their origins or broken taboos; many of the central figures are themselves the subject of prejudice or social exclusion. Our nearest genetic neighbours, chimpanzees, show many features of social behaviour, including the use of tools and purposeful occupation (Wood 1996, 2002). These purposeful occupations include attacking and killing other groups of chimpanzees. In arguing for the existence of occupational apartheid in the present global society, it cannot be pretended that had the pattern of social and technical development been different the processes of colonization would not have taken place. They were already happening in other parts of the world but it so happened that Europeans acquired the knowledge and were able to take advantage of the materials available to them to develop efficient weapons at a time of rapid social change. In the case of Britain, a long pattern of economic growth (Hobsbawm 1969), political circumstances and the convenience of a nearby island (Ireland) in the British archipelago in which to develop it favoured English colonialism in particular (Youings 1984, Foster 1989).

There are many examples of oppression arising from an occupation of territorial occupation. Throughout history and all across the globe, groups of people have competed for resources and, as a product of this competition, seen each other as different. While racism has been seen as a specifically Western phenomenon arising from Western cultural and political dominance (Fernando 1991, Malik 1996), the roots of occupational apartheid lie in this much older human characteristic of competing for limited resources, whereas on the whole occupational therapists tend to view occupation as something positive: 'Man, through the use of his hands as they are energized by mind and will, can influence the state of his own health' (Reilly 1962, p. 2).

It can also be a negative force. Occupations are the means by which we extract resources from the environment around us and deprive others of those resources, creating occupational injustices (Townsend & Wilcock 2004a,b). Although occupational therapists recognize a human right to occupation (World Federation of Occupational Therapists 2006), occupations are themselves resources that can be restricted to those in power (Steinberg 2003) – just as the right to mate and so have descendants is competed for among animals. Indeed, many of the arguments used to justify racial segregation or 'repatriation' in the UK and many other societies have been concerned with just this specific issue (Boxer 1973a, Arendt 1986, Ramdin 1987).

If access to occupation is a right (World Federation of Occupational Therapists 2006) then oppressive forms of occupation that can produce occupational apartheid need to be restricted. Nussbaum (2003) argued that some rights are more fundamental than others. To enable a society based on occupational justice, some rights even need to be actively restricted.

Conclusion

The consequences of conquest and domination have produced lasting damage over generations to the physical and mental health both of those who are oppressed and of those who have been the oppressors (Fanon 1990, Fernando 1991, Littlewood & Lippsedge 1993). Fanon (1990), for example, gives the example of a secret policeman engaged in torture who seeks psychiatric treatment because he begins to mistreat his family and asks whether there is a cure for a conscience. The racism that has resulted from a colonial past continues to provoke fear and violence in many postcolonial societies.

These occupations have also produced benefits. Since the earliest times, cultures have developed as a consequence of invasion and collision between different peoples (Sowell 1994,

Fernandez-Armesto 2000). As a result many of the occupational choices open to people are dependent on the heritage they have gained from the intermixing of peoples. Sowell (1994) maintains that at times groups of people have developed specific roles around local capabilities or needs, for example British technical expertise in the 19th century, Chinese and Jewish trading ability in many societies.

One occupational therapy activity, in the UK, has often been stereotyped as indicative of the inconsequence of the profession: making a cup of tea (Sachs 1990). In the UK, because of the variety of different cultural origins in her department, one researcher found 16 approaches to this simple daily activity of living (Fair & Barnitt 1999). Cooking and recipes are a particularly valuable indicator of cultural transference (see Ch. 20). Ortiz (1977), for example, in an edition of a book produced for an American and British audience, describes the global origins of Caribbean cooking; Hafner (1993) similarly offers culinary snapshots of the African continent. In the late 1960s Hobsbawm (1969, p. 321) was already reporting a 'plebeian and egalitarian' popular culture in the UK that reflected a global influence. Subsequent generations of the UK population have had flirtations with jazz, blues, soul and hip-hop from the black experience in the USA, ska and reggae from Jamaica and the incorporation of African and Asian influences into popular music. It is easy to be dismissive of this kind of crossover as a mere product of the global smorgasbord of culture, marketed as a novelty to a fickle public; in fact it is a continuation of the marketability of artefacts from other cultures that has continued from prehistoric times when humans first began to trade with each other the products of their occupations derived from materials found or developed in their own territory. Indeed, the cultural exchange masks a deeper exchange of knowledge that might be traced back to the fossilized origins of humanity itself.

It also masks the global trade in arms, such as the ubiquitous butterfly mines in conflict zones (Kronenberg & Pollard 2006). Many of the companies involved in developing weapons systems also have divisions that develop the entertainment systems on which we listen to blues, reggae, hip-hop and soul. Everyone knows really where they came from and how they are the uplifting products of the experience of some forms of occupational apartheid. We should actually listen to the music to which our feet are tapping. Let's take a critical look at the occupations of doing, being, belonging and becoming.

References

Arendt H 1986 The origins of totalitarianism. Andre Deutsch, London

Aristotle 1962 The politics (trans TA Sinclair). Penguin, Harmondsworth

Bardon J 1992 A history of Ulster. Blackstaff Press, Belfast

Bettelheim B 1970 The informed heart. Paladin, London

Bettelheim B 1992 Recollections and reflections. Penguin, Harmondsworth

Biko S 1987 I write what I like. Heinemann, Oxford

Bonfim V 2005 Once a street child, now a citizen of the world. In: Kronenberg F, Simó Algado S, Pollard N (eds) Occupational therapy without borders: learning from the spirit of survivors. Elsevier/Churchill Livingstone, Edinburgh: p 245–260

Boxer C R 1973a The Portuguese seaborne empire. Pelican, Harmondsworth

Boxer C R 1973b The Dutch seaborne empire. Pelican, Harmondsworth

Brogan H 1990 The Penguin history of the United States of America. Penguin, Harmondsworth

Bush M L 2004 Race, ethnicity and whiteness. Sage Race Relations Abstracts 29(4): 5–48

Cage A 2007 Occupational therapy with women and children survivors of domestic violence: are we fulfilling our activist heritage? A review of the literature. British Journal of Occupational Therapy 70: 192–198

Card C 2002 The atrocity paradigm, a theory of evil. Oxford University Press, New York

Checkland O, Checkland S 1989 Industry and ethos. Edinburgh University Press, Edinburgh

Creek J 2003 Occupational therapy defined as a complex intervention. College of Occupational Therapists, London

Creek J, Illot I, Cook S, Munday C 2005 Valuing occupational therapy as a complex intervention. British Journal of Occupational Therapy 68: 281–284

David E 1973 Spices, salt and aromatics in the English kitchen. Penguin, Harmondsworth

Ewans M 2002 European atrocity, African catastrophe: Leopold II, the Congo Free State and its aftermath. Routledge, London

Fair A, Barnitt R 1999 Making a cup of tea as part of a culturally sensitive practice. British Journal of Occupational Therapy 62: 199–205

Fanon F 1986 Black skins, white masks. Pluto, London

Fanon F 1990 The wretched of the Earth (trans C Farrington). Penguin, Harmondsworth

Fernandez-Armesto F 2000 Civilisations. Macmillan, London

Fernando S 1991 Mental health, race and culture. Macmillan/MIND, London

Foster R F 1989 Modern Ireland 1600–1972. Penguin, Harmondsworth

Fraser N (1997) Justice interruptus. Routledge, London

Gomberg P 2007 How to make opportunity equal: race and contributive justice. Blackwell, Oxford

Graeber D 2004 Fragments of an anarchist anthropology. Prickly Paradigm Press, Chicago, IL. Available online at: http://libcom.org/library/fragments-of-an-anarchist-anthropology-david-graeber; accessed 9 October 2007

Hafner D 1993 A taste of Africa. Hodder, London

Hammell K W 2004 Dimensions in meaning in the occupations of everyday life. Canadian Journal of Occupational Therapy 71: 296–305

Harding T 1991 Ethical issues in the delivery of mental health services: abuses in Japan. In: Bloch S, Chodoff P P (eds) Psychiatric ethics, 2nd edn. Oxford University Press, New York: p 473–491

Heal C, Allsop M 1986 Queer gear. Century, London

Hemming J 1983 The conquest of the Incas. Penguin, Harmondsworth

Herodotus 1972 The histories (trans A De Selincourt). Penguin, Harmondsworth

Hobsbawm E J 1969 Industry and empire: an economic history of Britain from 1750 to the present day. Pelican, Harmondsworth

Iwama M 2006 The Kawa Model: culturally relevant occupational therapy. Churchill Livingstone/Elsevier, Edinburgh

Kazez J 2007 The weight of things: philosophy and the good life. Blackwell, Oxford

Kristeva J 1991 Strangers to ourselves (trans L Roudiez). Columbia University Press, New York

Kronenberg F 1999 Street children: being and becoming. Unpublished research study, Hogeschool Limburg, Heerlen

Kronenberg F 2005 Occupational therapy with street children. In: Kronenberg F, Simó Algado S, Pollard N (eds) Occupational therapy without borders: learning from the spirit of survivors. Elsevier, Edinburgh: p 261–276

Kronenberg F, Pollard N 2005 Overcoming occupational apartheid, a preliminary exploration of the political nature of occupational therapy. In: Kronenberg F, Simó Algado S, Pollard N (eds) Occupational therapy without borders: learning from the spirit of survivors. Elsevier Churchill Livingstone, Edinburgh: p 58–86

Kronenberg F, Pollard N 2006 Political dimensions of occupation and the roles of occupational therapy. American Journal of Occupational Therapy 60: 617–625

Latey M 1972 Tyranny: a study in the abuse of power. Pelican, Harmondsworth

Littlewood R, Lippsedge M 1993 Aliens and alienists. Routledge, London

Luthuli A 1963 Let my people go. Faber, London

Malik K 1996 The meaning of race. Macmillan, London

Mandela N 1994 Long walk to freedom. Abacus, London

Manning C A W 1964 South Africa and the world: in defense of apartheid. Foreign Affairs, October: 135–149

Marcellinus A 1986 The later Roman Empire (trans W Hamilton). Penguin, Harmondsworth

Mason M 2000 Incurably human. Working Press, London

Mattingly C, Fleming M 1994 Clinical reasoning: forms of inquiry in therapeutic practice. FA Davis, Philadelphia, PA

Nussbaum M 2003 Capabilities as fundamental entitlements: Sen and social justice. Feminist Economics 9(2–3): 33–59

Ortiz E L 1977 Caribbean cookery. Penguin, Harmondsworth

Ortiz E L 2002 The book of Latin American cooking. Grub Street, London

Orwell G 1954 Nineteen eighty-four. Penguin, Harmondsworth

Parry J H 1973 The Spanish seaborne empire. Pelican, Harmondsworth

Ramdin R 1987 The making of the black working class in Britain. Wildwood House, Aldershot

Rawls J 1973 A theory of justice. Oxford University Press, Oxford

Reilly M 1962 Occupational therapy can be one of the great ideas of 20th century medicine. American Journal of Occupational Therapy 16: 1–9

Sachs A. 1990 The soft vengeance of a freedom fighter. Grafton, London

Siddle R 1999 From assimilation to indigenous rights: Ainu resistance since 1869. In: Fitzhugh W, Dubreuil C (eds) Ainu: spirit of a northern people. National Museum of National History, Smithsonian Institution and University of Washington Press, Washington, DC: p 108–115

Smith H C 2005 Feel the fear and do it anyway: meeting the occupational needs of refugees and people seeking asylum. British Journal of Occupational Therapy 68: 474–476

Sowell T 1994 Race and culture. Basic Books, New York

Steinberg S 1995 Turning back: the retreat from racial justice in American thought and policy. Beacon Press, Boston, MA

Steinberg S 2003 Nathan Glazer and the assassination of affirmative action. New Politics 9:3. Available online at:http://www.wpunj.edu/~newpol/issue35/steinberg35.htm: accessed 21 May 2007

Tacitus 1959 The annals of imperial Rome (trans M Grant). Penguin, Harmondsworth

Taylor S 2005 The complete cattle raid of Cooley/Táin bó Cualnge. Available online at: http://adminstaff.vassar.edu/sttaylor/Cooley/index.html; accessed 8 February 2008

Thucydides 1972 The history of the Peloponnesian war (trans R Warner). Penguin, Harmondsworth

Townsend E 1993 Occupational therapy's social vision. Canadian Journal of Occupational Therapy 60: 174–183

Townsend E, Wilcock A 2004a Occupational justice. In: Christiansen C, Townsend E (eds) Introduction to occupation: the art and science of living. Prentice Hall, Thorofare, NJ: p 243–273

Townsend E, Wilcock A 2004b Occupational justice and client centred practice: a dialogue. Canadian Journal of Occupational Therapy 71: 75–87

Whiteford G 2005 Globalisation and the enabling state. In: Whiteford G, Wright-St Clair V (eds) Occupation & practice in context. Elsevier Churchill Livingstone, Marrickville, New South Wales: p 349–361

Whitelock D 1972 The beginnings of English society. Pelican, Harmondsworth

Wicks A, Whiteford G 2005 Gender, occupation and participation. In: Whiteford G, Wright-St Clair V (eds) Occupation & practice in context. Elsevier Churchill Livingstone, Marrickville, New South Wales: p 197–212

Wilcock A 1998 An occupational perspective of health. Slack, Thorofare, NJ

Wilcock A 1999 Reflections on doing, being and becoming. Australian Occupational Therapy Journal 46: 1–11

Wood W 1996 The value of studying occupation: an example with primate play. American Journal of Occupational Therapy 50: 327–337

Wood W 2002 Ecological synergies in two groups of zoo chimpanzees: divergent patterns of time use. American Journal of Occupational Therapy 56: 160–170

World Federation of Occupational Therapists (2006) Position paper on human rights. Available online at: http://www.wfot.org/office_files/Human%20Rights%20Position%20Statement%20Final.pdf; accessed 9 October 2007

Youings J 1984 Sixteenth-century England. Pelican, Harmondsworth

Three sites of conflict and cooperation:
class, gender and sexuality

5

Dikaios Sakellariou, Nick Pollard

Abstract

This chapter discusses class, gender and sexuality. Although these elements have played an important role in the construction of a professional identity for occupational therapists, and often regulate access to opportunities for engagement in valued and dignified occupation, they have often been ignored in professional discourse. Groups of people can be subordinated through institutionalized practices, societal behaviours and political decisions. Class, gender and sexuality are elements of the occupational narratives therapists receive from their clients in the negotiation of assessment and the planning of intervention, and yet all three have to some extent been neglected in the discussion of the profession's concern with meaningful or purposeful occupation. These exclusions can be defined as sites of conflict and cooperation. The chapter concludes with a discussion on the direction of professional involvement so that it does not reinforce occupational injustices, deprivation or apartheid.

Introduction

A discussion of politics and access to occupation cannot afford to ignore the concept of diversity, which has only recently begun to enter the professional discourse of occupational therapy (Abreu & Peloquin 2004, Kirsh et al 2006, Trentham et al 2007). This signifies professional recognition of the influence that varying identities and subjective experiences can have on access to occupation.

Diversity is not merely a matter of ethnicity and gender (Awaad 2003, Iwama 2003, Harrell & Bond 2006, Kirsh et al 2006) but refers to a multitude of characteristics, including class, race, linguistic group, sexuality, disability status, age or marital condition, that can influence perceptions of the world, meaning of occupation and access to power. Being different in one or more characteristics from the dominant group in any context can lead to restricted access to services for groups of people. This is not just in terms of service availability but also applies to the quality of interactions with occupational therapists (see, for example, Kirsh et al 2006) because professionals can be unable to recognize nuances in the needs of clients from minority groups.

Diversity can limit access to what Rawls (1973, p. 62) refers to as the 'primary goods', including liberties, opportunities, wealth, food and education. Difference leads to the construction of the 'other', a conceptual category within which a specific characteristic is singled out and becomes the defining quality (Kristeva 1991). These 'otherisms' (Abreu &

Peloquin 2004, p. 354) can have a negative bearing on the establishment of collaborations not only within occupational therapy but also between therapists and other people they work with – community members, disabled people's organizations or other professionals for example. Limited access to primary goods can also create disadvantageous differences, such as class inequalities, which arise from the maldistribution of resources.

In this chapter we will critically consider three characteristics that are important in the formation of a personal identity and that often regulate access to opportunities for engagement in valued and dignified occupation. These are class, gender and sexuality.

It is perhaps surprising that class and gender are rarely considered together, particularly when many of the restrictions experienced by women are also experienced through class and/or sexuality (Skeggs 1997, Taylor 2007). People are classed, engendered and sexual beings all at the same time, all the time. These identities are constantly in operation. This is particularly important in professions, such as occupational therapy, that offer many women the possibility of leaving behind their working-class origins for the middle-class status and access to better earnings that go with professional education (Pollard & Walsh 2000). People seeking careers in occupational therapy are not motivated primarily by the earnings but by 'people-oriented factors – interests in being of service to the community and in helping people' (Meredith et al 2007, p. 240; see also Roney et al 2004). This evokes the social activist motivations of early occupational therapists, many of whom were working at a time when, because there was a surplus of women following the First World War, many sublimated their social expectations in a career of service (Nicholson 2007). Occupational therapy pioneers, along with those in nursing and social work, came from a class of women whose visions of social action were aimed at their working class contemporaries (Pollard & Walsh 2000).

Class, gender and sexuality present challenges to the holism espoused by occupational therapy. All three issues are an element of the occupational narratives we receive from our clients in the negotiation of assessment and the planning of intervention, and yet all three have in some way been neglected in the discussion of the profession's concern with meaningful or purposeful occupation. These exclusions can be defined as sites of conflict and cooperation (see Ch. 1). As yet, little is known about the diversity of the population of occupational therapists beyond the figures showing that in many Western countries most are white and female. It has long been assumed that many occupational therapists are middle class but widening access to educational opportunities has attracted entrants from lower income groups (Beagan 2007). As a consequence of these dominances it may be difficult for professionals, new career entrants and the clients they work with to challenge assumptions that frame the profession. As Beagan (2007) has discovered, for example, a perception that students from impoverished origins should pass middle-class occupational expectations has inhibited their development, and also poses a risk that similar concepts would be imposed in assessments and intervention with clients in practice.

Class, gender and sexuality operate and influence access to opportunities for engagement in occupation including income, wealth, liberties, education and food. These constitute the primary goods that Rawls (1973) asserts need to be distributed equally in a society. For clarity these three elements, class, gender and sexuality, will be examined separately, despite the reality that, far from being exclusive and independent, they are embedded in each other. The last part of the chapter will offer a synthesis of the observed inequality apparatus, using Fraser's (1997) concepts of distribution and recognition injustices.

Occupation in a classed society

The unequal distribution of wealth, access to education and the burden of disease and disability point to the existence of a class system of social stratification (Hartery & Gahagan 1998; see Chs 14, 19). Class is a rather blurred concept because of its complexity and variance across cultures but it is largely determined by and determines access to education, health and wealth (Pincus et al 1998, Field & Briggs 2001). For example, a study of the London Borough of Camden found that life expectancy across the borough varied by 10 years in a pattern mirroring wealth and poverty levels (Stafford & Marmot 2006).

Class refers to a hierarchical system of social stratification based on the possession of power, commonly associated with level of income and education in industrialized societies. The system of social classification used in many countries is mainly based either directly on these two elements or on paid occupation, which is in turn dependent upon education and is a defining factor for earnings (Hartery & Gahagan 1998). These criteria belie the complexity of perceptions of class, which go beyond one's bank account or job title. Class is also defined by the context within which people are acculturated, the geographical spaces they occupy, their social networks and finally how individuals and groups both see themselves and also perceive how others see them (see Chs 11, 13, 14, 19).

Perceived increased social mobility and more importantly the domination of public discourses by a middle-class perspective and the silencing of working-class voices have led to the illusion of a classless society (Wilson 1992), a Utopia where class does not matter. Identity has been proposed instead as an alternative that provides a more stable basis on which social connectedness can be developed. As the example of a working-class writing organization (Woodin 2005) shows, people often base their participation and belonging to a group upon the characteristic they feel has the most prominent role in the way they define and perceive their life (Chs 13, 14, 20).

Identities connected to gender, sexuality, race or disability provide a platform upon which a sense of belonging and support can be built. These can often be portrayed as exclusive identities, for example individuals may describe themselves as disabled *or* black *or* gay. Such identities can also operate exclusions, as Taylor's (2005a, 2007) study of working-class lesbians shows. Women in her study could not identify with a queer identity or a gay lifestyle, as these were grounded in a middle-class perspective. Individuals may be disabled *and* black *and* gay, and also possess aspects of their identity based on an experience of class. Identity is by definition inclusive of all the personal elements that make people who they are; one for example is both a sexual being and an individual living in a classed society (Taylor 2005a).

The normative ideal of the typical citizen as a middle-class, heterosexual, non-disabled person is an illusion, fed by the invisibility of those who do not fit in with it. People of working-class backgrounds do not often see their stories represented in the mass media, unless they are linked with issues of poverty and deprivation. White working-class women are represented or thought of as 'loud, excessive, drunk, vulgar, disgusting', as Skeggs (2005, p. 965) illustrated in her exploration of representations of white working-class women in England. Behind the association of working class with destitution and the presentation of the issue from a normative, capitalistic perspective lies the implication that belonging to the working class is a state most people should avoid and that, given the chance, working-class people would opt to elevate to the powerful middle class (Haylett 2003). Instead of pointing to a solution, this approach becomes part of the problem, as people become reluctant to claim a working-class identity for themselves. Thus a source of community connectedness and support derived from a common identity is lost. But, if working-class people are 'loud' and 'disgusting', their middle-class counterparts are 'boring'; thus problems of recognition and representation are not restricted in a single class (Skeggs 2005). Class embarrassment and subsequent class identity denial can be found across the classes. These problems of identity may actually threaten the coherency of some communities (Sayer 2002).

Numerous authors suggest that class correlates strongly with experiences of health (Marmot & McDowall 1986, Blaxter 1987, Vagerö & Lundberg 1989, Karlsen & Nazroo 2002, Krieger et al 2003, 2005). People belonging to lower socioeconomic classes carry a disproportionate burden of disease and disability, and die earlier (Drexler 2005). The causal explanation behind the link between class and inequalities in health has been shown to be multivariate, mainly centred along three axes, i.e. deprivation, social networks and behaviour patterns (Lundberg 1991). Lack of a sustainable income and lack of access to educational opportunities correlate with lack of exercise (Raudsepp 2006), obesity (Novak et al 2006), environmental injustice, i.e. living in areas with a disproportionately high burden of environmental pollution (Stephens et al 1999, Elliott et al 2004), and nutritional inequities often leading to unhealthy dietary habits (Travers 1996). People in such areas may be reluctant to demand a cleaner environment, since, as the pollution comes from local industries, this might threaten their jobs. Sometimes this can lead to tragic consequences, as in the case of the methyl mercury poisoning outbreak in south Japan in 1956. This affected the central nervous system of its victims with a condition since identified as Minamata disease (see www.nimd.go.jp/english/index.html, www6.ocn.ne.jp/~mf1997/index.html).

Poverty means that people often have to resort to inadequate housing solutions with no suitable heating or insulation as their resources need to be directed to more pressing needs such as food (Lawrence 2004). In a recent study Morris et al (2007) brought together existing evidence on requirements for housing, nutrition, exercise, psychosocial relations and medical care (but excluding rent, mortgage and council tax) for older people with the aim of establishing the minimum income for healthy living. This was estimated to be 50% higher than the state pension, which at the time of their study was £87.30 per week.

All these situations create inequalities in opportunity, which, through lack of basic resources, lead to increased vulnerability to disease, as people do not have access to education, healthy food or safe drinking water (Armelagos et al 2005). The uneven distribution of wealth both within and between countries under global capitalism often leads to micro- and macro-parasitic economic strategies. Through these a select elite of people or countries enjoy a disproportionately high fraction of resources at the expense of those in the lower socioeconomic strata (Armelagos et al 2005).

Social mobility decreased and disparities between the classes increased through the kind of capitalism that re-emerged during the 1980s. In this period economic policy retreated from state intervention in the economy and favoured allowing capital markets to determine their own level. These changes enabled shareholding and private equity companies, concerned primarily with profits, to increase wealth creation for their own members. Much of the wealth of this minority population came from the rest, with the result that the gap between rich and poor has increased (Orton & Rowlingson 2007). Recent studies in the UK have shown not only decreasing social mobility but also decreasing achievement among a large group of the population who have been ignored for several decades (Margo et al 2006). This section, white working-class boys, was a focus of concern in the 1960s (Holbrook 1964), when it was felt that the grammar-school system creamed off children who were educable from those who were not. A consequence of putting children through years of compulsory education in which little is expected of them has been that they raise their own children in turn with little expectation of the education system. However, this leaves them with few skills, and fewer abilities on which to base these skills, with which to gain jobs – or the kinds of job that earn more money (Margo et al 2006).

As the first post-Second World War generation became politicians in the UK in the 1980s and 1990s their peers were among the voters who elected for the retreat from the policies that had given them social mobility. Social mobility refers broadly to the facility with which people can move from one socioeconomic group, or class, to another, between generations. Thus a generation that is upwardly mobile experiences a better quality of life, based on economic measurements, than its parents. In the UK and the USA social mobility has been static for several decades, but in the UK generations born since 1970 have experienced more downward social mobility (Hartery & Gahagan 1998, Berube 2006, Margo et al 2006). In the UK the trend towards downward social mobility continues independently of the reduction in absolute poverty, because the gap is increased by the rich getting richer (Shaw et al 2005, Orton & Rowlingson 2007).

Downward social mobility is not purely economic in character but is influenced by the loss of social capital, access to facilities, poorer standards of health and education, and reduced life chances. It is sometimes concentrated in specific locations, since those who can do so will move out of poorer housing areas where, for example, there is an increased perception of crime (Berube 2006). Indeed, half of the people on low incomes appear to live in the most deprived fifth of areas of the UK (Palmer et al 2005). These areas often have higher levels of crime (Sampson et al 1997, Howe & Crilly 2001, Green et al 2002, Innes & Jones 2006), scarcer free and safe space where children can play (Kapasi 2006) and crime rates that deter older people from going out in their community (Green et al 2002). Taking into account the dearth of resources for socialization and play in poor communities it is not surprising that the literature suggests that it is not only personal socioeconomic position but also the prevalence of poverty in the community that is a contributing factor to poor health (Robert 1999). This lack of social opportunity means that occupational choices according to preference are made harder to make (Rebeiro 2000) and people can be occupationally deprived because of a nexus of social disadvantages, inequalities and environmental constraints (Whiteford 2000, Blanden & Gibbons 2006).

Social capital

Class is not necessarily fixed, since it is possible to move from one socioeconomic class to others. It also has a generational dimension. Putnam (2000) has described how people who grew up in the years of the baby boom after the Second World War enjoyed prosperity and a number of social measures that gave them easier access to occupational diversity through leisure. In the UK this was to lead to the rapid growth of higher education, investment in primary and secondary education, grants for students and welfare benefits. The consequence, for those who were able to take advantage of these changes, was that people were able to form many networks and learned to develop their personal, social and communication skills to facilitate themselves in achieving occupational goals and so gain in material wealth (Margo et al 2006). This rather intangible social network, for example knowing someone who can fix your car, do your plumbing, having friends on whom you can rely for support and to whom you can give support, is what Robert Putnam (2000), among others, has termed 'social capital'. Social capital depends on the ability of people to trust each other, to reciprocate actions for the benefit of each other and through this to experience a sense of cohesion and participation (Putnam 2000, Cummins 2006, Roberts & Chada 2006).

This sense of connectedness based on the idea of a shared class culture and identity is what makes examining social capital so important. It forms a largely untapped asset that can contribute to community development and creating a space where opportunities for engagement in occupation can be constructed (Isaksson et al 2007, Pollard et al forthcoming), for example through occupations such as volunteerism or civic involvement (see Chs 12–14).

Social capital provides a support network, social connections and a sense of safety for a community but it cannot regulate the inclusiveness of this community; in other words, those who belong to the community benefit while those who are outside either do not benefit or even are exploited through the very structures that provide support for other communities (Putnam 1993, Farmer et al 2003). As Poortinga (2006) observes, people can benefit from social capital only if they can access it.

While the link between increased social capital and population health appears to be positive the exact reason remains unclear (Whitehead & Diderichsen 2001, Henderson & Whiteford 2003, Folland 2007). Islam et al (2006) suggest that the extent to which people living in the same area will individually benefit from the existing social capital depends on personal variables, such as willingness to engage in community actions and participate in social networks (Poortinga 2006). Ability to use social capital therefore infers a competence that is acquired through exposure to it: 'those who have social capital tend to accumulate more' (Putnam 1993). Thus any effort to use this dynamic potential should create opportunities for inclusive access to it.

The development of social capital faces several challenges, according to Putnam (2000). One of the emblems of the new post-war prosperity was the television. More recently the wider availability of computers and entertainment systems based on them has created conditions where young people in particular spend a lot of time interacting with this equipment alone. This produces several effects, one of which is that people spend less time talking or doing other activities with each other. It has also replaced reading, as people rely on electronic media for news and information, an effect that has been significantly amplified through the availability of the Internet. Putnam (2000) has claimed that declining newspaper readership is associated with a decline in community engagement, although new Internet communities may be emerging.

Another influence was the redesigning of communities into areas for work, areas for shopping and leisure activities, and areas for living. Previously, in communities in the UK one could encounter every few streets a row of local shops, a few pubs and various community buildings such as church halls and scout huts. These were often the centres of villages that had been swallowed up by urban growth. Many areas have seen the demise of these resources and in newer housing estates facilities such as libraries are a car drive away. Although there are communities that retain strong ties with each other, many people choose or have to move away from their parental home to other towns in search of work or education. The increasing numbers of migrant populations and single parents are less connected to their neighbours in the surrounding community, and less able to access or be aware of local provision, much of which has been centred on the needs of traditional families (Stafford & Marmot 2006).

The changing working environment has also contributed to the demise of social capital. One of the factors that determines the location of companies needing unskilled workers is the price of local labour. Such employees tend to be recruited locally, while professional jobs are advertised in journals and papers on a national basis (Gibbons et al 2005). More of the unskilled job opportunities that have become available since the 1980s have been taken up by women, who have required the local, flexible, part-time nature of these opportunities in order to combine work with raising families, while more men have remained out of work. These new jobs lack training or career development opportunities and are often low paid, increasing a divergence in an already heavily gendered employment market (Bimrose et al 2003). This disparity is perhaps familiar to many occupational therapy departments, where locally recruited support workers work with therapists who may have originated from other parts of the country.

Consequently, says Putnam (2000), people invested their social capital in their workplace rather than in their communities. The increased suburbanization of jobs that Wilson (2003) observed means that people with no access to their own means of transportation may have to travel for a considerable time to work each day with less time spent in the local community. After work, it's easier to drive home, eat a meal in front of the TV and go to bed. There is less time to invest in playing with children, or even conversation. Human beings become more focused on work and material wealth, with poorer and less skilled workers servicing the leisure and producing the goods that improve the quality of life of those who have more money, professional skills and education (Gibbons et al 2005). In the UK, USA and, through the adoption of American working practices, across Europe people work more hours per week, often many unpaid hours, to maintain their jobs. Work-related stress and depression is a considerable social and health issue (Cooper 2007).

The construction of a space that values, respects and gives meaning to class identity can be an important asset for a community, serving as a resource for the building of more coherent communities and the strengthening of local cultures and identities, as suggested by the culture-led Newcastle/Gateshead regeneration project (Miles 2005). However, improvements in access to social capital cannot be addressed by policies that are aimed just at developing a neighbourhood. A raft of social, educational, health and community measures is required to improve the life chances of those affected by poverty (Gibbons et al 2005). The creation of opportunities for access to research and education can help change impressions of science as elitist and improve the educational and occupational prospects of young people (see for example the 'It's our Science, our Society, our Health' project, www.lshtm.ac.uk/pehru/ourscience). Participatory art projects can provide a safe space where people can build networks and can contribute to building social involvement and community cohesion (Matarasso 1997, Schmid 2005; see Chs 11, 13, 14, 20). They can bring people together and facilitate the development of a sense of pride in local cultures, a vital element for community participation and investment of time and effort in the community (Matarasso 1997, Schmid 2005). Community writing and publishing groups can provide access to educational experiences, networking opportunities and increased community participation (see Chs 13, 14, also, for example, QueenSpark, www.queensparkbooks.org.uk, and Exposure, www.exposure.org.uk). Other concerns need also to be addressed too in order to make social capital available to community members. Teenage pregnancy, for example, and consequently gender issues and sexual health, play a significant part in changing the occupational trajectories of young people and their access to opportunities for networking, education and occupation. These need to be sustained through educational initiatives.

Provision of facilities where people can connect meaningfully with each other is vital to the maintenance of social capital (Lowndes et al 2006, Margo et al 2006, Roberts & Chada 2006, Stafford & Marmot 2006; see Chs 11, 13–15, 20) but often the kinds of community and voluntary organization that people express their social capital through are unconnected with political structures (Lowndes et al 2006). A fundamental problem of community intervention has been that political structures can tend to be self-serving, particularly among entrenched traditional groupings or areas where there is no overall party control (Tait 2005, Lowndes et al 2006). Policies oriented to community development tend to be more rhetorical than practical, more inclined to make assumptions than to work with actual needs (Kapasi 2006, Lowndes et al 2006). Where more public consultation is in evidence there is more community involvement in developing local social organizations (Lowndes et al 2006). The declining involvement in political parties may point to an increasing perception that power is concentrated among a privileged group and does not connect with the occupational needs of the voters politicians claim to serve.

The same issue applies to occupational therapists. If occupational therapists themselves come from a very narrow base within the population, effective practice can happen only where practitioners are able to work from a principle of curiosity that is disposed to understanding and negotiating rather than assuming and interpreting the needs of the people therapists are working with (Stagnitti 2005).

Generating community involvement depends on a number of factors that are connected with motivation and capacity, supported by informal networks, reciprocity and the construction of shared goals that run across classes (Blokland 2002). People need resources and abilities to be able to develop community initiatives and sustain them through creating local organizations, but they may also need incentives to do so themselves rather than leaving it to officials from local government or public institutions (Lowndes et al 2006). Most importantly, a sense of at-homeness with the community is necessary, a sense that can be developed through the sharing of a common class identity or goal. Although physical communities based on the sharing of a identity based on sexuality or disability exist (see, for example, Pritchard et al 2002), most people do not live in such habitats. Moreover, even in communities structured around sexual identities or disability, dwellers often share a middle-class identity that gives them access to space and to the resources to choose their living environment, and this may be used to exclude others.

In the mediation of community resources, for example care facilities, occupational therapists may be among the officials who wield power and be perceived as agents of social control, outsiders to the community with whom they are working. As Hammell (2007) has indicated, the professional self-interest that occupational therapists may have in meeting the needs of their employers can stand in the way of this engagement and perpetuate an established and exclusive hierarchy (Farmer et al 2003). It takes time to establish the trust and built the social capital necessary to engage other community members in identifying and working towards their needs. Through their consistent engagement with a community, occupational therapists along with other health professionals can become assets for community sustainability and social capital, although it remains unclear whether they would use this potential for altruistic and not personal reasons (Farmer et al 2003).

Occupational therapy as a classed practice

Access to higher education is highly stratified by class and income, and people from working-class backgrounds are less likely to attend university (Hartery & Gahagan 1998, Palmer et al 2005). This can perpetuate poverty, as higher-paid jobs often require tertiary education.

Generally, occupational therapists have received a 3- or 4-year university education leading to a degree, whereas in some countries, such as Canada, a master's level qualification is now required for professional registration.

In many countries the majority of clients occupational therapists engage with are less likely to have had access to further education and often earn below-average incomes. In some countries where occupational therapists practise, however, occupational therapy will mostly be available through private health care and so will not be accessed by the most impoverished or possibly the most disabled groups of people (Ch. 7). In global terms most of the world's population of disabled people will be unable to access an occupational therapist and will not even have heard of one.

Being and becoming an occupational therapist involves participation in a distinct professional culture that is grounded in social class and gender divides and informs practice (Abberley 1995, Mackey 2007). Like many other health professions that are seen in gendered terms (e.g. some branches of psychiatry such as those dealing with children, learning difficulties and the mental health of the elderly (Pringle 1998)), and nursing (Diaski 2004), it has been argued that occupational therapists have been disempowered (Griffin 2001).

However, occupational therapists exercise power stemming from their status as members of a profession. This can be seen in the way occupational therapists construct their 'client', as illustrated by Abberley (1995). Their occupational perspective of health has yet to gain ground on the biomedical perspective of the medical profession to which they are allied; therefore therapists cannot claim neutrality (Mackey 2007). The benefits of occupational therapy are not well supported in research: most of the research methodologies that occupational therapists use are regarded as weak and often there is little interest in the outcomes (Pollard & Walsh 2000, Department of Health 2006). Mounting a robust challenge to this problem is hindered by a lack of research experience in the profession, itself a problem arising from the opportunities open to its gendered membership (Pollard & Walsh 2000, Meade et al 2005, Department of Health 2006). Even where the profession, has sought to gain status, for example the arguments during the 1990s in the UK over the ability of senior occupational therapists to act as care coordinators for mental health clients (Wilcock 2002), these trappings have often been bought at a price of increasing genericism. In some cases they have made occupational therapists more useful to a generic culture within the health system and have provided recognition, but not always. Medical practitioners have expressed concerns about such extensions to practice with regard to competence and litigation (Department of Health 2006), and in May 2007 the College of Occupational Therapists joined the Royal College of Nursing, the British Psychological Society and the trade unions Unison and Amicus in leaving the Mental Health Alliance campaign against a new Mental Health Bill, on the grounds that it had failed adequately to represent non-pharmacological interventions to the UK government. One of the key factors in the dispute was a question as to whether mental health professionals other than psychiatrists were capable of determining whether patients should be detained in care under the Act.

The organizations argued that the professionalism of their members was discounted by this decision. Occupational therapists have sought the power that goes with professional status and being an agent of social control (Wilcock 2002, Hammell 2004, 2007) but have often been unable to gain recognition of the specialized role they perform within the multidisciplinary teams in mental health settings (Peck & Norman 1999). One contributory factor may be that the availability of post-registration training is very much dependent on the resourcefulness of individual allied health professionals and their access to courses and restricted funding (Department of Health 2006).

Griffin (2001) has suggested that occupational therapists are reluctant to use power to gain recognition, favouring cooperation over conflict situations. The ensuing paradox is that, although occupational therapy is a profession, its disempowered status within the health care arena places it in an insecure position, not knowing with whom it is best to make alliances.

It's a man's world...engendered occupation

Gender is a cultural identity referring to patterns of behaviour commonly associated with biological sex. As such it cannot be seen as natural nor can it be fixed, but it is entangled in a constant dialectical relationship with the cultural setting or context where it occurs. Gender can be seen as a regulator for the behaviour of women and men, stipulating accepted, preferred and valued behaviours, attitudes and occupations (Loizos & Papataxiarchis 1991, Connell 1995).

Being a woman or man is a role that assumes certain obligations and enjoys specific privileges. Possession of the corresponding biological sex is only one of the criteria one has to fulfil in order to be rendered capable of being a man or a woman (MacWhannell & Blair 1998). While masculinity is embodied in the male body and its performance it is also a social practice (Wellard 2002, Beagan & Saunders 2005, Brickell 2005). Boys learn that their main goal in life is performing, 'getting the job done', dominating women (Connell 1995, Lazos 1997, Tepper 1999) and they grow up being trained in typical 'male' attributes such as toughness, physical activity, bravery, sexual vivacity, virility, independence, dominance, aggression and decisiveness, among others (Connell 1995, Tepper 1999). 'Real' men are not supposed to or expected to be weak, emotional or frail, sentimental or even sensual; these are all 'female' attributes and not acceptable for a man. This gender-role stereotyping can lead to occupational deprivation, as people are obliged to conform to societal expectations rather than their individual needs (Whiteford 2004).

Gender identity is not a fixed category; it is mutable. It can be deeply personal and can be invented and reinvented, constructed and re-constructed. We can thus talk of multiple gender identities: polymasculinity or masculinities instead of *the* masculinity. Although it is the prevailing discourse, a phallocentric and oppressive notion of masculinity cannot provide a coherent gender identity for the majority of men (O'Neill & Hird 2001). Murphy, drawing from his own experience as a quadriplegic, illustrates a striking disanalogy between this ideal and men's lived experiences: 'paralytic disability constitutes emasculation of a more direct and total nature' (Murphy 1990, p. 94).

The issue of gender is twofold. One side is represented by the regulation of behavioural patterns. Sexism, androcentrism (i.e. social conditions that favour male dominance) and power differentials constitute another often ignored or taken for granted aspect. The dominant normative conceptualization of gender favours male over female. The restrictions of access experienced by working-class people to primary goods, however one defines them, are also faced by women (Nussbaum 2002). The gender pay gap (Karamessini & Ioakimoglou 2007) and asset gap (Deere & Ross 2006, Warren 2006) have been well documented, although there remains controversy over the mechanisms through which they are constructed. Having limited access to material resources places women in disproportionately greater danger of poverty; indeed women are overrepresented among the poor. Their restricted access to basic resources such as education, housing and food further limits their chances of getting out of poverty.

Reduced income and assets translate into reduced power (Deere & Ross 2006). Without monetary resources women possess little negotiation power, cannot control their representations or the public discourse concerning them and have limited opportunity of exit from abusive situations. Women experience a disadvantage in access to resources and power, when compared with men. Men enjoy liberties, such as nonconsensual sex in wedlock, that may be socially sanctioned or even institutionalized through the absence of legislature and in effect limit the freedom of women. Gender justice cannot be pursued without limiting male freedom (Nussbaum 2003a). For example, if not limited, the right to sexual pleasure can lead to violence towards women, increased risk of unwanted pregnancy and contraction of sexually transmitted diseases (Oriel 2005). The very nature of gender inequality means that it is mostly men who hold the power to instigate change and any equality oriented programmes need to take this into consideration (Connell 2005).

Emancipation, which is structured around strategies of empowerment, is basic in attempts to address gender inequalities. This can be achieved through education; for Nussbaum (2003b) regulation of access to education plays a vital role in the construction of gender inequality. More women than men have not had access to education, and illiteracy is common. This reduces employment opportunities and denies women jobs that would provide financial independence and give them decision-making and action-taking power (Nussbaum 2003b). The intersection of gender and class cannot be ignored (Skeggs 2005, McDowell 2006). Knowledge of legal procedures and one's own rights, networking, lobbying and in effect being actively involved in political procedures are all largely dependent on literacy. Education gives women better knowledge of their body, the health risks they face and contributes to the development of negotiation power in issues of sexual health and violence (Grown et al 2005). Women with higher incomes generally feel safer and participate more in community activities, since a sense of safety is also important for civic participation (Caiazza 2005).

Being denied occupations or being constrained in their participation, women often face what Wicks and Whiteford (2005, p. 202) call 'occupational tensions'. The restructuring of economic policies in many countries has given women access to paid employment but in part-time, low-paying and undervalued jobs. Disparities between the genders are perpetuated by the unrecognized domestic labour that remains the remit of women (Warren 2006).

The construction of a feminine profession

While occupational therapy's feminine values and underpinning philosophies have been problematized, for example the recognition of restrictions in gendered social expectations for women and consequently for men in a profession perceived as feminine (Meade et al 2005), the gendered aspect of both the profession and occupation is complex (Pollard & Walsh 2000, Taylor 2003, Wicks & Whiteford 2005). Occupational therapy is both contained within and tries actively to engage with dominant male power structures operating in health and social care services and in the broader social, cultural and political context, but female occupational therapists are dissatisfied with their lack of opportunities for career development (Meade et al 2005). Male occupational therapists appear to gain promotion more quickly than their female colleagues and exercise a disproportionate influence in the profession (Meade et al 2005). In professions where numbers of women are proportionately high turnover is also high, a correlation that is associated with their traditional domestic roles in childcare (Pollard & Walsh 2000). Occupational therapy has a tradition of flexibility in which people have been able to find work according to their requirements. For some it has offered a professional career without the pressures of needing to gain advancement (Frank 1992), although more recent concerns around continuing professional development and changes to pay structures may be changing this perception.

In the USA and the UK occupational therapy originated among middle-class women seeking a professional career, some of whom might be described as early feminists through their connections with the suffragette movement and the radical politics of figures like William Morris and John Ruskin (Wilcock 2002, Wicks & Whiteford 2005; see Ch. 7).

In Britain, according to Trollope (1994), many such women were missionaries with Christian purpose, not so much persuaded that women should boldly take on a male-ordered world, more that they could quietly show the way by good example. Pearsall (1983, p. 521) remarks of Octavia Hill, an important ancestor of the occupational therapy family, that she sublimated her sexuality to an idealized 'do-gooding', effective but tending to distort 'life as it is' (p. 522). While Elizabeth Casson was one of the first women to qualify as a doctor, and some of the ideas early occupational therapists espoused came from the somewhat utopian socialist Arts and Crafts movement led by John Ruskin and William Morris (Wilcock 2002, e.g. Ruskin 1862, Morris 1890), the challenges they presented to the establishment were necessarily contained within professional boundaries. They sought to work within, to accommodate and be accommodated rather than to confront.

In order to establish themselves and their profession, occupational therapy pioneers sometimes had to make do with scant resources, particularly during the Second World War. However, compromises made in training and resources undermined the status of the profession within health services (Townsend 1998, Wilcock 2002).

Early in the development of the profession most occupational therapists were employed in psychiatric settings. From the 1960s increasing numbers of occupational therapists in the UK worked in physical medicine, eventually far outweighing those employed in mental health. The profession felt itself under increasing pressure to justify itself through an evidence base but chronically lacked investment in education and preparation for research, which undermined these efforts (Wilcock 2002). The core domestic activity was seen as less scientific and important even though domestic assessment suites were built in many UK hospitals at this time (Pollard & Walsh 2000, Wilcock 2002). Much occupational therapy intervention was perceived by other professionals as low status, of little practical value or not meeting patients' needs for occupational fulfilment (Hamlin et al 1992, Hammell 2004, Clark 2007). In psychiatry occupational therapists have sometimes been seen as rather selective, choosing to work with more able clients who offered less challenging behaviours (Clark 2007). Feminist critiques suggest that occupational therapists have accepted their representation as feminine, and their concern with domestic and craft activities reinforced the stereotypical view of their status as women. This may derive from patterns of socialization into different forms of leisure and work activity (Taylor 2003) but it is upheld, for example, in schoolchildren's perception of occupational therapy as a female career (Miller & Hayward 2006).

The lack of research expertise in the profession continues to be a problem (Department of Health 2006). Occupational therapists rarely produce the kind of results that can be interpreted in generalizable ways and sometimes, it is argued, maintain a perception that the complexity of occupation cannot be reduced for research purposes (Duncan et al 2007). This presents an ethical problem, because it means that therapists are unable to articulate their competence or the basis for their opinions in their role as advocates. Consequently they may at least risk failing in their duties through not having the knowledge to meet the demands of client-centredness, although some have even ignored clients' needs (Wright-St Clair 2001, Atwal & Caldwell 2003). Occupational therapy has not proved itself sufficiently indispensable to health care to secure resources, whether this is demonstrated through never having sufficient staff to cover annual leave or therapists finding their opinions dismissed when clients are being discharged before their ability to manage at home has been properly assessed (e.g. Lymbery 2002, Atwal & Caldwell 2003).

While the initial postwar enthusiasm for the profession generated purpose-built facilities, for much of its later history, especially in psychiatry, occupational therapy has got along in inadequate accommodation – such as wooden huts (our experience) or just 'living out of cupboards'. Therapists scrounged waste materials or asked for donations to bolster tight budgets and relied heavily on craftspeople and non-professional support workers supervised by smaller numbers of trained staff (Townsend 1998, Wilcock 2002). Sometimes these people have appeared more pragmatic and open to engaging clients in relevant and fulfilling occupations than the therapists themselves (Hammell 2004, Clark 2007).

It might be argued that, had the social construction of occupational therapy profession been more gender and class balanced, it might have been less craft and more work-process centred. For example, this is suggested by Clark's (2007) slightly dismissive anecdotes of rather genteel occupational therapists at Fulbourn hospital. Many anecdotes of the personal resourcefulness of professionals in getting suitable resources counter these views (Wilcock 2002, Breines 2005, Schmid 2005). Of course, work-based approaches are not exclusively male (e.g. Thibeault 2002); if there have been tendencies towards feminine characterization of activities (Bracegirdle 1991, Pollard & Walsh 2000) this has not necessarily proved a barrier to client-centred practice (Sumsion & Smyth 2000).

Even though most occupational therapists are women, the profession has not taken on a feminist ideology. Discussions from a feminist base have been limited (Ch. 7) or else hesitant. Kelly (1996) debated whether the profession was feminist or feminine, and Pollard & Walsh (2000) subsequently explored whether there was a valuable maternal principle operating in the way occupational therapists maintain a safe therapeutic space in which clients can explore their recovering abilities. Valuable as this may be, it reflects an aspect of the occupational therapist as a female 'carer' (Wright-St Clair 2001), subject through gender stereotyping to a patriarchically defined alliance with medicine, bound to remain so constrained as long as the majority of occupational therapists are women in a male-ordered world (MacWhannell & Blair 1998).

The reason why a feminine principle of caring or nurturing is derided in a masculine environment is because it threatens the idea of male autonomy, which is held to be the basis of leadership skills (Scheidt 1998). Thus the gendered majority of occupational therapists, often mothers, working part-time or taking leave around childcare needs, often contributing the second income to family finances, reflect the asymmetry of child rearing and domestic aspects of traditional gender relationships. They are allied health care workers, handmaidens to medicine, without the autonomy of men or male doctors to whom their career development is sacrificed (Pollard & Walsh 2000).

Gender is an important determinant of the delivery of occupational therapy, its access to resources and its ability to meet both the ethical demands of professional authority and the needs of disabled people. We have seen how, over the history of occupational therapy (Ch. 7), a particular perspective on occupation developed, centred on productive occupation through craft, work, domesticity and leisure (Breines 2005) but, comprehensive as this picture appears to be, it still overlooks some of the key areas of need experienced by clients.

Sexuality

Sexuality refers to sexual desires, choices and behaviours, in short to sexual identity (Weeks 2003). Historically it was largely constructed and is still commonly perceived as a purely personal issue, connected with individual choices and desires. Thus any attempt to recognize inequalities or move the debate to a political level was dismissed (Richardson 2004). It was basically assumed that 'sexual desire is natural and automatic and heterosexual and universal' (Gagnon & Parker 1995, p. 12). The gay liberation movement of the 1970s, informed by left-wing movements of the time, put the issue back in the political agenda. It explicitly connected the sexual with the political, asking for a deconstruction of the canonistic dichotomies of sexualities and gender. The movement called instead for people to have the right to determine their own sexuality (Robinson 2003).

Sexuality is regulated through the axes of gender and class and operates in the social organization of society, as evidenced through the heteronormativity (i.e. reinforcing heterosexuality as a social norm) of institutions like marriage, church, work and even the health professions, including occupational therapy, as Jackson's study illustrates (Jackson 2000, Weeks 2003, Röndahl et al 2006, Danby 2007). Whom we have sex with, what we do with our bodies and how we get erotic pleasure are all socially and politically regulated issues (Weeks 2003). Conceptions of what is permissible change over time and influence access to full citizenship rights. Taylor's (2005a,b) account of the discussion around the repeal of Section 28/2a (which prohibited the promotion of homosexuality by local authorities) in Scotland is telling of the limitations that social insularity can impose on citizenship.

Sexuality gives meaning to occupations (Jackson 1995); it also influences access to occupation, through discriminatory practices, exclusion, limited access to public discourse, fear and legislation that either fails to protect or actively refuses rights (Weeks 2003). For example, the pay gap between homosexuals and heterosexuals can be traced back to the discrimination homosexual people encounter in homophobic work environments (Brown 1998).

Sexuality is inseparable from class and gender (Skeggs 2001, Weeks 2003, Taylor 2005a, 2007), for example in its exploitation as a commodity (Nyanzi et al 2005). Such transactions commonly have male purchasers and female vendors (their power differential is mainly constructed on grounds of gender) but roles can be reversed when power differentials are based on class and access to wealth (Nyanzi et al 2005). Gay sexualities are often constructed and perceived as middle class. Working-class lesbian women and homosexual men can feel excluded from gay establishments and have different access to resources from their middle-class peers (Taylor 2005a, 2007, Oswin 2007).

One product of the short-lived and incoherent radical gay movement is the understanding of sexuality as a personal matter. This has cultivated notions of normalization, or what Oswin (2007, p. 656) calls 'homonormativity', through institutions such as gay marriage, which is maintained in order to achieve integration within a heterosexual society (Richardson 2005). This politics of assimilation or social conformity perpetuates the dominant discourses of class, sexual and gender dichotomy. The production of the 'normal' gay can only lead to further marginalization of people who do not, or do not want to, fit into this rhetoric (Taylor 2007).

Sexuality as an occupational area and a source of inequalities in access to opportunities for engagement in occupation has been ignored in professional discourses of occupational therapy (Couldrick 1998, Harrison 2001, Sakellariou & Simó Algado 2006a, Pollard & Sakellariou 2007), despite suggestions of both the relevance of sexuality in individuals' occupational life and the legitimacy of sexuality as an area of professional concern (see, for example, Jackson 1995, Birkholtz & Blair 1999, Kingsley & Molineux 2000, Williamson 2000, Bergan-Gander & von Kürthy 2006, Sakellariou & Sawada 2006, Sakellariou & Simó Algado 2006a,b). Disabled people are often regarded as asexual, denied the right to express themselves sexually or to have a sexual identity (Shakespeare et al 1996, Stoner 1999, Sakellariou 2006). Although disabled people place a high priority on sex and sexual expression and feel that these unaddressed issues constitute a major barrier to their participation in society, occupational therapists remain reluctant to deal with sexuality (Couldrick 2005, Parritt 2006, Sakellariou & Simó Algado 2006a, Basson 2007, Pollard & Sakellariou 2007).

Professionals or care workers sometimes think that it is better to avoid the challenges that may arise when people form sexual relationships (Pollard & Sakellariou 2007). It can seem safer to stick with procedural concerns rather than engage in interactive issues. If people with learning disabilities develop sexualized behaviours this may make them prone to abuse by workers, relatives or people in the wider community. Dealing with these situations can be difficult where clients are unable to see the consequences, for example that they are being exploited or are at risk of abuse. Sexual abuse has often been noted in psychiatric contexts and can also be an issue for people with physical disabilities (Shakespeare et al 1996).

These significant concerns are also connected with the need to protect and maintain the client–worker relationship. Stoner (1999) describes how health and social care workers have occasionally misunderstood requests to facilitate severely impaired clients in meeting their sexual needs as being asked to participate. Even where workers are willing to assist people to have sex their peers may regard this as unprofessional or conflicting with their personal beliefs. In Denmark social care can include work that enables disabled people to have sexual experiences (Smith 2006) but this may be unethical in countries where prostitution is connected with crime, slavery, exploitation and sexually transmitted disease (Pollard & Sakellariou 2007).

Although clinical practice concerning relationships and sexual functioning are the concern of specialist branches of medicine and counselling, these issues are also the everyday working experience of occupational therapists and other health and social care professionals. The knowledge and professional development that uphold clinical specialisms such as occupational therapy count for little if it is unable to work with the needs reasonably expressed by its clients. Client-centredness is challenged if people with disabilities are not given the choice and opportunity for negotiating their own healthy sexual relationships on the assumption of asexuality, or because professionals do not want to discuss it. Sexuality is a central element of Western culture; consequently some clients may give sex a very high priority in their daily lives and identity (Couldrick 2005, Smith 2006). While the experience of disability frequently impacts on the negotiation of sexual aspects of relationships that people may have found very significant, other people who have lived with disability all their lives may simply want to participate in the experience that people around them are clearly able to share in their own lives. Denying the opportunity to discuss what is significant to an individual amounts to occupational apartheid and occupational injustice (Sakellariou & Simó Algado 2006b).

Acknowledging the sociopolitical construction of sexuality and its importance in people's everyday lives necessitates structural changes in the basis of the profession and not only in the attitudes of individual therapists. It is not enough to talk about the sexual issues of disabled people without exploring the contexts where these arise and without challenging the canonistic representations of sexuality. Occupational justice may be found in the deconstruction of the hegemonic position that favours one sexuality over the other.

Closing the divide; affirmation or transformation?

Class, gender and sexuality are all sources of various forms of social, economic, political or occupational injustice. They regulate access to education, social capital, financial resources, employment and health care. This in turn leads to decreased life opportunities and an increased burden on health and well-being through the two axes of distribution and recognition (Fraser 1997). Distribution refers to the predominantly economic injustice stemming from the unequal allotment of resources through marginalization, exploitation and deprivation. Its impact is far-reaching and creates multiple disadvantages.

A prime example of injustice structured on mechanisms of distribution is class (Fraser 1997). People are usually acculturated within the class in which they were born, and this determines their access to resources such as education, health care and food. Class is commonly recognized to be a structured, social convention that is the basis of the construction and maintenance of societies. It is structured around a notion of production and profit and consequently serves as the sanctioned form of dominance (Graeber 2004). This makes possible the existence of the multiple classes that are necessary to sustain social structures and human occupations based on economic exploitation (Haylett 2003).

The cultural construction of class is fundamental in the formation of the subordination of working-class discourses (Bernans 2002, Skeggs 2005, Tait 2005, Taylor 2007; see Chs 13, 14). These issues of recognition are usually secondary to the problem of access to resources; they are important side effects of limited opportunities for representation amid dominant cultural values. In other words, unequal distribution forms the basis for misrecognition or even non-recognition and an apparent silence in the articulation of working-class perspectives (Morley & Worpole 1982; see Ch. 14). Schematically put, the limited economic power of working-class people makes them vulnerable to misrepresentation; they are not poor because they are *depicted* as loud, vulgar or lazy. The issues of both economics and cultural representation need to be challenged in order to address class inequality (Haylett 2003).

Gender and sexuality are cultural identities that are also conceived in terms of a fixed normality. This is maintained through the construction of mechanisms designed to avert difference, such as sexism and homophobia, or through the promotion of androcentrism and heteronormativity. There is an implicit dichotomy between occupational behaviours that are accepted and perceived as normal and those that at best are tolerated. Tolerance further reinforces the existing dichotomy and infers the presence of a *tolerator*. As one participant in Taylor's study of working-class lesbians put it, however, 'I don't want to be fucking tolerated, do you know what I mean, I want to exist equally along with everybody else' (Taylor 2005a, p. 488).

Women and gay people find their experiences subjugated, silenced, misrepresented and excluded from public discourse (Sayer 2002). They are disrespected and devalued, having to live in a society replete with androcentric and heteronormative institutions (Fraser 1997). The cultural devaluation of their subjective and occupational experience of gender and sexuality operates in two ways, through both its denial and its location in an accepted order (Weeks 2003). These issues of misrecognition and misrepresentation lead to economic and other injustices (Fraser 1997). Women receive less money than men for the same job, domestic labour is systematically devalued, gay people are denied jobs or access to institutions such as marriage that secure a degree of financial security and state benefits. Thus, in the case of gender and sexuality, injustices of distribution can be seen as secondary to injustices of recognition.

However, injustices in distribution are significant in the misrecognition of women and gay people; societies are androcentric and heteronormative because heterosexual men have more power over other groups of people. Thus they are occupationally favoured in being able to exercise more political power and having better access to public discourses. Maldistribution of resources among the classes can be traced back to the ideological construction of the worker–employer relationship in capitalistic economic systems (Bernans 2002). Although they are presented separately here, issues of distribution and recognition operate together, often in unexpected ways. Skeggs' (1999, 2005) research, for example, illustrates how straight white working-class women can be misrecognized in gay spaces or how gay women can be made to feel unwelcome in lesbian venues when their sexuality is contrasted with that of the straight women occupying the same space (Skeggs 2001). Taylor's (2007) research shows how working-class lesbians are misrecognized in gay scene spaces and are thus denied a sense of connection with spaces specifically structured around the notion of a common sexuality. It becomes obvious that identities are embedded and spaces are not only gendered or sexualized but also classed. This is fertile ground for occupational injustices; it can easily be surmised that the outcomes of such denials of doing, being, becoming and belonging may produce detrimental consequences for occupational balance and health.

Recognizing the divide is one issue, closing it is another. Affirmation and transformation are the two approaches examined by Fraser (1997) as potential solutions to the issues of recognition and distribution. Affirmation refers to action directed to presenting differences as equal, but distinct, realities. Affirmative action seeks to reallocate resources within the existing system of production and to provide relief to those who experience deprivation and limited access to them (Fraser 1997). This strategy can be seen as mainstreaming discourses of class, gender and sexuality, without challenging dichotomies. It suggests that groups need to be kept clearly defined in their demarcated spaces in order to increase their visibility and ensure access to resources and recognition. Most programmes carried out by non-governmental organizations on gender equality focus on strategies that, while improving the economic position of women, do little to address the underlying inequalities (Bessis 2003). Similar criticism is made of attempts to mainstream gay and lesbian sexualities because they connect to traditionally patriarchic institutions such as marriage (Richardson 2004, 2005).

In contrast with affirmative action's concern with unjust outcomes, transformation challenges the origins of established institutional structures, such as gender division, canonistic sexuality and class stratification (Fraser 1997). Resources are not reallocated but the system of production is challenged. Gay sexualities are not mainstreamed or tolerated; instead the construction of the sexuality discourse around an axis of normativity is deconstructed. Sexuality, along with gender, becomes a fluid identity. This was the aim of several of the first radical gay organizations such as the Gay Liberation Front, Lavender Menace and Front Homosexuel d'Action Révolutionnaire (see Radicalesbians 1970, London Gay Liberation Front 1971, Guerin 1983; for an exploration of the link between homosexuality and the revolutionary left, see Berry 2003, Robinson 2003).

The main difference, then, is about accepting or denying the constructed dichotomies in our understanding of the human occupations connected with class, sexuality and gender. The answer to this is to ask ourselves what direction action should take for effective practice that does not reinforce occupational injustices, deprivation or apartheid. Although occupational therapists may be led to believe that affirmative action might offer some 'easy wins' and identifiable outcomes, these are rarely sustainable. In reality, affirmative action serves to provide an illusion of equality and perpetuates injustices.

Conclusion

The enactment of full citizenship is realized through access to political discourse (Arendt 1958/1998, Tait 2005). Debates on class, gender and sexuality are ultimately debates on citizenship: about who has it, who doesn't and what to do in order to gain it (Chs 1, 2). Groups of people can be subordinated through institutionalized practices, societal behaviours and political decisions. Their access to political discourse and power to influence it through their own representations in public discourses is restricted (Chs 1, 3, 4, 11, 14, 15, 18–20). Class, gender and sexuality are among the elements that are perceived in a hierarchical dichotomy and thus provide fertile ground for discrimination in the allocation of resources for health, education and liberty (Chs 14, 18, 19). This compromises opportunities for access to meaningful and dignified occupation and to chances to develop occupational literacy.

References

Abberley P 1995 Disabling ideology in health and welfare – the case of occupational therapy. Disability and Society 10: 221–232

Abreu B, Peloquin S 2004 Embracing diversity in our profession. American Journal of Occupational Therapy 58: 353–360

Armelagos G, Brown P, Turner B 2005 Evolutionary, historical and political economic perspectives on health and disease. Social Science and Medicine 61: 755–765

Arendt H 1958/1998 The human condition. University of Chicago Press, Chicago, IL

Atwal A, Caldwell K 2003 Ethics, occupational therapy and discharge planning: four broken principles. Australian Occupational Therapy Journal 50: 244–251

Awaad T 2003 Culture, cultural competency and occupational therapy: a review of the literature. British Journal of Occupational Therapy 66: 409–413

Basson R 2007 Sexuality in chronic illness: no longer ignored. Lancet 369: 350–352

Beagan B L 2007 Experiences of social class: learning from occupational therapy students. Canadian Journal of Occupational Therapy 74: 125–133

Beagan B, Saunders S 2005 Occupations of masculinity: producing gender through what men do and don't do. Journal of Occupational Science 12: 161–169

Bergan-Gander R, von Kürthy H 2006 Sexual orientation and occupation: gay men and women's lived experiences of occupational participation. British Journal of Occupational Therapy 69: 402–408

Bernans D 2002 Merely economic? Surplus extraction, maldistribution and misrecognition. Rethinking Marxism 14: 49–66

Berry D 2003 For a dialectic of homosexuality and revolution. Paper delivered at the 'Socialism and Sexuality: Past and Present of Radical Sexual Politics' conference held in Amsterdam, 3–4 October 2003. Available online at: www.iisg.nl/~womhist/socandsex.html; accessed 2 September 2007

Berube A 2006 Overcoming barriers to mobility: the role of place in the United States and the UK. In: Delorenzi S (ed) Going places: neighbourhood, ethnicity and social mobility. Institute for Public Policy Research, London: p 12–28

Bessis S 2003 International organizations and gender: new paradigms and old habits. Signs: Journal of Women in Culture and Society 29: 633–647

Bimrose J, Green A, Orton M et al 2003 Improving the participation of women in the labour market: Coventry and Warwickshire. Institute for Employment Research, Coventry

Birkholtz M, Blair S 1999 'Coming out' and its impact of women's occupational behaviour – a discussion paper. Journal of Occupational Science 6: 1–7

Blanden J, Gibbons S 2006 The persistence of poverty across generations: a view from two British cohorts. Policy Press, Bristol. Available online at: www.jrf.org.uk; accessed 1 September 2007

Blaxter M 1987 Evidence on inequality in health from a national survey. Lancet 2: 30–33

Blokland T 2002 Neighbourhood social capital: does an urban gentry help? Some stories of defining shared interests, collective action and mutual support. Sociological Research Online 7(3). Available online at: http://www.socresonline.org.uk; accessed 2 September 2007

Bracegirdle H 1991 The female stereotype and occupational therapy for women with depression. British Journal of Occupational Therapy 54: 193–194

Breines E B 2005 Occupational therapy activities for practice and teaching. Whurr, London

Brickell C 2005 Masculinity, performativity, and subversion. Men and Masculinities 8: 24–43

Brown C 1998 Sexual orientation and labor economics. Feminist Economics 4(2): 89–95

Caiazza A 2005 Don't bowl at night: gender, safety and civic participation. Signs: Journal of Women in Culture and Society 30: 1608–1631

Clark D H 2007 The story of a mental hospital: Fulbourn 1858–1983. Available online at: http://www.human-nature.com/free-associations/clark/index.html; accessed 15 August 2007

Connell R 1995 Masculinities. University of California Press, Berkeley, CA

Connell R 2005 Change among the gatekeepers: men, masculinities, and gender equality in the global arena. Signs: Journal of Women in Culture and Society 30: 1802–1825

Cooper G 2007 Mental wellbeing at work. International Journal of Public Health 52: 131–132

Couldrick L 1998 Sexual issues: an area of concern for occupational therapists? British Journal of Occupational Therapy 61: 493–496

Couldrick L 2005 Sexual expression and occupational therapy. British Journal of Occupational Therapy 68: 315–318

Cummins J 2006 Measuring social capital in Camden. In: Khan H, Muir R (eds) Sticking together: social capital and local government. The results and implications of the Camden social capital surveys of 2002 and 2005. Institute for Public Policy Research, London: p 31–37

Danby C 2007 Political economy and the closet: heteronormativity in feminist economics. Feminist Economics 13(2): 29–53

Deere C, Ross C 2006 The gender asset gap: what do we know and why does it matter? Feminist Economics 12(1): 1–50

Department of Health 2006 Extending the practice of allied health professionals in the NHS. Department of Health, London

Diaski I 2004 Changing nurses' dis-empowering relationship patterns. Journal of Advanced Nursing 48: 43–50

Drexler M 2005 Health disparities and the body politic. Harvard School of Public Health, Boston, MA. Available online at: http://www.hsph.harvard.edu/disparities/book/index.html; accessed 8 June 2007

Duncan E, Paley J, Eva G 2007 Complex interventions and complex systems in occupational therapy: an alternative perspective. British Journal of Occupational Therapy 70: 199–206

Elliott M, Wang Y, Lowe R, Kleindorfer 2004 Environmental justice: frequency and severity of US chemical industry accidents and the socioeconomic status of surrounding communities. Journal of Epidemiology and Community Health 58: 24–30

Farmer J, Lauder W, Richards H, Sharkey S 2003 Dr John has gone: assessing health professionals' contribution to remote rural community sustainability in the UK. Social Science and Medicine 57: 673–686

Field K S, Briggs D J 2001 Socio-economic and locational determinants of accessibility and utilization of primary health-care. Health & Social Care in the Community 9: 294–308

Folland S 2007 Does 'community social capital' contribute to population health? Social Science and Medicine 64: 2342–2354

Frank G 1992 Opening feminist histories of occupational therapy. American Journal of Occupational Therapy 46: 989–999

Fraser N 1997 Justice interruptus. Routledge, London

Gagnon J, Parker R 1995 Introduction. In: R Parker, J Gagnon (eds) Conceiving sexuality. Routledge, New York: p 3–16

Gibbons S, Green A, Grenn P, Machin S 2005 Is Britain pulling apart? Area disparities in employment, education and crime. University of Bristol, Bristol. Available online at http://www.bris.ac.uk/Depts/CMPO/workingpapers/wp120.pdf; accessed 12 October 2007

Graeber D 2004 Fragments of an anarchist anthropology. Prickly Paradigm Press, Chicago. Available online at: http://libcom.org/library/fragments-of-an-anarchist-anthropology-david-graeber; accessed 1 August 2007

Green G, Gilbertson JM, Grimsley MFJ 2002 Fear of crime and health in residential tower blocks, a case study in Liverpool, UK. European Journal of Public Health 12: 10–15

Griffin S 2001 Occupational therapists and the concept of power: a review of the literature. Australian Occupational Therapy Journal 48: 24–34

Grown C, Gupta G, Pande R 2005 Taking action to improve women's health through gender equality and women's empowerment. Lancet 365: 541–543

Guerin D 1983 Homosexualité et révolution. Bibliothéque Libertaire. Available online at: http://kropot.free.fr/Guerin-homorev.htm; accessed 3 September 2007

Hamlin R, Black L, Kathryn M, Froelich J, MacRae N 1992 Feminism: an inclusive perspective. American Journal of Occupational Therapy 46: 967–970

Hammell K W 2004 Dimensions in meaning in the occupations of everyday life. Canadian Journal of Occupational Therapy 71: 296–305

Hammell K W 2007 Client-centred practice: ethical obligation or professional obfuscation? British Journal of Occupational Therapy 70: 264–266

Harrell S, Bond M 2006 Listening to diversity stories: principles from practice in community research and action. American Journal of Community Psychology 37: 365–376

Harrison J 2001 'It's none of my business': gay and lesbian invisibility in aged care. Australian Occupational Therapy Journal 48: 142–145

85

Hartery T, Gahagan T 1998 Social stratification and social class. In: Jones D, Blair S, Hartery T, Jones R K (eds) Sociology and occupational therapy. Churchill Livingstone, Edinburgh: p 29–40

Haylett C 2003 Culture, class and urban policy: reconsidering equality. Antipode 35: 55–73

Henderson S, Whiteford H 2003 Social capital and mental health. Lancet 362: 505–506

Holbrook D 1964 English for the rejected, training literacy in the lower streams of the secondary school. Cambridge University Press, Cambridge

Howe A, Crilly M 2001 Deprivation and violence in the community: a perspective from a UK Accident and Emergency Unit. Injury 32: 349–351

Innes M, Jones V 2006 Neighbourhood security and urban change, risk, resilience and recovery. Joseph Rowntree Foundation, York. Available online at www.jrf.org.uk; accessed 8 June 2007

Isaksson G, Lexell J, Skär L 2007 Social support provides motivation and ability to participate in occupation. Occupational Therapy Journal of Research 27: 23–30

Islam K, Merlo J, Kawachi I, Lindström M, Gerdham U 2006 Social capital and health: does egalitarianism matter? A literature review. International Journal of Equity in Health 5. Available online at: www.equityhealthj.com/content/5/1/3; accessed 28 August 2007

Iwama M 2003 The issue is: toward culturally relevant epistemologies in occupational therapy. American Journal of Occupational Therapy 57: 582–588

Jackson J 1995 Sexual orientation: its relevance to occupational science and the practice of occupational therapy. American Journal of Occupational Therapy 49: 669–678

Jackson J 2000 Understanding the experience of noninclusive occupational therapy clinics: lesbians' experiences. American Journal of Occupational Therapy 54: 26–35

Kapasi H 2006 Neighbourhood Play and community action. Joseph Rowntree Foundation, York. Available online at www.jrf.org.uk; accessed 8 June 2007

Karamessini M, Ioakimoglou E 2007 Wage determination and the gender pay gap: a feminist political economy analysis and decomposition. Feminist Economics 13(1): 31–66

Karlsen S, Nazroo J 2002 Relation between social discrimination, social class, and health among ethnic minority groups. American Journal of Public Health 92: 624–631

Kelly G 1996 Feminist or feminine? The feminine principle in occupational therapy. British Journal of Occupational Therapy 59: 2–6

Kingsley P, Molineux M 2000 True to our philosophy? Sexual orientation and occupation. British Journal of Occupational Therapy 63: 205–210

Kirsh B, Trentham B, Cole S 2006 Diversity in occupational therapy: experiences of consumers who identify themselves as minority group members. Australian Occupational Therapy Journal 53: 302–313

Krieger N, Chen J, Waterman P, Rehkopf D, Subramanian S 2003 Race/ethnicity, gender, and monitoring socioeconomic gradients in health: a comparison of area based socioeconomic measures – the public health disparities geocoding project. American Journal of Public Health 93: 1655–1671

Krieger N, Chen J, Waterman P, Rehkopf D, Subramanian S 2005 Painting a truer picture of US socioeconomic and racial/ethnic health inequalities: the public health disparities geocoding project. American Journal of Public Health 95: 312–323

Kristeva J 1991 Strangers to ourselves (trans L Roudiez). Columbia University Press, New York

Lawrence G 2004 Housing, health and wellbeing: moving forward. Reviews on Environmental Health 19: 161–176

Lazos G 1997 I seksoualikotita os aksia stin sughroni Ellada [Sexuality as a value in modern Greece]. Delfini, Athens

Loizos P, Papataxiarchis E 1991 Introduction. In: Loizos P, Papataxiarchis E (eds) Contested identities; gender and kinship in modern Greece. Princeton University Press, Princeton, NJ: p 3–25

London Gay Liberation Front 1971 Manifesto. Russel Press, Nottingham. Available online at: http://www.fordham.edu/halsall/pwh/glf-london.html; accessed 1 September 2007

Lowndes V, Pratchett L, Stoker G 2006 Locality matters: making participation count in local politics. Institute for Public Policy Research, London

Lundberg O 1991 Causal explanations for class inequality in health – an empirical analysis. Social Science and Medicine 32: 385–393

Lymbery M 2002 Transitional residential rehabilitation: what helps to make it work? Building Knowledge for Integrated Care 10: 42–48

McDowell L 2006 Reconfigurations of gender and class relations: class differences, class condescension and the changing place of class relations. Antipode 38: 825–850

Mackey H 2007 'Do not ask me to remain the same': Foucault and the professional identities of occupational therapists. Australian Occupational Therapy Journal 54: 95–102

MacWhannell D, Blair S 1998 Sex, gender and feminism. In: Jones D, Blair S, Hartery T, Jones R K (eds) Sociology and occupational therapy. Churchill Livingstone, Edinburgh: p 55–65

Margo J, Dixon M, Pearce N, Reed P 2006 Freedom's orphans: raising youth in a changing world. Institute for Public Policy Research, London

86

Marmot M, McDowall M 1986 Mortality decline and widening social inequalities. Lancet 2: 274–276

Matarasso F 1997 Use or ornament? The social impact of participation in the arts. Comedia, Stroud, Gloucestershire

Meade I, Brown G T, Trevan-Hawke J 2005 Female and male occupational therapists: a comparison of their job satisfaction level. Australian Occupational Therapy Journal 52: 136–148

Meredith P, Merson K, Strong J 2007 Differences in adult attachment style, career choice and career satisfaction for occupational therapy and commerce students. British Journal of Occupational Therapy 70: 235–242

Miles S 2005 Understanding the cultural 'case': class, identity and the regeneration of NewcastleGateshead. Sociology 39: 1019–1028

Miller L, Hayward R 2006 New jobs, old occupational stereotypes: gender and jobs in the new economy. Journal of Education and Work 19: 67–93

Morley D, Worpole K 1982 The republic of letters. Comedia/MPG, London

Morris J, Wilkinson P, Dangour A, Deeming C, Fletcher A 2007 Defining a minimum income for healthy living (MIHL): older age, England. International Journal of Epidemiology 36: 1300–1307

Morris W 1890 News from nowhere. Available online at: http://www.marxists.org.uk/archive/morris/works/1890/nowhere/nowhere.htm; accessed 29 June 2007

Murphy R 1990 The body silent. WW Norton, New York

Nicholson V 2007 Singled out: how 2 million women survived without men after the First World War. Viking, London

Novak M, Ahlgren C, Hammarström A 2006 A life-course approach in explaining social inequity in obesity among young adult men and women. International Journal of Obesity 30: 191–200

Nussbaum M 2002 Women and the law of peoples. Politics, Philosophy and Economics 1: 283–306

Nussbaum M 2003a Capabilities as fundamental entitlements: Sen and social justice. Feminist Economics 9(2): 33–59

Nussbaum M 2003b Women's education: a global challenge. Signs: Journal of Women in Culture and Society 29: 325–354

Nyanzi S, Rosenberg-Jallow O, Bah O, Nyanzi S 2005 Bumsters, big black organs and old white gold: embodied racial myths in sexual relationships of Gambian beach boys. Culture, Health and Sexuality 7: 557–569

O'Neill T, Hird M J 2001 Double damnation: gay disabled men and the negotiation of masculinity. In: Backett-Milburn K, McKie L (eds) Constructing gendered bodies. Palgrave, New York: p 204–223

Oriel J 2005 Sexual pleasure as a human right: harmful or helpful to women in the context of HIV/AIDS? Women's Studies International Forum 28: 392–404

Orton M, Rowlingson K 2007 A problem of riches: towards a new social policy research agenda on the distribution of economic resources. Journal of Social Policy 36: 59–77

Oswin N 2007 Producing homonormativity in neoliberal South Africa: recognition, redistribution, and the equality project. Signs: Journal of Women in Culture and Society 32: 549–669

Palmer G, Carr J, Kenway P 2005 Monitoring poverty and social exclusion 2005. Joseph Rowntree Foundation, York. Available online at: www.jrf.org.uk; accessed 7 June 2007

Parritt S 2006 Secrecy, taboos and catch 22s. Disability Now, May. Available online at: www.disabilitynow.org.uk/timetotalksex/feat_may_2006.htm; accessed 1 September 2007

Pearsall R 1983 The worm in the bud, the world of Victorian sexuality. Penguin, Harmondsworth

Peck E, Norman I 1999 Working together in adult community mental health services: exploring inter-professional role relations. Journal of Mental Health 8: 231–242

Pincus T, Esther R, DeWalt D A, Callahan L F 1998 Social conditions and self-management are more powerful determinants of health than access to care. Annals of Internal Medicine 129: 406–411

Pollard N, Sakellariou S 2007 Sex and occupational therapy: contradictions or contraindications? British Journal of Occupational Therapy 70: 362–365

Pollard N, Walsh S 2000 Occupational therapy, gender and mental health: an inclusive perspective? British Journal of Occupational Therapy 63: 425–431

Pollard N, Sakellariou D, Kronenberg F (forthcoming) Community development. In: Molieux M, Curtin M, Supyk J (eds) Occupational therapy and physical dysfunction, 6th edn. Elsevier Churchill Livingstone, Edinburgh

Poortinga W 2006 Social capital: an individual or collective resource for health? Social Science and Medicine 62: 292–302

Pringle R 1998 Sex and medicine. Cambridge University Press, Cambridge

Pritchard A, Morgan N, Sedgley D 2002 In search of lesbian space? The experience of Manchester's gay village. Leisure Studies 21: 105–123

Putnam R 1993 The prosperous community: social capital and public life. American Prospect 13, Spring. Available online at: http://xroads.virginia.edu/~HYPER/DETOC/assoc/13putn.html; accessed 1 September 2007

Putnam R 2000 Bowling alone, the collapse and revival of American community. Simon & Schuster, New York

Radicalesbians 1970 The woman-identified woman. Know, Pittsburgh. Available online at: http://scriptorium.lib.duke.edu/wlm/womid/; accessed 1 September 2007

Raudsepp L 2006 The relationship between socio-economic status, parental support and adolescent physical activity. Acta Paediatrica 95: 93–98

Rawls A 1973 A theory of justice. Oxford University Press, Oxford

Rebeiro K 2000 Client perspectives on occupational therapy practice: are we truly client-centred? Canadian Journal of Occupational Therapy 67: 7–14

Richardson D 2004 Locating sexualities: from here to normality. Sexualities 7: 391–411

Richardson D 2005 Desiring sameness? The rise of a neoliberal politics of normalization. Antipode 37: 515–535

Robert S 1999 Socioeconomic position and health: the independent contribution of community socioeconomic context. Annual Review of Sociology 25: 489–516

Roberts J, Chada R 2006 What's the big deal about social capital? In: Khan H, Muir R (eds) Sticking together: social capital and local government. The results and implications of the Camden social capital surveys of 2002 and 2005. Institute for Public Policy Research, London: p 25–30

Robinson L 2003 Carnival of the oppressed: the angry brigade and the Gay Liberation Front. University of Sussex Journal of Contemporary History 6, August. Available online at: www.sussex.ac.uk/history/documents/lr.pdf; accessed 11 October 2007

Röndahl G, Innala S, Carlsson M 2006 Heterosexual assumptions in verbal and non-verbal communication in nursing. Journal of Advanced Nursing 56: 373–381

Roney A, Meredith P, Strong J 2004 Attachment styles and factors affecting career choice of occupational therapy students. British Journal of Occupational Therapy 67: 133–141

Ruskin J 1862 Unto this last. Available online at: http://en.wikisource.org/wiki/Unto_This_Last; accessed 14 October 2007

Sakellariou D 2006 If not the disability, then what: barriers to reclaiming male sexuality following spinal cord injury. Sexuality and Disability 24: 101–111

Sakellariou D, Sawada Y 2006 Sexuality after spinal cord injury: the Greek male's perspective. American Journal of Occupational Therapy 60: 311–319

Sakellariou D, Simó Algado S 2006a Sexuality and occupational therapy: exploring the link. British Journal of Occupational Therapy 69: 350–356

Sakellariou D, Simó Algado S 2006b Sexuality and disability: a case of occupational injustice. British Journal of Occupational Therapy 69: 69–76

Sampson R, Raudenbush S, Earls F 1997 Neighborhoods and violent crime: a multilevel study of collective efficacy. Science 277: 918–924

Sayer A 2002 What are you worth? Why class is an embarrassing subject. Sociological Research Online 7(3). Available online at: http://www.socresonline.org.uk; accessed 7 June 2007

Scheidt S D 1998 Great expectations: challenges for women as mental health administrators. In: Levin B L, Blanch A K, Jennings A (eds) Women's mental health services. Sage, Thousand Oaks, CA: p 55–74

Schmid T (ed) 2005 Promoting health through creativity. Whurr, London

Shakespeare T, Gillespie-Sells K, Davies D 1996 The sexual politics of disability. Cassell, London

Shaw M, Smith G, Dorling D 2005 Health inequalities and New Labour: how the promises compare with real progress. British Medical Journal 330: 1016–1021

Skeggs B 1997 Formations of class and gender. Sage, London

Skeggs B 1999 Matter of place: visibility and sexualities in leisure spaces. Leisure Studies 18: 213–232

Skeggs B 2001 Femininity, class and mis-recognition. Women's' Studies International Forum 24: 295–307

Skeggs B 2005 The making of class and gender through visualizing moral subject formation. Sociology 39: 965–982

Smith A D 2006 Torben the Dane demands a very social service. Observer, 1 January. Available online at: http://observer.guardian.co.uk/international/story/0,,1676217,00.html; accessed 5 July 2007

Stafford M, Marmot M 2006 Social capital and health in Camden. In: Khan H, Muir R (eds) Sticking together: social capital and local government. The results and implications of the Camden social capital surveys of 2002 and 2005. Institute for Public Policy Research, London: p 38–44

Stagnitti K 2005 The family as a unit in post-modern society: considerations for practice. In: Whiteford G, Wright-St Clair V (eds) Occupation and practice in context. Elsevier Churchill Livingstone, Marrickville, New South Wales: p 213–229

Stephens C, Bullock S, Scott A 1999 Environmental justice: rights and means to a healthy environment for all. London: Economic and Social Research Council, Global Environmental Change Programme. Available online at: www.foe.co.uk/resource/reports/environmental_justice.pdf; accessed 15 June 2007

Stoner K 1999 Sex and disability: whose job should it be to help disabled people make love? Eye Weekly December 8. Available online at: www.eye.net/issue/issue_08.12.99/news/sex.html; accessed 7 June 2006

Sumsion T, Smyth G 2000 Barriers to client centredness and their resolution. Canadian Journal of Occupational Therapy 67: 15–21

Tait V 2005 Poor workers' unions, rebuilding labor from below. South End Press, Cambridge, MA

Taylor J 2003 Women's leisure activities, their social stereotypes and some implications for identity. British Journal of Occupational Therapy 66: 151–158

Taylor Y 2005a The gap and how to mind it: intersections of class and sexuality. Sociological Research Online 10(3). Available online at: http://www.socresonline.org.uk; accessed 6 June 2007

Taylor Y 2005b Real politik or real politics? Working-class lesbians' political awareness and activism. Women's Studies International Forum 28: 484–494

Taylor Y 2007 'If your face doesn't fit it...': the misrecognition of working class lesbians in scene space. Leisure Studies 26: 161–178

Tepper M 1999 Letting go of restrictive notions of manhood: male sexuality, disability and chronic illness. Sexuality and Disability 17: 37–52

Thibeault R 2002 Muriel Driver memorial lecture: in praise of dissidence: Anne Lang-Etienne (1932–1991). Canadian Journal of Occupational Therapy 69: 197–204

Townsend E 1998 Good intentions overruled: a critique of empowerment in the routine organization of mental health services. University of Toronto Press, Toronto

Travers K 1996 The social organization of nutritional inequities. Social Science and Medicine 43: 543–553

Trentham B, Cockburn L, Cameron D, Iwama M 2007 Diversity and inclusion within an occupational therapy curriculum. Australian Journal of Occupational Therapy 54: S49–S57

Trollope J 1994 Britannia's daughters, women of the British empire. Pimlico, London

Vagerö D, Lundberg O 1989 Health inequalities in Britain and Sweden. Lancet 2: 35–36

Warren T 2006 Moving beyond the gender wealth gap: on gender, class, ethnicity, and wealth inequalities in the United Kingdom. Feminist Economics 12(1): 195–219

Weeks J 2003 Sexuality. 2nd edn. Routledge, London

Wellard I 2002 Men, sport, body performance and the maintenance of 'exclusive masculinity'. Leisure Studies 21: 235–247

Whiteford G 2000 Occupational deprivation: global challenge in the new millennium. British Journal of Occupational Therapy 63: 200–204

Whiteford G 2004 When people cannot participate. In: Christiansen C, Townsend E (eds) Introduction to occupation: the art and science of living. Pearson Education, Upper Saddle River, NJ: p 221–242

Whitehead M, Diderichsen F 2001 Social capital and health: tip-toeing through the minefield of evidence. Lancet 358: 164–165

Wicks A, Whiteford G 2005 Gender, occupation and participation. In: Whiteford G, Wright-St Clair V (eds) Occupation and practice in context. Elsevier Churchill Livingstone, Marrickville, New South Wales: p 197–212

Wilcock A 2002 Occupation for health, volume 2: a journey from prescription to self health. College of Occupational Therapists, London

Williamson P 2000 Football and tin cans: a model of identity formation based on sexual orientation expressed through engagement in occupations. British Journal of Occupational Therapy 63: 432–439

Wilson E 1992 A very British miracle, the failure of Thatcherism. Pluto Press, London

Wilson W 2003 Race, class and urban poverty: a rejoinder. Ethnic and Racial Studies 26: 1096–1114

Woodin T 2005 Muddying the waters: changing class and identity in a working-class cultural organization. Sociology 39: 1001–1018

Wright-St Clair V 2001 Caring: the motivation for good occupational therapy practice. Australian Occupational Therapy Journal 48: 187–199

Political challenges of holism: heteroglossia and the (im)possibility of holism

6

Dikaios Sakellariou, Nick Pollard

Abstract

Holism is a popular concept in occupational therapy but its meaning is not always clear. Therapeutic encounters incorporate a whole array of perspectives and voices: those of the therapist, client, other therapists and professionals, and the client's social network. This chapter (the title of which is paraphrased from Beetham 2002) challenges the notion of holism as a fixed competence and discusses it as a disciplined process of knowing how to know that which matters or navigate successfully within complex situations. The authors use the concept of heteroglossia to refer to the diverse perspectives each of the actors may have and how these impact upon their interactions. The chapter concludes with the limitations presented to holism by internal and external factors.

Heteroglossia refers to the hierarchically structured multiple discourses that operate within a society. These multiple discourses are interconnected and are grounded in the diverse cultural discourses operative in every society, informing the interactions between the different actors.

Holism pertains to an open process of developing analytical reasoning skills rather than developing a fixed set of knowledge or competence. Holism thus refers to a disciplined process of knowing how to know that which matters or navigating successfully within complex situations.

> I've had enough
> I'm sick of seeing and touching
> Both sides of things
> Sick of being the damn bridge for everybody
> [...]I do more translating
> Than the Gawdamn UN

Rushin 1983

A common understanding of needs and wishes, constraints, resources and construction of the conflict and cooperation situation needs to be reached before solutions can be negotiated. This gives rise to mechanisms that can be described as a political practice of occupational therapy, which regulate communication between therapists, people who face disabling situations, managers or other community members. The suggestion of a political practice, which implies different viewpoints among the actors, may seem to contradict the implications of the all-inclusive holism that is held to be central to occupational therapy. However, therapists and the people they work with often inhabit different worlds in the broader political environment (see Chs 5, 9, 10, 12, 14–19) and a mechanism is needed to bridge the communication gaps that may arise. This chapter will critically examine holism and present some challenges to it that limit its usefulness and inclusive nature. The Bakhtinian concept of heteroglossia is explained and proposed as an alternative mechanism to holism that can lead to more effective communication.

It allegedly took two paradigm shifts for the profession of occupational therapy to return to its humanistic philosophical roots. (For a discussion of the concept of paradigm shifts see Kuhn 1996.) Starting as a socially and politically informed approach to addressing issues of access to occupation, occupational therapy soon allied itself with the medical profession and adopted a biomedical paradigm (Ch. 7). A second change in focus and priorities emerged in the 1980s with a gradual move towards enabling occupation rather than medical rehabilitation as the overarching aim of occupational therapy interventions (Creek 1997, Wilcock 1998a). This brought an interest in holism, a concept used with increasing frequency within the profession. Holism was developed as a stream of philosophy and as a cosmotheory by the South African philosopher and politician Jan Smuts (1926) during the scientifically prolific inter-bellum period. Smuts believed that reductionism could not adequately explain the phenomena and procedures observed in society and in the natural world.

Holism expressed an antithesis to the positivist mode of enquiry, which set out to determine the nature of the world by isolating elements and studying them. Smuts called for a heterarchical, subjective understanding of the world that took account of the complex synergies that operate between its components. These, in turn, are parts within a greater whole: the physical and social world, which cannot be understood by merely breaking them up into their elements. Taking a holistic view means exploring interacting wholes in their totality, i.e. as parts of the larger context. The Merriam Webster Online Dictionary (2007) defines holism as 'a theory that the universe and especially living nature is correctly seen in terms of interacting wholes (as of living organisms) that are more than the mere sum of elementary particles'. Holism impacted on the thinking of occupational therapy through the influence it exerted upon the development of general systems theory (Wilcock 1998a).

Holism in occupational therapy

Creek (1997, p. 29) said that occupational therapists have a 'concern with the whole person, who has a past, present and future, functioning within a physical and social environment', a definition that appears to be congruent with Smuts' conceptualization of holism. As one of the fundamental tenets of occupational therapy, holism is accepted as an axiom and rarely questioned, yet professional understandings of it appear to vary. Therapists are uncertain of the nature of holism and how it can best be applied to actual practice (Finlay 2001). This polyphony regarding the meaning and the importance of holism might account for its inadequate application in clinical practice.

Although authors such as Wilcock (1998a) and Townsend (Townsend & Wilcock 2004a,b) have indicated the traditional nature of occupational therapy's concern with social and community factors in health and occupational balance, in practice it appears that holism in occupational therapy is often restricted to an individualistic and professionally constrained understanding of the persons occupational therapists work with. Therapists who accord themselves the credentials of holism as long as they interact with clients as whole persons have often overlooked human interactions with the greater social, political, economic environment in all its cultural diversity. One example of this is the way therapists enact policy and organizational directives even when they appear to conflict with clients' interests in a disabling and disempowering way (Hammell 2007). Holism as therapists define it, is not always the same as the way clients experience it.

Holism without a context?

Dickie and colleagues (2006) argue that an emphasis on the individual experience is inherent in many definitions of occupation in occupational therapy. Although they interact through occupation, individuals and their contexts are often seen as two distinct entities. Context is not simply where the individual is located or occupation takes place but, rather, it can be seen as an active and vital component; individual and context are engaged in a dialectical relationship through occupation, each informing and shaping the other.

Dualistic conceptualizations of holism might have served occupational therapy well when it still accepted a role restricted within a biomedical paradigm. They may prove inadequate where occupational therapists act as 'agents of change' (Pollard et al 2005, Sinclair 2005), rather than agents of social control (Hammell 2004) in a world facing gross disparities in access to occupation that are often the outcome of deep sociopolitical processes (Chs 5, 10, 17, 19). Holism pertains to all aspects of the occupational therapy process, implying an acknowledgement and understanding of the contextual nature of occupation. While holism, client-centred practice and occupation-based intervention are acknowledged as basic mandates of occupational therapy practice (College of Occupational Therapists 2005), there is often conflict between the delivery of practice objectives and organizational demands (House of Commons Health Committee 2006). Often the client comes third in this contest (Hammell 2007).

These beliefs should ideally be engaged in a dialectical relationship with professional practice where they can inform and guide each other so that they are mutually congruent; otherwise, as Owen and Holmes argue (1993, p. 1694), holism becomes merely the means for achieving a 'veneer of academic and moral respectability'. As Hammell (2007) points out, there is a distinction between acting as an advocate for the client's needs and responding to organizational pressures by acting as a gatekeeper to resources, especially when policy appears contradictory, even 'chaotic' (House of Commons Health Committee 2006, Mandelstam 2007, p. 227). Some of these dangers were detailed by Abberley's (1995) analysis of holism as a construct to avert guilt. It serves to remove the culpability for a potential failure from therapists and attribute it to the complex nature of the situation. Holism is linked to the process or the form of intervention but not to the outcome, which may depend on factors such as client motivation. Therapists complain of the lack of resources or funding to develop occupational therapy knowledge but do not acknowledge where occupational therapy has not met clients' expectations because of its own failings. Abberley (1995) argues that holism is a stratagem to retain authority and power within the client–therapist relationship while justifying unsuccessful interventions on the basis that 'it's impossible to do everything'. Hammell (2007, p. 263) says that 'the impotence of the profession's claims to have clients' interests at its core … [and]…passive acquiescence to the role of resource gatekeeper' indicate the redundancy of the claim of being client-centred.

Theory–practice dissonance

If the focus of the profession is self-serving (Hasselkus 2002) this presents a serious challenge to its claim to holism. Holism is not about a requirement of achieving a set or finite level of knowledge but an open process of developing analytical reasoning skills. When applied to practice these should enable focus on those factors that demand action. Holism thus refers to a disciplined process of knowing how to know that which matters or navigate successfully within complex situations.

This discussion indicates a gap between the professional holism theory and actual occupational therapy practice (McColl 1994, Finlay 2001). The theory is split from the practice of the profession and occupation, and individuals from their context. Yet occupation and context do not inhabit distinct spheres of experience (Whiteford & Wright-St Clair 2005). To use Arendt's (1958/1998) critique of dualism, occupational therapy can be seen to be expressed through two conditions, the *activa* of practice and the *contemplativa* of theory, which have evolved to become mutually exclusive. In other words, the holism postulated by occupational therapy theory is often not informed by practice and thus does not transpire into interventions, while practice is not always prepared effectively to translate theory into action.

According to the American Occupational Therapy Association (2002, p. 610) 'occupational therapists ... focus on assisting people to engage in daily life activities that they find meaningful and purposeful'. The American Occupational Therapy Foundation envisaged a society where occupational therapists would:

> *have as an internalized mandate of occupational therapy the promotion of equal opportunity for access to resources needed for full societal participation and the promotion of inclusion of all individuals in participation. The therapist perceives the reduction of poverty; the stabilization of the population; the achievement of a sustainable, natural environment; and the empowerment of women as problems that fall within the practice domain of occupational therapy insofar as these problems relate to the domain of societal health.*
>
> Gillette 2002, p. 700 (emphasis added)

Arguably, these mission statements reveal the holistic perspective of the respective professional bodies, a holistic perspective that goes beyond the confines of the therapeutic relationship and takes into account the broad underlying reasons for restrictions on access and engagement in occupation. Hammell (2007, p. 266) asks whether the profession and its individual members are currently working towards those aims in practice or merely expressing 'good intentions'.

Many people whose access and engagement in meaningful occupation is disrupted or is at risk of being disrupted could benefit from occupational therapy services, as evidenced by many of the contributing authors to this book and others (Watson & Swartz 2004, Kronenberg et al 2005). The Well Elderly Study carried out by an interdisciplinary team from the University of Southern California evidenced the benefits of occupational therapy for healthy elderly individuals (Jackson et al 1998), while the New Stories/New Cultures after-school enrichment programme demonstrated how occupation-based interventions can equip young people from low-income urban neighbourhoods with the necessary skills to navigate the social world effectively (Frank et al 2001).

Most occupational therapists work with people who face certain clearly defined biomedical conditions, get a referral and can afford occupational therapy services. Stories of vulnerable and at-risk populations, whose access to occupation is often compromised, still remain largely unheard within the profession. Poor people, healthy elderly individuals, refugees and asylum seekers are among the groups of the population who may experience a state of occupational apartheid or injustice with a pervasive impact on their quality of life (Sussenberger 1998). Such people often fall through the cracks of health care systems or manage to elude them altogether. An alternative view might be that health care systems are sometimes able to avoid identifying the needs of clients who may require more assistance than they can pay for. Consequently, occupational therapists are sometimes unaware of the occupational risk factors these people may be facing, are not empowered to engage with them or face considerable difficulties in doing so (Chs 15, 17, 19). This represents a paradox for a profession that maintains that its focus is on access to occupation rather than on a mechanistic view of health.

Health in occupational therapy literature is conceptualized as 'a state of complete physical, mental and social well-being, not merely the absence of disease or infirmity' (World Health

Organization 2001). If human occupation is about expressing the self through doing, being, becoming and belonging (Wilcock 1998b, Hammell 2004), it follows that something so apparently natural to the purpose of human life as occupation should be a right. The implication is that, just as Nietzsche says that humanity is the goal of humanity, humans should be enabled to do, and be, and so become (Nietzsche 1986). It is not merely that humans express themselves as they are, but as they have the potential to be.

Such a proposal might be considered an expression of occupational justice. However, humans generally live alongside other humans and other organisms that also do, are, and become in ways that are meaningful to them. Inevitably the interests of humans in expressing their right to occupation will come into conflict with the purposes of others. Nietzsche's (1986) vision of humanity is that it should continually test its strength and look forward but it seems intolerant of those unable to keep in step, is enviable of others who achieve successes and tries to restrict them.

This continual balancing on an equilibrium that humans are always trying to upset to their own advantage over others is one of the problems facing occupational therapists who want to present occupation as a benign concept. Occupation is 'the act of occupying; possession; the state of being employed or occupied; the time during which a country etc, is occupied by enemy forces; that which occupies or takes up one's attention; one's habitual employment, profession, craft or trade' (Chambers Dictionary, Kirkpatrick 1983, p. 874). The implication of possession (especially of that which previously had no owner) follows from the verb to occupy. Therefore occupation implies complex relationships between what a person does or people do and the environment, whether it is a raw environment or territory that previously belonged to others. To occupy something may produce the result that access to it may be restricted to others through the concept of ownership and prior right.

Occupation is therefore inextricably linked with a political, social, economic and environmental set of purposes. Occupational justice for one individual or set of people may produce occupational injustices for others. Therefore the utilitarian principle of an occupational equality is undermined by the result of human occupation as a producer of inequality: the poor, vulnerable and those in other disabling circumstances, many of them living in the world's richest economies, cannot afford to exercise *their* occupational rights.

The heteroglossic world

Occupational therapy operates in a complex world comprised of interconnected parts rather than segregated entities. This pertains as much to the development and process of occupational therapy within a multiprofessional and multiservice environment as to the nature of the occupational engagement and performance issues people bring in their interactions with occupational therapists.

To illustrate this multifactorial discourse we make use of the Bakhtinian concept of heteroglossia (Bakhtin 1981/1995, p. 218). Heteroglossia refers to the presence of 'another's speech in another's language', for example the presence of multiple perspectives within a novel, those of the author and those of the protagonists. These multiple discourses are interconnected and are grounded in the diverse cultural discourses operative in every society, which in turn are termed social heteroglossia (Kroeger 2005). In an analogy with the textual construction of a novel, where heroes are situated in interactions initiated by the author and act within preset boundaries, social actors operate within an inescapable dominant cultural discourse. These multiple 'languages', the diverse perspectives of the various actors together with the scripts, beliefs and attitudes present in society, comprise the social whole that is the setting of human action. Occupational therapy was constructed and functions within this heteroglossic context and both occupational therapists and the people therapists work with are acculturated into different social discourses, parts of a diverse whole.

The various vantage points from which people view the world, their different perspectives and the different 'languages' they speak are intertwined in relationships of power. Some 'languages' do not need any translation to make people understand them: they express experiences that are widely recognized as representative of society as a whole. Some others have been marginalized and the realities they communicate need to be reframed according to the rules of the dominant discourse (Beetham 2002; see Chs 5, 14). This chapter opened with a poem written in 1981 by Donna Kate Rushin, an African American woman. She poignantly illustrates how the burden of reframing and translating experiences often falls upon those with less power to influence public discourses. Their experiences often remain unknown unless they can engage in a continuous process of explanation.

The construction of a common language does not resolve this injustice as it both perpetuates power differentials (communications take place according to the norms and experiences of a dominant group) and also excludes people whose experience cannot be understood according to these conventions (Beetham 2002). The 'nothing about us without us' mantra so often expressed by disability rights advocacy groups indicates the need to listen to other narratives and interpret them as they are experienced by the people who live them, and not for what they represent to the people who listen to them (Franits 2005).

This entails an acceptance of heteroglossia and the development and application of mechanisms to make sense of it. In practice the achievement of any deep understanding would be very complex, even impossible. The heteroglossic aspect of action is also complicated by variations in the order of the narratives that make it up. Each individual's narrative depicts a cycle of events, causes and motivations that may ultimately be interrelated, directly or less directly (Ricoeur 1984). For example, one of the tasks of the therapist may be to collect together accounts of an event from a client, carers and professional colleagues, looking for points of consistency and inconsistency in order to develop a treatment plan. However, this composite history can only be partial. It may have to take into account the narratives of an employing organization or the development of policy in order that treatment is effectively implemented. These narratives may not have been considered in the others, although they may come to exert an effect on their future development. In evaluating any outcomes all those involved in composing the various narratives around an experience, for example of illness or disability, are engaged in analysing not just actions but a course of events, for which each individual will continue to maintain their own narrative. These histories are characterized by collapsing or expanding certain details, the progress of events and even their linearity in the course of the story according to their importance for the individual narrator.

Earlier, the impossibility of attaining a complete knowledge or applying a complete practice was criticized as a means of diverting the experience of failure in therapy. In one sense, the holistic practitioner is an unattainable myth. On the other hand, as an ideal, it can remind therapists of the need continually to develop their skills, knowledge and through them respect for the variety of the heteroglossic context of occupation. The development of a heteroglossic cultural awareness would inform theory and practice and enable therapists effectively to 'translate' and make sense of the various contexts within which occupational therapy operates and the multiple interactions that influence the process of the profession.

Good (1994) introduced the term 'semantic networks' to indicate that disease was grounded within 'diverse meanings, voices and experiences' (p. 171). Engagement in occupation is the product of interconnected social processes, in consequence of which its meaning is also multifaceted. Therapeutic encounters incorporate a whole array of perspectives and voices: those of the therapist, client, other therapists and professionals, the client's social network, including partners, relatives, friends and the voice of the client's employer. All these are ingrained within the specific cultural setting where interactions take place. The experience of the client is a synthesis of all these voices, as demonstrated in the Case Study below, and many more. This wider chorus includes the voices of administrators and case managers who decide what kind of treatment the person is entitled to, the voices of politicians who can, for example, determine a universal design policy to enable all people to interact with the physical environment, and the voices of legislators who set the framework for the rights and responsibilities of citizens. In this complex interplay any vantage point offers a unique synthesis of these voices but they cannot be heard all at once. A technician setting up microphones to record a choir is aware that poor positioning of the equipment will be detrimental to the balance of the sound.

It may be supposed that the therapist is in a key position to synthesize all the voices but may not be empowered to make the most effective judgements even when these are indicated by best practice. The voice of an administrator may carry more volume than that of a client. Policy aimed at large numbers of people may overwhelm the vocalization of need by one individual. The volume of clinical evidence may in some cases produce discordant perspectives of best practice.

Case Study

Mr A was a man in his early fifties who was referred to occupational therapy services by his consulting physician 3 years after having experienced a cerebrovascular accident (CVA) that had resulted in left-sided hemiplegia. The reason for the referral was persistent spasticity in the left upper limb, in spite of treatment with botulinum toxin A. During these 3 years Mr A had not received any rehabilitation services, either as an inpatient or an outpatient. Although he had medical insurance and the financial resources to seek medical services not covered by his insurance plan he had not received adequate information about his options for rehabilitation.

When he first met the occupational therapist Mr A expressed frustration over the spasticity of his arm. He accepted help from a domestic helper for most activities of daily living, including dressing and undressing, personal hygiene and going to the toilet. This was not an area of concern for him. He did not participate in cooking, cleaning or shopping occupations. Throughout this period Mr A had maintained employment as a professor in a large university, although he had to step down from his duties as the head of that university following the CVA. Since he could not drive, he depended on somebody being available to drive him to and from the university once or twice a week to hold his seminar and meet with his students. He felt that his status among his peers had suffered as a result of his hemiplegia and he avoided socializing with them.

Mr A was married and had two adult children who had left home to study. Mr A's wife had become increasingly frustrated by her husband's dependence upon her and believed he 'did not want to get well'. Two years after the CVA, she decided to separate and asked Mr A to move out of the house. After his separation Mr A returned to his parental home to live with his mother and a live-in domestic helper in her eighties who had been living with the family for many decades. Both women were overprotective of Mr A and thought he should not do anything for himself lest his situation worsen, a view shared by Mr A himself. Mr A had had a large social network but withdrew from it, believing that he would be a burden. He spent most of his waking hours engaged in writing and reading from his bed, since there was no study room in his parental home. Although Mr A could walk using a cane, he avoided going out except for medical appointments and teaching engagements. His reluctance was compounded by the uneven pavements, often occupied by vehicles, and heavy traffic in the densely populated urban area where he lived.

We can therefore see that Mr A's experience as a stroke survivor was multifaceted. Mr A's CVA existed within complex semantic networks and was the product of the interactions between many interconnected voices and factors. He had not been informed of his treatment options; his wife thought he did not want to get better; he and his carers thought that he had to be careful not to exacerbate his condition and he felt that he was a burden to others; the university had retained him in employment but on reduced duties; Mr A felt that his status was also reduced. The restrictions Mr A experienced in his engagement in occupation emanated from these interconnected elements. With the historical hindsight we have as readers of this case study it is possible to propose that with a different interplay of voices to inform Mr A of treatment possibilities at an earlier stage he might have experienced different outcomes.

The dissonance between theory and practice that is increasingly being observed in the profession indicates a conflict between beliefs and actions and an inadequate synthesis of these diverse and divergent voices (Molineux 2004, Forsyth et al 2005). If practice and knowledge occur in a dialectical relationship, as Higgs and Titchen (2001) note, then the communication channels between these two interconnected elements of occupational therapy often appear to have been disrupted. Creating an opening for holistic practice requires the establishment of safe and adaptable communication mechanisms across the spectrum of the political actors in occupational therapy.

Who is disabled?

A holistic view of persons and occupations changes the way disability is defined. Wood and colleagues (2005) stated that impaired body structures do not equal impaired occupational engagement, a position that is also expressed from a disability rights perspective (Mason 2001; see Ch. 14). Consequently, a person with an impairment who has access to occupation and is not restricted in terms of occupational engagement should not be considered disabled in occupational terms. It is not the fact of impairment by itself but the 'dominance of one person over another that . . . turns impairment into disability' (Kelly 2001, p. 396).

The importance of biomedical conditions that a person may experience is not dismissed but as long as this situation does not bar a person from engagement in meaningful occupation it does not need to be a disabling one. People and their occupations are seen as integral components of their contexts rather than merely interacting (but distinct) parts. For the profession this not only affects the basis for accepting referrals and making interventions but also the directions in which occupational therapists are being impelled. In addition to assessing people on social benefits for their capacity for work, or for compensation following injury, occupational therapists work in preventive and primary care, which aims to anticipate the issues that can lead to disability.

Paraphrasing Radomski (1995, p. 487) there is more to disability than not being able to put on your pants. Many people have neither a diagnosed illness nor an impairment yet are none the less marginalized and their participation in meaningful occupation is compromised as a product of their marginalization (Chs 5, 16, 18). If occupational therapists reconceptualize disability as a predominantly social phenomenon and define it in occupational terms, then disability will not be thought of as a passive, permanent state arising from within and because of the individual. Such views have been used to discriminate against people and identify them as the problem, whereas the focus should be on the sociopolitical reality that determines their situation (Kielhofner 2005).

Disability can be viewed as a dynamic process that is created through the interaction of social actors with their context (Sakellariou 2006). It is the 'product of interconnections' between the multiple, heteroglossic discourses within which disability is situated (Good 1994, p. 171). We can see disability being constructed every day: when wheelchair users do not have access to appropriate transportation, when children do not have access to the educational opportunities of their choice because of lack of financial resources and when people do not take employment for fear of losing their benefits. These examples all present situations that may lead to disability, i.e. a long-term disruption of occupational participation. Such disabling situations result from factors such as the inaccessibility of physical places, lack of employment, patronizing behaviours or racism. Any member of a community may encounter them, although individuals who do not correspond to the normative ideal of the average citizen as a white, middle-class, heterosexual and able-bodied male may be more at risk of experiencing them (Olshansky et al 2005). These disabling situations are not natural, inevitable events but are perpetrated, whether intentionally or not, by persons and societies and have a deep impact on the occupational choices open to people.

It is not possible to attribute these influences to one oppressive group or individual or another. As has been argued, occupations occur in social contexts that are the product of many elements. Thus, if some people do not go out because they feel at risk of attack from other people in their neighbourhood, this occupational restriction may arise because there is a genuine risk or because the local paper has printed several accounts of incidents, leading to an exaggerated perception of that risk. If some people develop a criminal regard for those who are more vulnerable as prey, it is probable that they themselves have a narrow and impoverished vision of their own occupational potential. In other words, positive opportunities to do, be, become and belong are not available or appear too challenging. It is possible that gaining access to positive opportunities is out of their control, or that crucial information or support necessary to enable them has not been present (see Case Study below).

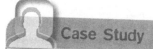

Case Study

The teenage son of an African American family living below the poverty line is likely to attend poorly resourced educational facilities (Sussenberger 1998), to have reduced leisure opportunities (Shinew et al 2004) and be exposed to violence (Selner-O'Hagan et al 1998). Living in impoverished neighbourhoods has been found to contribute to high-school drop-out (Vartanian & Gleason 1999), adoption of violent behaviour and delinquency (Tolan et al 2003) and reduced self-rated health status (Cagney et al 2005). This boy may not be able to envisage a realistic and satisfying occupational trajectory for himself in the future; thus the experience of poverty and its associated stigma, combined with a lack of appropriate social and community policies, may lead to him becoming a gang member.

By providing a sense of belonging to a group and a time structure, gang membership may represent a productive occupation for youth with limited opportunities for engagement in meaningful occupation (Snyder et al 1998). This trajectory further exposes young people to greater risk of exposure to drugs, alcohol and other substance abuse, casual sexual contact and sexually transmitted diseases, greater likelihood of contact with the police, being thrown out of their parental homes, disrupted home life and a combination of circumstances that may impact detrimentally on their mental health. They may be unable to develop more appropriate social skills that will equip them for work or the take-up of positive social opportunities, and because of their gang association and their experience of alcohol and drug abuse they may be socially excluded from positive peer influence because other people will want to protect themselves from the possibility of being victims of crime. They are more likely to experience negative self-esteem and to continue to maintain some of these negative habituations in adult life. Many of these may contribute to continued poor health, poverty, poor access to health care and reduced life expectancy. Culturally embedded representations of African American men lead to misrecognition and negative stereotyping; as Fanon argues black people need to operate in a white man's world (Fanon 1986, Malik 1996), i.e. a world defined by Western cultural definitions (Friedman 1994). Misrecognition can precipitate communal experiences of occupational apartheid, as opposed to individual experiences of occupational injustice, as other groups of people deny opportunities to them in preference to young men from other racial groups, for example for employment or education. We see that lack of resources, and the influence of the neighbourhood, both associated with income level, may exert a powerful influence on the occupational choices available or perceived as available to young people. Personal volition is not dismissed. It is not the aim of this example to depict a predetermined occupational trajectory but to show the impact the sociopolitical context can have on access to occupation and how these two should really be seen as a whole.

The growing issue of political, economic and environmental refugees and their marginalized experiences in the host countries in which they arrive has given impetus to this, particularly since the disabling experiences resulting from the traumatic events that often precipitate their migration have often been under-recognized. Although preventive approaches to disability can be regarded as having a separate focus in poverty and other social aspects of life, none the less because they are in anticipation of detrimental effects to the body they are still concerned with a narrowly defined idea of health. Disability, however, is a product of a dynamic social process.

Challenges to holism

Monoglossia

The inadequate application of holism in occupational therapy is in part the result of the dominant middle-class and female character of the occupational therapy profession in many (but not all) countries, and the origins of the underpinning philosophies and supporting practices in a Western, white paradigm (Kirsh et al 2006; see Chs 5, 7). To this we should add the difficulty that people with disabilities have had in entering the profession and the subsequent further reduction in the variety of perspectives that could inform theory and practice within the profession (Velde 2000, Sivanesan 2003). Despite the origins of occupational therapy in social action, its development as a profession has necessarily depended on certain privileges that its members and professional bodies have sought to maintain (Hammell 2007). Its place in the hierarchical order of health and social care professions has been constructed within and shaped by the dominant cultural discourse. Although occupational therapists point to their differences with aspects of this discourse, for example in their holistic principles and concern with health through occupation, they have none the less had to collaborate with other more powerful elements of this culture in order to maintain their professional status (Hammell 2007). The development of leadership skills among occupational therapists has been described as 'match[ing] their behaviour to the situational expectations of the organization: to find the "best fit", to influence their followers and to facilitate strategic change in order to sustain effectiveness' (Stewart 2007, p. 233, citing Morden 1997). There is nothing in this about leaders advocating client-centredness in the face of organizational objectives. The demand that occupational therapy leaders are there to serve 'the NHS's vision of the future' (Stewart 2007, p. 233) is rather empty given that health services are constantly changing. While this is inevitable as health care demands change with the population, many of the changes in health services in the UK have been administrative or structural (House of Commons Health Committee 2006). They have used up resources that might have been applied to the implementation of policy such as 'Our Health, Our Care, Our Say' (Department of Health 2006) in setting up and paying off executive committees, corporate logos and the rolling out of new corporate visions (House of Commons Health Committee 2006).

Positioning according to organizational demand has led to the development of a monoglossic discourse; in other words, occupational therapy is largely monocultural in its reflection of the dominant elements of the structures that accord it a place among them because no other discourse is held to be appropriate unless it meets with these interests. A dominant, white, Western, middle-class perspective seems to inform practice and this has led to limited appreciation of the importance for human occupation of different experiences and cultural beliefs (Awaad 2003, Iwama 2005, 2006). Occupational therapy purportedly deals with the whole person to enable engagement in occupation, but this whole person seems to consist only of the elements therapists (under the aegis of organizational directives) feel are appropriate. People from dominant language groups, who are often monoglot because of their cultural privilege, expect other people to accommodate their linguistic poverty (Beetham 2002). Occupational therapy tends to be exported from the dominant cultures of the Western world; consequently even where it is practised in non-Western contexts many of the ideas and tools of occupational therapy are imported rather than indigenous. In recent years, this mismatch of theory and practice context has been challenged in the specific cultural contexts of Brazil (Barros et al 2005) and Japan (Iwama 2003, 2005, 2006, Kondo 2004, Odawara 2005) and in the cultural diversity of Western societies (Crabtree 2000, Whiteford & Wilcock 2000, Chiang & Carlson 2003 and many of the contributors to this book).

Occupational therapy's position that therapy is client-centred and directed towards the whole person is also increasingly being challenged both within the profession (Hasselkus 2002, Hammell 2007) and by clients as to the nature of client-centred practice (Maitra & Erway 2006). Occupational therapists have appropriated the cultural discourse of therapy and the client–therapist interaction is regulated on the basis of the values of occupational therapy. The term 'occupation' has been employed in a symbolic way to describe a central element of occupational therapy but both signifier (i.e. occupation) and its meaning (i.e. forms of activity that constitute 'occupation') are selected by occupational therapists. Inevitably there is a conflict with holism. If within a service the range of occupational activities that are used as treatment media is limited, this serves to constrain the options for both clients and perhaps the remit of the therapists offering them. Not only is access to occupational therapy services then regulated by non-holistic criteria but the appropriate use of occupational media themselves can also be limited by a reductionist approach to those activities that can be assessed within a department. Clients' needs for occupation are related to their specific context. Even a simple meaningful activity can have complex outcomes that are not always readily assessed with standardized measures, but this does not mean that they lack clinical importance (Breines 2005, Bannigan 2007, Hocking 2007).

Divergent values become problematized in varying degrees. People find that their experiences are not always acknowledged within either the professional or official discourse of occupational therapy or therapists' employers, to the extent that the legitimacy of professional practice is challenged (Abberley 1995, Hasselkus 2002, Hammell 2007). Kirsh et al (2006) found that sexual and cultural identities are sometimes not recognized and respected in therapy, leading to inadequate therapeutic interactions and to a questioning of the intentions of occupational therapy. Experiences of gender (Pollard & Walsh 2000), spirituality (Belcham 2004) and sexuality (Couldrick 2005, Sakellariou & Simó Algado 2006) are often ignored in the process of occupational therapy, leading to plausible questions regarding the nature of holism as implemented in practice and the relevance of the profession to the lives and needs of the people it serves (Ch. 5). Talking about his experience of rehabilitation (occupational therapy being part of it), Murphy, a cultural anthropologist who became gradually paralysed as a result of a tumour developing around his vertebrae, said that 'there was nothing at all in my rehabilitation that prepared me for the psychological and social challenges I would face' (Murphy 1990, p. 56), while the physicist Stephen Hawking reported that 'I have not received much help from people calling themselves occupational therapists' (Hawking 1996, p. 27).

Theory–practice–context complex

Theory and practice need to be unitary enough to be recognized as occupational therapy irrespective of the setting yet context-specific to be sensitive to the particular, heteroglossic cultural discourses within which they will be implemented. This complexity points to the difficulty of obtaining standards that can be applied both globally and locally. Standards and resolutions that have been developed in one occupational therapy body may be difficult to apply wholesale in another; global standards may be locally inapplicable. For example, tenets such as independence and autonomy, which are considered to be central in the process of occupational therapy, are interpreted in different ways in different cultures (Whiteford & Wilcock 2000, Tamaru et al 2007: see Ch. 17). A theory–practice gap is not always a problem of inadequate utilization of theory in practice; sometimes the problem is a theory being unable to recognize the practice (Steward 1996).

Furthermore, education and continuing professional development is frequently constrained within the time resources allocated to it. Although there may be demands to insert more material on the political nature of occupation into the curriculum and a holistic perspective of the occupational therapy process, this often forces the question of what it should replace. Courses need to be attractive to applicants, they have to offer equivalent value to other degrees in terms of content, students have to be able to take them without accruing more debt than they will be able to pay off easily at the end, and the courses have to offer a coherent education for practice. Although some students seem to be satisfied with their career choices (Meredith et al 2007), if occupational therapy education does not have the means to provide a critical and analytical discourse on the role of the profession within a complex system of health and social care hegemony then it is arguably difficult for new practitioners to visualize how to develop their role and efficiently navigate in that system over the course of their careers. They will lack the means to work around pressures that restrict and narrow the scope of their practice or that divert them into generic roles (Chs 1, 7). The recent move to master's level registration requirement that has occurred in Canada and the USA and is being discussed in several other countries, including the UK, might indicate the need occupational therapists feel to consolidate their role within a complex environment.

The big, bad world

Challenges to holistic practice come not only from within the profession but also from the broad political context within which occupational therapy operates. These are often shared with other professions and can be in the form of the erosion or specialization of role as a result of organizational demands (Hocking & Nicholson 2007), competition for limited resources within health services and difficulties in connecting practice to an evidence base (Schmid 2005, Bannigan 2007). One result of this is that other health professionals have simply not heard or had the chance to listen to the occupational therapy story (Peck & Norman 1999). Practitioners may be unable to contextualize the importance of the work they are doing or feel ill equipped to meet the challenges that impact on the delivery of interventions. Occupational therapists face the risk of becoming gap fillers, as Fortune (2000) observed.

All professional groups encounter humiliations that compromise their effectiveness in practice (Owen 2002). Occupational therapists need to be clear about good practice and to avoid being drawn into situations that compromise their expertise. As Bannigan (2004, p. 147) asserted, 'occupational therapy is not a leisure pursuit'; occupational therapists need to have a practice that is informed by theory and a theory that is responsive to practice needs. Otherwise, the risk of losing our professional identity will never be too far away (Duncan et al 2007).

Occupational therapists traverse a dilemma at the edge of the hole in holism, between having a concept that is either too vague or too narrow (Hammell 2004) and is constantly changing in shape. Duncan et al (2007) have argued that one of the problems with the profession's pursuit of holism is the presentation of itself as an intervention that is so complex that it cannot be adequately researched, but Bannigan (2007) suggests that this need not be a concern if complexity is accepted. If it is recognized that knowing all the answers is impossible and that changes or outcomes are often related to wider contextual situations, it is possible to construct research around these boundary issues or attempt to define an 'event horizon' in which they occur. In order to remain within the limits of the event horizon, rather than being thrown out to the periphery or sucked into the black hole, professionals have to present concepts that are recognizable even though they may not address all the needs of the profession. The event horizon is a zone of complexity that operates in several dimensions, for example: between being understood and not being understood and so gaining or not gaining appropriate referrals; between being community or hospital focused; between being oriented to the client and being oriented to the care team. Syntheses need to be found that will allow the profession to enact its holistic mandate while at the same time remaining recognizable as a professional entity by other stakeholders. This will arise from engagement in the doing of practice, the prime professional purpose and its explication, but can emerge only if it is accepted that the boundaries are permeable, fuzzy and in flux rather than concrete. It is this quality that makes them available to research, debate and negotiation.

References

Abberley P 1995 Disabling ideology in health and welfare – the case of occupational therapy. Disability and Society 10: 221–232

American Occupational Therapy Association 2002 Occupational therapy practice framework: domain and process. American Journal of Occupational Therapy 56: 609–639

Arendt H 1958/1998 The human condition. University of Chicago Press, Chicago, IL

Awaad T 2003 Culture, cultural competency and occupational therapy: a review of the literature. British Journal of Occupational Therapy 66: 409–413

Bakhtin M 1981/1995 Heteroglossia in the novel. In: Dentith S (ed) Bakhtinian thought: an introductory reader. Routledge, London: p 195–224

Bannigan K 2004 Occupational therapy is not a leisure pursuit. British Journal of Occupational Therapy 67: 147

Bannigan K 2007 Making sense of research utilisation. In: Creek J, Lawson-Porter A (eds) Contemporary issues in occupational therapy, reasoning and reflection. John Wiley, Chichester: p 189–216

Barros D D, Ghirardi M, Lopes RE 2005 Social occupational therapy: a socio-historical perspective. In: Kronenberg F, Simó Algado S, Pollard N (eds) Occupational therapy without borders: learning from the spirit of survivors. Elsevier Churchill Livingstone, Oxford: p 140–151

Beetham M 2002 Speaking together: heteroglossia, translation and the (im)possibility of the just society. Women's Studies International Forum 25: 175–184

Belcham C 2004 Spirituality in occupational therapy: theory in practice? British Journal of Occupational Therapy 67: 39–46

Breines E B 2005 Occupational therapy: activities for practice and teaching. Whurr, London

Cagney K, Browning C, Wen M 2005 Racial disparities in self-rated health at older ages: what difference does the neighborhood make? Journal of Gerontology 60B: S181–S190

Chiang M, Carlson G 2003 Occupational therapy in multicultural contexts: issues and strategies British Journal of Occupational Therapy 66: 559–567

College of Occupational Therapists 2005 Code of ethics and professional conduct. College of Occupational Therapists, London

Couldrick L 2005 Sexual expression and occupational therapy. British Journal of Occupational Therapy 68: 315–318

Crabtree J 2000 What is a worthy goal of occupational therapy? Occupational Therapy in Health Care 12: 111–126

Creek J 1997 The knowledge base of occupational therapy. In: Creek J (ed) Occupational therapy and mental health, 2nd edn. Churchill Livingstone, Edinburgh: p 27–45

Department of Health 2006 Our health, our care, our say: a new direction for community services. Stationery Office, London

Dickie V, Curtchin M, Humphry R 2006 Occupation as transactional experience: a critique of individualism in occupational science. Journal of Occupational Science 13: 83–93

Duncan E, Paley J, Eva G 2007 Complex interventions and complex systems in occupational therapy: an alternative perspective. British Journal of Occupational Therapy 70: 199–206

Fanon F 1986 Black skin, white masks (trans C Markman). Pluto Press, London

Finlay L 2001 Holism in occupational therapy: elusive fiction and ambivalent struggle. American Journal of Occupational Therapy 55: 268–276

Forsyth K, Summerfield Mann L, Kielhofner G 2005 Scholarship of practice: making occupation-focused, theory-driven, evidence-based practice a reality. British Journal of Occupational Therapy 68: 260–268

Fortune T 2000 Occupational therapists: is our therapy truly occupational or are we merely filling gaps? British Journal of Occupational Therapy 63: 225–230

Franits L 2005 Nothing about us without us: searching for the narrative of disability. American Journal of Occupational Therapy 59: 577–579

Frank G, Fishman M, Crowley C, Blair B et al 2001 The new stories/new cultures after-school enrichment program: a direct cultural intervention. American Journal of Occupational Therapy 55: 501–508

Friedman J 1994 Cultural identity and global process. Sage, London

Gillette N 2002 The Foundation – a vision of society in the 21st century. American Journal of Occupational Therapy 56: 699–700

Good B 1994 Medicine, rationality, and experience. Cambridge University Press, Cambridge

Hammell K W 2004 Dimensions in meaning in the occupations of everyday life. Canadian Journal of Occupational Therapy 71: 296–305

Hammell K W 2007 Client-centred practice: ethical obligation or professional obfuscation? British Journal of Occupational Therapy 70: 264–266

Hasselkus B R 2002 The meaning of everyday occupation. Slack, Thorofare, NJ

Hawking S 1996 Striving for excellence in the face of disabilities. In: Zemke R, Clark F (eds) Occupational science: the evolving discipline. F A Davis, Philadelphia: p 27–30

Higgs J, Titchen A 2001 Rethinking the practice–knowledge interface in an uncertain world: a model for practice development. British Journal of Occupational Therapy 64: 526–533

Hocking C 2007 The romance of occupational therapy. In: Creek J, Lawson-Porter A (eds) Contemporary issues in occupational therapy, reasoning and reflection. John Wiley, Chichester: p 23–40

Hocking C, Nicholson E 2007 Occupational for occupational therapists: how far will we go? In: Creek J, Lawson-Porter A (eds) Contemporary issues in occupational therapy, reasoning and reflection. John Wiley, Chichester: p 41–54

House of Commons Health Committee 2006 Changes to primary care trusts. Second report of session 2005–06. Stationery Office, London

Iwama M 2003 [Illusions of universality: the importance of cultural context in Japanese occupational therapy] (in Japanese). OT Janaru 37: 319–323

Iwama M 2005 Occupation as a cross-cultural construct. In: Whiteford G, Wright-St Clair V (eds) Occupation and practice in context. Elsevier Churchill Livingstone, Marrickville, New South Wales: p 242–253

Iwama M 2006 The Kawa Model, culturally relevant occupational therapy. Elsevier Churchill Livingstone, Edinburgh

Jackson J, Carlson M, Mandel D, Zemke R, Clark F 1998 Occupation in life-style redesign: the USC Well Elderly Study occupational therapy program. American Journal of Occupational Therapy 52: 326–336

Kelly M 2001 Disability and community: a sociological approach. In: Albrecht G, Seelman K, Bury M (eds) The handbook of disability studies. Sage, Thousand Oaks, CA: p 396–411

Kielhofner G 2005 Rethinking disability and what do to about it: disability studies and its implications for occupational therapy. American Journal of Occupational Therapy 59: 487–496

Kirkpatrick E M (ed) 1983 Chambers twentieth century dictionary. W & R Chambers, Edinburgh

Kirsh B, Trentham B, Cole S 2006 Diversity in occupational therapy: experiences of consumers who identify themselves as minority group members. Australian Occupational Therapy Journal 53: 302–313

Kondo T 2004 Cultural tensions in occupational therapy practice: considerations from a Japanese vantage point. American Journal of Occupational Therapy 58: 174–184

Kroeger J 2005 Social heteroglossia: the contentious practice or potential place of middle-class parents in home–school relations. Urban Review 37: 1–30

Kronenberg F, Simo Algado S, Pollard N 2005 Occupational therapy without borders: learning from the spirit of survivors. Churchill Livingstone, Edinburgh

Kuhn T 1996 The structure of scientific revolutions. University of Chicago Press, Chicago, IL

McColl A 1994 Holistic occupational therapy: historical meaning and contemporary implications. Canadian Journal of Occupational Therapy 61: 72–77

Maitra K, Erway F 2006 Perception of client-centered practice in occupational therapists and their clients. American Journal of Occupational Therapy 60: 298–310

Malik K 1996 The meaning of race: race, history and culture in western culture. Macmillan Press, London

Mandelstam M 2007 On the bandwagon? British Journal of Occupational Therapy 70: 227

Mason M 2001 Incurably human. Working Press, London

Meredith P, Merson K, Strong J 2007 Differences in adult attachment style, career choice and career satisfaction for occupational therapy and commerce students. British Journal of Occupational Therapy 70: 235–242

Merriam Webster Online Dictionary (2006) Available online at: http://www.m-w.com; accessed 13 October 2007

Molineux M 2004 Occupation in occupational therapy: a labour in vain? In: Molineux M (ed) Occupation for occupational therapists. Blackwell, Oxford: p 1–14

Murphy R 1990 The body silent. WW Norton, New York

Nietzsche F 1986 Human, all too human: a book for free spirits (trans RJ Hollingdale). Cambridge University Press, Cambridge

Odawara E 2005 Cultural competence in occupational therapy: beyond a cross-cultural view of practice. American Journal of Occupational Therapy 59: 325–334

Olshansky E, Sacco D, Braxter B, Dodge P et al 2005 Participatory action research to understand and reduce health disparities. Nursing Outlook 53: 121–126

Owen J 2002 Management stripped bare. Kogan Page, London

Owen M, Holmes C 1993 'Holism' in the discourse of nursing. Journal of Advanced Nursing 18: 1688–1695

Peck E, Norman I 1999 Working together in adult community mental health services: exploring inter-professional role relations. Journal of Mental Health 8: 231–242

Pollard N, Walsh S 2000 Occupational therapy, gender and mental health: an inclusive perspective? British Journal of Occupational Therapy 63: 425–431

Pollard N, Alsop A, Kronenberg F 2005 Reconceptualising occupational therapy. British Journal of Occupational Therapy 68: 524–526

Radomski M V 1995 There is more to life than putting on your pants. American Journal of Occupational Therapy 49: 487–490

Ricoeur P 1984 Time and narrative, vol. 1 (trans K McLaughlin, D Pellauer). University of Chicago Press, Chicago, IL

Rushin D 1983 The bridge poem. In: Moraga C, Anzaldúa G (eds) This bridge called my back: writings by radical women of color, 2nd edn. Kitchen Table, Women of Color Press, New York, p xxi. Available online at: http://www.neiu. edu/~lsfuller/Poems/bridge.htm: accessed 17 August 2007

Sakellariou D 2006 The disabler, the disablee and their context: a tripartite view of disability. British Journal of Occupational Therapy 69: 49

Sakellariou D, Simó Algado S 2006 Sexuality and disability: a case of occupational injustice. British Journal of Occupational Therapy 69: 69–76.

Schmid T 2005 Promoting health through creativity: an introduction. In: Schmid T (ed) Promoting health through creativity, for professionals in health, art and education. Whurr, London: p 1–26

Selner-O'Hagan M, Kindlon D, Buka S 1998 Assessing exposure to violence in urban youth. Journal of Child Psychology and Psychiatry 39: 215–224

Shinew K, Floyd M, Parry D 2004 Understanding the relationship between race and leisure activities and constraints: exploring an alternative framework. Leisure Sciences 26: 181–199

Sinclair K 2005 Foreword. In: Kronenberg F, Simó Algado S, Pollard N (eds) Occupational therapy without borders: learning from the spirit of survivors. Elsevier Churchill Livingstone, Oxford: p xiv

Sivanesan N 2003 The journey of a visually impaired student becoming an occupational therapist. British Journal of Occupational Therapy 66: 568–570

Smuts J 1926 Holism and evolution. Available online at: http://www.archive.org/details/ holismandevoluti032439mbp: accessed 13 October 2007

Snyder C, Clark F, Masunaka-Noriega M, Young B 1998 Los Angeles street kids: new occupations for life program. Journal of Occupational Science 5: 133–139

Steward B 1996 The theory/practice divide: bridging the gap in occupational therapy. British Journal of Occupational Therapy 59: 264–268

Stewart L P 2007 Pressure to lead: what can we learn from the theory? British Journal of Occupational Therapy 70: 228–234

Sussenberger B 1998 Socioeconomic factors and their influence on occupational performance. In: Neistadt M, Blesedell Crepeau E (eds) Willard & Spackman's occupational therapy, 9th edn. Lippincott Williams & Wilkins, Philadelphia, PA: p 67–79

Tamaru A, McColl M, Yamasaki S 2007 Understanding independence: perspectives of occupational therapists. Disability and Rehabilitation 29: 1021–1033

Tolan P, Gorman-Smith D, Henry D 2003 The developmental ecology of urban males' youth violence. Developmental Psychology 39: 274–291

Townsend E, Wilcock A 2004a Occupational justice and client centred practice: a dialogue. Canadian Journal of Occupational Therapy 71: 75–87

Townsend E, Wilcock A 2004b Occupational justice. In: Christiansen C, Townsend E (eds) Introduction to occupation: the art and science of living. Prentice Hall, Thorofare, NJ: p 243–273

Vartanian T, Gleason P 1999 Do neighborhood conditions affect high school dropout and college graduation rates? Journal of Socio-Economics 28: 21–41

Velde B P 2000 The experience of being an occupational therapist with a disability. American Journal of Occupational Therapy 52: 183–188

Watson R, Swartz L 2004 Transformation through occupation. Whurr, London

Whiteford G, Wilcock A 2000 Cultural relativism: occupation and independence reconsidered. Canadian Journal of Occupational Therapy 67: 324–336

Whiteford G, Wright-St Clair V 2005 Occupation & practice in context. Elsevier Churchill Livingstone, Marrickville, New South Wales

Wilcock A 1998a An occupational perspective of health. Slack, Thorofare, NJ

Wilcock A 1998b Reflections on doing, being and becoming. Canadian Journal of Occupational Therapy 65: 240–256

Wood W, Hooper B, Womack J 2005 Reflections on occupational justice as a subtext of occupation-centered education. In: Kronenberg F, Simó Algado S, Pollard N (eds) Occupational therapy without borders: learning from the spirit of survivors. Churchill Livingstone, Edinburgh: p 378–388

World Health Organization 2001 Basic documents, 43rd edn. World Health Organization, Geneva

Practice

SECTION 3

107

PRACTICE

The final section of this book begins with an important historical and global review of occupational therapy practice by Gelya Frank and Ruth Zemke. This chapter gives a thorough perspective of the social transformational purpose that many in the profession are endeavouring to reassert as the core of intervention. Frank returns with other colleagues at the end of the section to explore the application of some of these principles in a historical project with Native Americans of the Tule River Tribe.

In order to facilitate navigation through the range of examples of occupational therapy as a social and political practice that follow, the chapters have been grouped loosely into themes. The first chapters explore transformational practice in educational contexts. Beck and Barnes review the use of the pADL framework in the context of a student community project at a homelessness centre, while Boggis explores the use of the same framework and occupational justice concepts in developing student awareness of health disparities and making the connection between personal and public ethics. A student placement with an indigenous community in north-eastern Australia stimulated Paluch, Boltin and Howie's discussion of occupational justice and political factors affecting interventions with aboriginal groups.

The next group of chapters concerns work on projects with specific communities. They are examples of 'emergent narrative' (Mattingly 2000, p. 205), arising from the immediacy of the interaction between individuals, communities and environmental factors. While some of these have been sponsored by occupational therapists, others have involved occupational therapists as volunteers, and the emphasis of the chapter is on the value and meaning of community-based occupation as a contribution to community development. Georgian occupational therapists Kapanadze, Despotashvili and Skhirtladze describe an arts project with street children that exceeded the expectations of all involved, Coleman, Kirby and Kirby give an account of a befriending network established through an evangelical organization in Sheffield, UK. McNulty describes the genesis of a mental health users' arts group in Sleaford, UK. However, community developments, while good in themselves, are not enough unless they produce other sustainable effects for social change and occupational empowerment. Abel, Clarke and Parks relate the experience of an online community publishing project that addressed the topics of education, class, social participation and disability from US and UK perspectives. Although this chapter does not use the language of occupational therapy, it is included as an illustration of the kind of interdisciplinary community action and collaboration with disabled people that students – and perhaps student occupational therapists – can bring about. It is an example of the application of the ideas set out in Sections 1 and 2, parallels occupational literacy and derives in part from some of the same experiences of community publishing that contributed to these chapters. The main theoretical model for this practice was contained mostly in a 20-year-old anthology (Morley & Worpole 1982) and the shared experience of its members. In some ways it resembles the development of poor workers unions in the USA, and was similarly situated outside both pedagogy and culture norms, being rarely written down and objectively described (O'Rourke 2005, Tait 2005, Woodin 2005a,b,c, 2007) Tracking down evidence of this kind of activity is frequently difficult and the historical evidence is often ephemeral, yet, as the authors have argued (particularly in Ch. 2), the occupation of political action at community level is the key to larger-scale movements. Abel et al contribute a Gramscian analysis of this activity and conclude that one of the key factors in enabling social participation and bringing further transformational outcomes from this is the role of activist 'legislators' who ensure that expressions of intent are pursued, looking at how the experiences of people with disabilities highlighted through this exercise will inform changes to future educational practice.

The diverse social consequences of global migration drive the next group of chapters. Davies, Wilson, Mitchell, and Opacich, Lizer and Goetsch explore different occupational dimensions of minority cultures in Western societies. In a personal account Davies reveals the professional conundrums and individual challenges that UK occupational therapists find in meeting people in their communities who are denied asylum and become stateless, highly vulnerable people, experiencing occupational apartheid in a European democracy. Wilson gives a clear account of the establishment of Occupational Opportunities for Refugees and Asylum Seekers (OOFRAS), an Australian non-governmental organization, while Mitchell describes the issues of working with a refugee community across the mutual discovery of cultural boundaries in rural Australia. Opacich, Lizer and Goetsch give a detailed account of the establishment and provision of a community service for the backstretch community in the US horse racing industry, people moving according to the demands of their work and because of this and their minority background having little access to health resources. Again, this is significant precisely for the reason that such initiatives composed of community-based actions involving many people are often difficult to record. Once they have ceased to be current these experiences can quickly become lost to history (Tait 2005). While evidencing of community development in the long term may be a matter of analysing historical data, the immediate perception of what has been done, how it was done and the part that individuals and communities took is crucial to enabling others to imagine what they might do with their communities.

In the final chapters of the section we return to the experiences of indigenous people, this time amongst Native Americans. Heyman-Hotch and Frank and her colleagues offer two perspectives, one of occupational alienation and the other concerning an affirmative history project with the Tule River Tribe that helped tribal elders to meet long-standing tribal goals through a set of history-making occupations, while also having a positive effect on communication among families in the tribe and between generations. The section concludes with a reprised problematization of holism, context and the uncertainty of knowledge as elements in the political setting for occupational therapy.

References

Mattingly C 2000 Emergent narratives. In: Mattingly C, Garro L C (eds) Narrative and the cultural construction of illness and healing. University of California Press, Berkeley, CA: p 181–211

Morley D, Worpole K (eds) 1982 The republic of letters. Comedia, London

O'Rourke R 2005 Creative writing, education culture and community. NIACE, Leicester

Tait V 2005 Poor workers' unions: rebuilding labor from below. South End Press, Cambridge, MA

Woodin T 2005a Building culture from the bottom up: the educational origins of the Federation of Worker Writers and Community Publishers. History of Education 34: 345–363

Woodin T 2005b 'More writing than welding': learning in worker writer groups. History of Education 34: 561–578

Woodin T 2005c Muddying the waters: changes in class and identity in a working class cultural organization. Sociology 39: 1001–1018

Woodin T 2007 'Chuck out the teacher': radical pedagogy in the community. International Journal of Lifelong Education 26: 89–104

Occupational therapy foundations for political engagement and social transformation

Gelya Frank, Ruth Zemke

Introduction

An international movement in occupational therapy has been forming that embraces political engagements and social transformation. This paper attempts to frame some historical, theoretical and interdisciplinary foundations to support its growth. Some signs of the movement include the surge of attention to community-based rehabilitation at the World Federation of Occupational Therapists meeting in Cape Town, in 2004, resulting in affirmation of occupational injustice and occupational apartheid as valid problems for occupational therapy practice (World Federation of Occupational Therapists 2004). The European Network of Occupational Therapy in Higher Education has been working inclusively to build the occupational therapy profession from the ground up in the Republic of Georgia and other former Soviet republics in the Balkan and Caucasian regions (see www.enothe.hva.nl). At least two landmark collections of essays have already appeared in English (Watson & Swartz 2004, Kronenberg et al 2005).

Definition of key occupational therapy concepts related to politics and social change

Occupation 'In occupational therapy, occupations refer to the everyday activities that people do as individuals, in families and with communities to occupy time and bring meaning and purpose to life. Occupations include things people need to, want to and are expected to do.' (Approved by World Federation of Occupational Therapists Executive, July 2007)

   Occupational therapy 'is based on the belief that the need to engage in occupation is innate and is related to survival, health, well-being, and life satisfaction. Occupational therapy, therefore, is a profession whose focus is on enabling a person (i.e. individual client) or a group of persons (i.e. group, community or an organization client) to access and participate in activities that are meaningful, purposeful, and relevant to their lives, roles and sense of well-being' (American Occupational Therapy Association Statement on Practice 2000, p. 3).

Continued

Occupational injustices 'exist when participation is barred, confined, segregated, prohibited, undeveloped, disrupted, alienated, marginalized, exploited or otherwise devalued' (Townsend & Whiteford 2005, p. 112).

Occupational apartheid refers to 'the segregation of groups of people through the restriction or denial of access to dignified and meaningful participation in occupations of daily life on the basis of race, color, disability, national origin, age, gender, sexual preference, religion, political beliefs, status in society, or other characteristics. Occasioned by political forces, its systematic and pervasive social, cultural and economic consequences jeopardize health and wellbeing as experienced by individuals, communities and societies' (Kronenberg & Pollard 2005a, p. 67).

These events constitute a 'movement' because the ideas and activities have arisen independently and heterogeneously, operating through social networks, rather than from any single, centralized source (McAdam et al 1996, Diani & McAdam 2003). The small-scale demonstration and outreach projects associated with this movement mainly flourish as alternatives to formal institutions, cropping up outside national health systems and private health insurance reimbursement. Occupational therapists initiate such projects or ally with them in local communities, and the projects often rely on donations of funds and of professional expertise, or on micro-credits and volunteered labour (Yunis & Jolis 2003). Non-governmental organizations, corporate philanthropy or university-based research initiatives provide sponsorship. Some non-governmental organizations are humanitarian and secular; others have a religious mission. These projects engage individuals and communities in occupations to expand their capacity and quality of participation in larger social, economic and political structures.

Without doubt, the movement emerging in occupational therapy intersects with other global movements at this time (Keck & Sikkink 1998; Tarrow 2005). This is readily indicated by the phrase 'without borders' used by the Occupational Therapy Without Borders project, which evokes the 1999 Nobel Peace Prize-winning organization, Doctors Without Borders (Médecins Sans Frontières 1997). Occupational therapy is one of several professions to develop a 'without borders' outreach. The terms used to identify the demonstration projects in the occupational therapy movement, however, reflect the profession's uneasy alliance with biomedicine and its institutions. South African occupational therapist Ruth Watson (2004) suggests the phrase 'community and population development' for opportunities to engage in meaningful occupations among 'immigrant and migrant populations, homeless people, refugees, people in war-torn regions, and historically disadvantaged individuals, groups and communities who live in poverty' (p. 6). Brazilian occupational therapist Sandra Maria Galheigo (2005) and colleagues (Barros et al 2005) use the rubric 'social occupational therapy' for their approach to problems that fall outside the social welfare system. These occupational therapists reach beyond biomedicine and treating pathology to address disparities in occupational choices, which in turn are associated with disparities in health and well-being.

Addressing this set of concerns – the unevenness of global wealth, differentials in the protection of human rights and obstacles to the exercise of personal agency and political power – represents an upheaval in thinking and action within the occupational therapy profession. The overall thrust is radical but not unprecedented. We believe that interdisciplinary foundations and collaborations will help to strengthen the capacity of occupational therapy to influence social change. This was certainly the case during the progressive era in the USA, when the founding of occupational therapy was itself a social reform. It is too early to tell whether or not the profession per se will move in the direction of political engagements and social transformation. Perhaps these areas will remain outside mainstream practice. We take the position that the ideas motivating the movement are important enough to be introduced to all occupational therapy students so they may make informed choices about becoming agents of change.

In this chapter, we employ concepts, theories and methods from several disciplines to consider how current issues in occupational therapy internationally relate to larger trends on the world stage. We examine the early political roots of the occupational therapy profession in the USA to raise questions for further discussion: What kinds of knowledge are relevant and useful for occupational therapy approaches to social transformation? What competencies will occupational therapists need to practise in social and political arenas? Should the profession try to specialize education and treatment in these areas of practice? How can knowledge from other disciplines help inform the directions to take? Finally, we offer a practice model for occupational therapy's engagement in social and political goals.

Occupational therapy in the world system

World system and dependency theories help to explain the distribution of occupational therapy around the world today and something about its content (Frank 1967, Wallerstein 1974, 1980, 1989, 2004). According to statistics compiled by the World Federation of Occupational Therapists, most occupational therapists are located in the USA and Europe (Townsend & Whiteford 2005; Table 7.1). The USA heads the list in number of members reported by national associations. Japan ranks second, which may reflect the impact of the USA on academic and medical institutions there after the Second World War. The Japanese Ministry of Health and Welfare established the first occupational therapy school in 1963 with a teaching staff mostly of occupational therapists from the USA (Japanese Association of Occupational Therapists website, www.jaot.or.jp/e-history.html).

American and British (i.e. Anglophone) influence on occupational therapy worldwide is especially striking after grouping membership in national associations by linguistic/cultural and regional spheres (Table 7.2). While various cultures and civilizations employed

Table 7.1 • Occupational therapy national associations ranked by size, c. 2004

Rank	Country	Members
1	USA	35692
2	Japan	20226
3	UK	14482
4	Germany	c. 11000
5	Sweden	9302
6	Canada	7500
7	Denmark	6198
8	Australia	3500
9	Netherlands	3312
10	Norway	2734

Data adapted from Townsend & Whiteford (2005), based on sources compiled by the World Federation of Occupational Therapists (WFOT). WFOT data are compiled from the reports of membership among national occupational therapy associations. Because accreditation and membership requirements vary from country to country, WFOT's numbers do not necessary reflect parallel data and may under-report numbers of practising occupational therapists in a specific country. For example, the American Occupational Therapy Association is made up of about 37000 members but, according to the AOTA website, the actual workforce includes more than 100000 practitioners, including occupational therapists and occupational therapy assistants.

Table 7.2 Selected linguistic-cultural, regional and national traditions at the start of the 21st century

Linguistic or regional sphere	Influence	National tradition	Current membership
Anglophone	American	**USA**	**57 413**
		USA	35 692
		Japan	20 226
		Republic of China (Taiwan)	744
		Republic of Korea	505
		Philippines	246
	British	**UK**	**29 659**
		UK	14 482
		Canada	7500
		Australia	3500
		India	1912
		South Africa	1287
		Hong Kong	c. 800
		Singapore	158
		Bermuda	20
Scandinavia			**19 794**
		Sweden	9302
		Denmark	6198
		Norway	2734
		Finland	1426
		Iceland	134
Western Europe			**16 925**
		Germany	c. 11 000
		Netherlands	3312
		France	978
		Belgium	735
		Spain	540
		Portugal	250
		Italy	110
Latin America	Spanish		**921**
		Venezuela	500
		Chile	250
		Argentina	171
	Portuguese		**890**
		Brazil	890

Data from Townsend & Whiteford (2005), based on World Federation of Occupational Therapists sources. Data are lacking for most of Latin America and numbers for Chile and Argentina seem under-reported. Assignment of countries to a particular linguistic or regional sphere is for this chapter and is not intended to preclude regrouping the data for further analyses.

occupational approaches to health from ancient times, the professionalization of occupational therapy is recent and closely tied to the emergence of the UK and the USA as industrial powers in the 19th and early 20th centuries (Wilcock 2001, 2002). Allied victories in the First and Second World Wars lent these powers even greater economic strength and strategic global influence. These facts help to explain the impact of American and British occupational therapy on the profession, given that most national associations, including those in Europe, were established after the Second World War (World Federation of Occupational Therapists website, www.wfot.org). As Kronenberg and Pollard noted in an address to the American Occupational Therapy Association (AOTA): 'Globally, the AOTA represents the single largest national community of occupational therapy practitioners, and the volume of literature, research, and tools it generates significantly influences the thinking, the practice, education and research of occupational therapy practitioners all over the world' (Kronenberg & Pollard 2006, p. 617).

World system theory holds that, although national, traditions of professions and academic disciplines may vary according to local circumstances, their distribution and development are not random. Academic disciplines are formed and undergo transformation within systems of power. This phenomenon has been explored recently in the discipline of anthropology and the subdiscipline of medical anthropology (Krotz 1997, Cardoso de Oliveira 2000, Kuwayama 2004, Ribeiro & Escobar 2006; also see Baer et al 2004, Saillant & Genest 2006). Contributors to this conversation focus on framing anthropological scholarship and theories to reflect and respond to local realities around the globe. The same kind of effort is taking place among Japanese occupational therapy scholars, who are reworking theories about human occupation, originally framed and published in English, to make sense in Japanese culture (Kondo 2004, Iwama 2005, Odawara 2005; see also Zemke 2004). In Singapore, where occupational therapy was established in the 1930s under colonial British aegis, similar concerns are also emerging (Yang et al 2006). These examples signal a need for comparative and critical histories of the occupational therapy profession in various countries, regions and linguistic–cultural spheres.

Chapters by Brazilian occupational therapists Galheigo (2005) and Barros, Ghirardi and Lopes (2005) in the book *Occupational Therapy Without Borders* can help to illustrate issues concerning the production and circulation of professional knowledge in the world system. Galheigo and her colleagues cite Portuguese translations of European and North American thinkers including sociologist Erving Goffman (USA), philosophers Jean-Paul Sartre and Michel Foucault (France), and neo-Marxist theorist Antonio Gramsci (Italy). They are able to balance this roster of 'imports' with references to Brazilian educator Paulo Freire (1970), a major contributor to world discourse with his Marxist-inflected 'pedagogy of the oppressed'. The authors also rely on a critical Brazilian literature published in Portuguese in sociology, social medicine, the history of psychiatry and occupational therapy focused on the issue of deinstitutionalization. The deinstitutionalization approach, however, originated in the North with Norwegian scholar Bengt Nirje's theory of 'normalization' and subsequent publications by German-born American scholar Wolf Wolfensberger (1975, 1996).

While Galheigo and her colleagues' work reflects the resilience of Brazilian intellectual resources, particularly the radical tradition associated with Paulo Freire, the occupational therapy literature published in Portuguese remains mostly inaccessible to scholars elsewhere in the world. Libraries in the USA, for example, do not tend to subscribe to Brazilian or Portuguese journals, nor is the work generally translated. Local debates are muted on the world stage, such as the following: should Brazilian occupational therapists prioritize science-driven clinical issues to meet standards in the North, and use their resources to develop evidence-based practice? Or should they prioritize politically driven conditions in cities such as São Paulo, Brasilia and Rio de Janeiro, or indigenous and rural areas such as Amazonias or Mato Grosso (Nick Pollard, personal communication, 2007)?

The situation is equally or more acute with regard to the Spanish-speaking countries of Latin America. Limited access in the North to Spanish-language literature impoverishes world discourse among occupational therapists because Spanish is the predominant national language in Central and South America. The data reported by the World Federation of Occupational Therapists on the number of occupational therapists in Latin America are sketchy (Table 7.2). Yet Latin America presents some of the most important occupational challenges in the world related to development policies because the gap in income between rich and poor is among the highest in the world (World Bank website, www.worldbank.org). According to the World Bank, Latin America is the most highly urbanized developing area: about 77% of the population lives in cities. The rate of urban growth means that the cost of meeting basic needs is also rapidly increasing, along with demands on environmental and natural resources (World Bank website). From 1990 to 2005, Latin America had the highest percentage of private investment in infrastructure among developing regions in the world. As we will discuss later, under current neoliberal policies of international development, private investment carries particular risks to a population concerning the distribution of wealth and the provision of public services. Income inequality in the region worsened in this period, as reported by the World Bank in 2003, with the richest one-tenth of the population earning 48% of the total income, while the poorest tenth earned only 1.6%.

Given such data, it is not difficult to see how the hegemony of the USA and Europe in the world system is not simply a matter of prestige. The production and circulation of knowledge has both an ideological and a material base. On the ideological side, peer review based on established Eurocentric standards results in the reproduction of such knowledge in published research and promotion of faculty in academic institutions around the world. On the material side, disciplines flourish when there is economic support for education and the proliferation of academic institutions such as universities, professional schools, libraries and laboratories. There must be salaries for faculty, resources to support research, graduate programmes, equipment and opportunities to publish. But in developing countries resources such as these are often hard to come by. Consequently, there is a tendency to rely on importing knowledge and expertise from the North and to use academic knowledge to support wealth-producing rather than poverty-eliminating initiatives.

Optimistically, globalization may offer new opportunities for exchange to occur internationally (Ribeiro & Escobar 2006). Computers and Internet access may allow diverse national and local sectors to define their own interests, needs and contributions (see, for example, the Open Access Initiative of the Open Society Institute at the Soros Foundation: www.soros. org). Realistically, however, most scholars and professionals will need to keep up with western European and American discourses to remain viable players in the global circulation of knowledge. This factor has become more pronounced since the end of the Cold War (the Berlin Wall was torn down in 1989; the Soviet Union was dissolved in 1991). The Cold War was characterized by a polarizing counterplay of Soviet Russian ideological and scholarly influences in the world against those of the 'West'. This dynamic has been only partly replaced by focus on a new dynamic of conflicts between 'Western democracies' and militant Islamic nationalist movements that challenge the secularization of values associated with capitalist expansion.

What defines the 'world system'? How did it come about, and can it be changed? Introduced by sociologist Immanuel Wallerstein (1974, 1980, 1989, 2004), world system theory holds that the economies of the so-called First, Second and Third Worlds are part of a single world system that can be said to have emerged in or by the 17th century. This process, sometimes called 'modernization', proceeded from Europe's colonial expansion into the Americas, Asia and Africa (see Ch. 4). The result of modernization was a division of labour and markets structured with a 'core' of wealth and power existing in relation to a less wealthy and powerful 'periphery'. The core is mainly identified with the northern hemisphere (the North) and the periphery with the southern hemisphere (the South). Kronenberg and Pollard (2006) consequently call for occupational therapists to recognize that only a small percentage of the world's population, about 6%, owns 60% of the world's wealth, and those people tend to live in the North.

In terms of intellectual sources, Wallerstein draws on the historical materialism of Karl Marx, the broad cultural approach of French historian Fernand Braudel and Wallerstein's own research on postcolonialism and development in Africa. One of the most important areas of contemporary anthropological theory and research has been to explore and challenge the assumption that 'modernization' imposes secular values and cultural uniformity throughout the world – the so-called 'Americanization' or 'McDonaldization' of world cultures (Zemke 2003). The consensus among anthropologists, however, is that cultural diversity takes new forms rather than disappearing (see, for example, the essays in Ong & Collier 2005). Consequently, it is important to pay attention to local and emergent conditions, making use of anthropological and other scholarship that can serve occupational therapy internationally (Frank & Zemke 2006, Frank et al 2008, Frank et al forthcoming).

A corollary to world system theory, 'dependency theory', holds that developed nations actively, if not always consciously, promote the dependence of poorer nations through various policies and initiatives. These nations (the North) exert control through economics, media, politics, banking and finance policies, education and all aspects of human resource development. This theory was worked out with special reference to Chile and Brazil in the 1960s by Andre Gunder Frank (1967), who served as Professor of Sociology and Economics at the University of Chile, where he was involved in reforms under the government of Salvador Allende. Frank noted that attempts by the dependent nations to resist the influences of dependency often result in economic sanctions and military invasion and control. He later experienced this himself in Chile when Allende's government was toppled by a coup d'état in 1973 with support from the USA. The pattern was replayed the following decade in Nicaragua and El Salvador.

Through globalization policies such as the North American Free Trade Agreement (NAFTA), the periphery sells its products and labour at low prices on the world market but buys the core's products at comparatively high prices. These practices create relatively stable structures of inequality internationally. 'Semiperiphery' buffer zones such as China and India serve simultaneously as core to the periphery and as periphery to the core. Some observers suggest that the valence of world power is shifting again to Asia, after centuries of Eurocentrism (Frank 1998). World system theory holds that the expansion of capitalism eventually commodifies all things, everywhere, including human labour, natural resources, land and human relationships. The effect on human occupation in the sense of how people live their everyday lives is pervasive. Not infrequently, wars are fought as a direct or indirect consequence of the structuring of global markets and development. Control of oil in the Persian Gulf was a key factor in the First Gulf War in 1991 and, many claim, important in the current American-led war in Iraq, begun in 2003.

The academic sector offers a place where an analysis of occupational therapy in the world system can flourish within interdisciplinary exchanges. Such conversations can provide conceptual tools for practice in specific local contexts. Conversely, occupational therapists engaged in practice oriented toward social change can contribute important new knowledge. We quote Kurt Lewin, a social psychologist and refugee to the USA from Nazi Germany, who was interested in participant action research and its relationship to building democratic institutions. Kurt Lewin argued that 'the best way to understand something is to try to change it' (Greenwood & Levin 1998, p. 19).

In summary, the role of the USA and the UK in world politics and world trade seems to account for the proliferation of occupational therapy as a profession and much about its content. The dominance of the medical rehabilitation model internationally is linked to this set of influences (Gritzer & Arluke 1989). In other words, the development of occupational therapy on the world stage has been closely tied to the circulation of Western biomedicine after the Second World War. The broad scope of the Anglophone sphere helps to account also for the rapid spread of occupational science, an academic discipline founded at the University of Southern California in 1989. The acceptance of occupational science can be seen not only in the founding of the *Journal of Occupational Science*, published in Australia, and in associations in the English-speaking world such as the Society for the Study of Occupation: USA (www.sso-usa.org) and the Australasian Society of Occupational Scientists (asos.nfshost.com) but also in associations of occupational scientists in Japan and Taiwan (Zemke 2003).

We offer below a political history that helps to contextualize the limited social analysis and the absence of political analysis in the early occupational science literature (Yerxa et al 1990, Clark et al 1991). We suggest that American occupational therapy turned away from the political and reformist tendencies of its founding years. Few analyses of gender, class and race, for example, have appeared in the professional literature of this predominantly female profession, quite in contrast with nursing, teaching and social work (Frank 1992). It does not surprise us that critical discourses calling for political engagement by occupational therapists have originated outside the USA – in Canada, Australia, New Zealand, the UK, the Netherlands, Spain, Brazil, South Africa and elsewhere.

> ## Professional development requires audacious values and critical assessment of local conditions
>
> As contributors to the founding of occupational science, we feel that occupational science is worthy on its own merits. Chief among these merits is the establishment of a distinctive knowledge base about the core concept of 'occupation'. Not only does such a knowledge base provide new directions for treatment but, in the most basic logistical manner, it was essential for the legitimation and survival of occupational therapy in the academy (Abbott 1988). We note that occupational science continues to evolve (Zemke & Clark 1996) and that criticism, including self-criticism, is productive for the discipline. Although the University of Southern California chose to grant degrees in occupational science, not many others have followed. However, we observe that occupational scientists' 'naming and framing' a discipline has affected the research as well as practice direction in the field of occupational therapy.

Precedents for political engagement and social reform: Hull House activism and occupational therapy's road not taken

Occupational therapy's origins in the USA during the progressive era (1890–1920) were political, at least among those founders associated with Chicago's Hull House (Table 7.3). Key figures such as Julia Lathrop, Adolf Meyer and Eleanor Clarke Slagle were engaged initially in efforts to reform treatment of the mentally ill. They believed that the deplorable conditions of the urban poor were causing an increase in otherwise preventable mental illnesses. They worked on improving clinical settings, the treatment of patients with mental illness and the social conditions from which the patients came and to which they returned. Building on previous histories of the profession, it is possible to reconstruct how Pragmatist philosophy, the Arts and Crafts Movement, the Mental Hygiene Movement and the Settlement Movement were more closely intertwined with socialism and democratic political reform than has perhaps been realized (Breines 1986, Levine 1986, 1987). In this light, the Arts and Crafts Movement, for example, was not simply an aesthetic revival or a hobbyist fad for personal renewal but an array of strategies to realign lopsided relationships among owners, workers and consumers (Lears 1981, Boris 1986; also see Levine 1987).

Table 7.3 American occupational therapy's emergence in Chicago in relation to pragmatism, politics and social reform

Date	Event
1889	**Jane Addams** and **Ellen Gates Starr** found Hull House Settlement in Chicago on Christian Socialist principles after visiting London's Toynbee Hall
1891–3	Socialist Labor Party member **Florence Kelley** moves to Hull House in 1891 and makes it a centre of labour reform; her research with other Hull House women into the sweat shops in Chicago's garment industry leads to the Illinois Factory Act 1893. **Kelley** then appointed Chief Factory Inspector for Illinois by reform Governor John Peter Altgeld

Date	Event
1893–5	Social reformer **Julia Lathrop** begins investigation of Illinois State mental hospitals and other institutions; mentors and works with psychiatrist **Adolf Meyer** at Illinois State Hospital in Kankakee to achieve asylum reforms including state examinations for interns and appointment of women physicians
1894	**John Dewey** appointed chair of departments of Philosophy, Psychology and Pedagogy, University of Chicago; his political thinking expands, while travelling there, by newspaper accounts of workers' cooperation during the Pullman Strike in Chicago. He founds the Dewey Laboratory School at the university the following year and, 2 years later, becomes a trustee of Hull House
1902	Hull House resident **Florence Kelley** helps gain passage of the federal Pure Food and Drug Act 1902
1903	**Jane Addams**, **Florence Kelley** and others at Hull House establish the Women's Trade Union League. Union meetings often held at Hull House and members of the settlement helped support workers during industrial disputes. As a result, some wealthy people withdraw their support from Hull House
1905	**John Dewey** leaves Chicago for Columbia University in New York City
1908	**Eleanor Clarke Slagle** takes the first course organized by **Julia Lathrop** and **Rabbi Emil Hirsch** at the Chicago School of Civics and Philanthropy to train craft teachers to work with mental patients
1910	**Adolf Meyer** moves from Chicago to Baltimore to direct the new Phipps Psychiatric Clinic at Johns Hopkins Medical School
1913	**Eleanor Clarke Slagle** moves to Baltimore for 2 years to become Director of Occupations under psychiatrist **Adolf Meyer** at the Phipps Clinic
1915	**Slagle** organizes and directs Henry B. Favill Memorial School of Occupations in Chicago, teaching courses in Curative Occupations and Recreation that continue **Lathrop** and **Hirsch's** work; **Jane Addams** attends first Congress of Women's International League for Peace and Freedom in the Hague in an effort to deter US involvement in the First World War
March 1917	**Eleanor Clarke Slagle** and colleagues found National Society for the Promotion of Occupational Therapy in Clifton Springs, NY
August 1917	US Surgeon General recruits occupational therapists (reconstruction aides) to serve in the First World War
1919	American women gain the right to vote by constitutional amendment
1920	Vocational Rehabilitation Act resolves a conflict between the US Veterans Administration (under the US Surgeon General) and civilian vocational counsellors. The VA's role is restricted to medical rehabilitation ('prevocational phase'). Consequently, occupational therapy's scope of practice becomes defined as medical not vocational
1923	Henry B. Favill School closes when war-related need for occupational therapists ends. **Eleanor Clarke Slagle** becomes Director of Occupational Therapy for the New York State Mental Hygiene Commission until her death in 1942

We can read occupational therapy's emergence in Chicago as a case study that exemplifies how movements for social change work through networks, collaborations and political action. After the profession was officially founded in 1917, however, occupational therapy took a different road, leaving its activist roots behind. Occupational therapy allied itself with the US military and the American Medical Association (AMA), two of the most powerful but also conservative institutional sectors in the country (Starr 1982). Early contributors to the professional literature were mainly physicians, who sought to explain scientifically the effects of occupation on the individual organism (Gordon 2002).

Jane Addams and Ellen Gates Starr founded the Hull House Settlement in 1889, on the Christian Socialist model of Toynbee Hall in East London, which they had visited (Addams 2002a). The idea of an urban 'settlement' referred to the work of educated, service-minded young people who lived together along cooperative principles to serve the disenfranchised surrounding poor immigrant or minority community (Addams 2002a). Laissez-faire capitalism in the USA was then at its height (Zinn 2003). Rapid industrialization had resulted in an unprecedented acquisition of wealth and power by a small sector of the population – sometimes referred to as the 'robber barons'. Immigration policies resulted in a massive influx of mostly unskilled labour from the margins of Europe. Internal migration brought African Americans from the rural south to the northern cities, while the US Supreme Court decision in the case of Plessy v Ferguson (1896) upheld 'separate but equal' legislation. A 'closed-door' policy at the national level kept out new Asian immigrants while racial discrimination targeted those already in the country. The parallels with issues today at the start of the 21st century are difficult to overlook.

Political engagement means seeking alliances and making choices

Sharp political contradictions resulted in difficult choices for the Hull House activists. As Zinn (2003) notes, President Theodore Roosevelt's wing of the Republican Party, known as the Progressives, initiated American aggression and imperialism in the Spanish American War (1898), resulting in acquisition of the Philippines, Puerto Rico, Guam and, for a period, Cuba. Yet, the same Progressive Republicans were the standard-bearer of many of the reforms sought by the Hull House activists, including the Pure Food and Drug Act of 30 June 1906, which provided for inspection of meat products and forbade the manufacture, sale or transportation of adulterated food products or poisonous patent medicines. The USA made a further, decisive shift to intervene in international affairs with its entry and later victory in the First World War (1914–1918). Of the Hull House activists, Jane Addams voted for the Progressive Party in some elections and the Socialist Party in others. Ellen Gates Starr and Florence Kelley were socialists. Florence Kelley (1859–1932) joined Hull House in 1891 and remained until 1899, when she moved to Lillian Wald's Henry Street Settlement on New York's Lower East Side, a hub of reform on a par with Hull House. According to US Supreme Court Justice Felix Frankfurter, Kelley 'had probably the largest single share in shaping the social history of the USA during the first 30 years of this century…playing a powerful if not decisive role in securing legislation for the removal of the most glaring abuses of our hectic industrialization following the Civil War' (quoted in Sklar 1985, p. 658).

Addams and Starr initially focused on aesthetic ideals fostered by the critic John Ruskin's essays decrying the abuses associated with industrialism. His book, *The Stones of Venice* (Ruskin 2007), first published in 1850–1853, was the bible of the Arts and Crafts Movement. Very soon, Addams and Starr realized that more focused political engagement was needed. Active issues on the Hull House agenda included passage of laws and policies to provide a minimum wage, 40-hour working week, overtime pay, safe working conditions, workers' compensation and childcare (Addams 1930, 1990, 2002b,c). The Hull House residents, who were mostly educated women and who lived cooperatively, worked to organize unions; participate in strikes; improve public sanitation; establish well-baby clinics, public baths and gymnasiums; gain political rights for immigrants; and secure voting rights for women. Addams' participation in antimilitarist protest during the First World War resulted in the formation of the Women's International League for Peace and Freedom and the American Civil Liberties Union.

Other burning issues addressed by Hull House activists included securing legislation to protect the public from toxins in the environment, guarantee the quality of food and drugs, establish special courts for juvenile offenders, and reform prisons and state mental institutions.

In the Hull House context, occupational therapy emerged from Julia Lathrop's efforts to reform the Illinois state mental institutions (Addams 2004). State mental hospitals existed at this time, but not public or private health insurance. Consequently, there was no reimbursement for treatment of individual patients or clients outside commitment to such institutions. Although these were public, tax-supported institutions, they were mainly places of last resort where poor people with criminal histories, alcoholism, chronic mental illness, antisocial behaviour, depression or reactive psychoses were thrown together indiscriminately (Meyer 1948a). Hull House's innovative programmes were initially supported by private wealth funnelled through personal and corporate philanthropy. The Hull House reformers worked to pass laws to regulate industrial and urban conditions, targeting the sites where injuries and illnesses occurred in order to prevent them.

Lathrop's years at Hull House, from 1890 to 1909, focused on visiting social welfare institutions throughout Illinois and promoting reforms in public institutions for the insane, indigent, delinquent and children. Beginning in 1893, Lathrop, 35 years old, served as the first woman member of the Illinois State Board of Charities, a position she used eventually to introduce reforms such as the appointment of female physicians to state hospitals and removal of the insane from state workhouses. That same year, 1893, Lathrop met Adolf Meyer, the 26-year-old Swiss doctor of neurology and psychiatry who had just received an appointment as pathologist at the Illinois Eastern Hospital for the Insane at Kankakee. Lathrop introduced Meyer to Hull House and its approach to social issues.

As a former student of Adolf Meyer later noted, 'Miss Lathrop came as a visitor for the State Board of Charities and Correction, open-minded, deeply concerned in her work and interested in Meyer as a European who could answer her questions about social service abroad, particularly child welfare (20 years later she became the first head of the Federal Children's Bureau). She introduced him to Jane Addams, another vibrant woman who was doing a share of the world's work, and to Governor Altgeld. When Meyer slipped and injured himself on a visit to the fair, Miss Lathrop had him put up for a week at Hull House, which was an excellent point of orientation in sociology' (Lief 1948, p. 49).

Lathrop and Meyer forged an enduring alliance (Lief 1948). In 1894, Meyer responded to a public address by the well known psychiatrist, S. Weir Mitchell, who charged that doctors in mental hospitals were unscientific in their methods and had failed to contribute useful information about the insane. Meyer wrote an angry rebuttal to the new, reform-oriented Governor John Peter Altgeld to suggest that the Governor invite the hospital workers to write reports. He enlisted the help of Julia Lathrop, who induced the Governor to give the Illinois hospital physicians a chance to express their own views and visions. As a result, the Illinois State Board published a compilation of the reports, which allowed Meyer to disseminate his studies at Kankakee, in which he combined pathology and case histories, and to propose innovative methods for interviewing patients.

Lathrop used the published reports to persuade the Illinois State Board in 1895 to hold competitive examinations for medical internships in state mental hospitals, the first policy of its kind in the USA – and Meyer was appointed as an examiner (Lief 1948). Later that year, Meyer accepted a position at the State Lunatic Hospital at Worcester, Massachusetts, where he remained for the next 7 years. Much of his work focused on reorganizing how records were kept on patients, which improved classification and statistical analysis and allowed him to demonstrate that most mental illnesses were capable of amelioration. In 1902, Meyer moved to Manhattan to take a position coordinating pathological work at all 13 of New York State's mental hospitals, introducing new methods of assessing and categorizing symptoms and acquiring the reputation of 'having transformed the state's insane asylums into mental hospitals' (Lief 1948, p. 101).

While in New York, in 1907–1909, Meyer collaborated with Clifford W. Beers to establish the National Committee for Mental Hygiene, with Julia Lathrop among the small group of about a dozen founders (Meyer 1948c). Their agenda was to launch a public campaign for asylum reform following publication of *A Mind that Found Itself*, Beers' (1908) account of the horrific treatment he had received in mental institutions while treated for manic depression. Meyer's political thinking from this period comes through in a talk he gave in Baltimore in 1909, titled 'The Problem of the State in the Care of the Insane'. Meyer used statistics to demonstrate variations in the incidence and prevalence of mental illness by class, region and cultural environment. He argued that mental illness was rising and that it was related to stressful urban conditions that undermined the well-being of vulnerable populations. He wrote in support of greater public investment to improve mental health in and outside of the asylums and in favour of early treatment to prevent chronic mental problems:

> Not only must the state or the public provide for the best possible medical treatment and for the physical welfare and comfort of its large number of patients, but it must strive to make its institutions centers of progress, which must be concerned not only with meeting the emergencies of the day, but with the more far-reaching problems of prophylaxis and of stemming the tide of increase. The institutions for the insane must indeed become the nucleus of a far-reaching work for social and individual mental hygiene and mental readjustment.
>
> Meyer 1948a, p. 320

Meyer's commitment to public services made his decision difficult when in 1908 he was offered the position of director of the new psychiatric clinic at Johns Hopkins University, a private institution. 'For the past 15 years,' his former student and biographer Alfred Lief (1948) wrote,

> Meyer had been in state service. He preferred a state hospital system to private hospitals. Here was an offer from 'one of the foremost medical centers established and supported by private enterprise'. How would he harmonize his orientation toward serving the community with the fact of functioning in an organization munificently endowed to pursue specialties and not having to wait for public appropriations?
>
> Lief 1948, p. 336

Meanwhile, Julia Lathrop continued to work on institutional reforms and helped to establish the first court in the USA for juvenile offenders, in 1899, to distinguish their treatment under the law from that of adults charged with similar crimes. In addition to her other activities, she worked with Jane Addams, John Dewey and others to organize the Chicago School of Civics and Philanthropy in 1908, where they offered a 2-year programme in social work. The establishment of the Chicago School of Civics and Philanthropy represented the latest stage of development of social work education in Chicago, beginning with lectures by Addams, Dewey and others at the Chicago Commons, founded in 1894. In 1895, the Chicago Commons became home to the newly established School of Social Economics, with minister and social work educator Graham Taylor as president. It offered the earliest social work courses in the USA. The programme grew into the nation's first year-long social work education programme, the Social Science Center for Practical Training in Philanthropic and Social Work, established in 1903.

Five years later, in 1908, the institution's name changed again and became the Chicago School of Civics and Philanthropy. Under the continued leadership of Reverend Graham Taylor, the School offered for the first time a 2-year programme. This was the programme, built with contributions from Lathrop, Adams and Dewey, in which future leader of occupational therapy Eleanor Clarke Slagle enrolled. She was a woman then widowed, or possibly divorced, about 40 years old, from a politically connected Republican family in Upper New York State. Slagle's mentor Julia Lathrop served as vice president of the Chicago School. Among its trustees were Jane Addams and philanthropist Julius Rosenwald, heir to the Sears-Roebuck fortune. In 1920, the School merged to become a graduate school at the University of Chicago, the School of Social Service Administration (School of Social Service Administration, University of Chicago website, www.ssa.uchicago.edu/aboutssa/history/tour1c.shtml).

Julia Lathrop, influenced by Clifford Beers' (1908) account of his self-recovery as a mental patient and having helped to found the National Committee for Mental Hygiene, collaborated with Rabbi Emil Hirsch to introduce a training course in occupations for hospital attendants at the Chicago School of Civics and Philanthropy. Eleanor Clarke Slagle was enrolled in this course, called 'Invalid Occupations'. In 1910, after Adolf Meyer decided to move to Johns

Hopkins University, he asked Julia Lathrop to recommend a social worker who was trained in the use of occupations with mental patients to help him set up the clinic. Meyer later recalled: 'When we opened the Phipps Clinic for action, Miss Lathrop was able to lend us Mrs Slagle as the model...in the service of therapy' (Meyer 1922, quoted in Breines 1986, p. 106).

Histories of occupational therapy: True? Valid? Official? Mythical? Alternative?

The writing of history is tied so closely to human values and intentions that it must be seen in 'the sociocultural and political framework in which it is practised' (Iggers 1997, p. 18). Official histories of institutions (nation states, professions, businesses, etc.) often identify an official founder and a defining event, among a number of founders and events. In the USA, this figure is Eleanor Clarke Slagle. Yet many facts concerning Slagle's life are fragmentary, even the year of her attendance at Julia Lathrop's course on invalid occupations at the Chicago School of Civics and Philanthropy: 1911 (Quiroga 1995) or 1908 (Dunton 1947, Breines 1986). Psychiatrist and cofounder of the National Society for the Promotion of Occupational Therapy, William Rush Dunton Jr, mistakenly identified the 1908 course as the first ever in occupational therapy. But the first course was actually offered by a nurse, Susan Tracy, on the East Coast in 1906 (Breines 1986). In his well known 1922 address, Meyer gave tribute to his wife and collaborator, Mary Potter Meyer, a social worker and classmate of Slagle, as a founder of occupational therapy (Lief 1948; also Breines 1986). The American Occupational Therapy Association honours a member of the profession each year with the Eleanor Clarke Slagle Award. Why not also an Adolf Meyer Award for Transactional Mental Health? A Jane Addams Award for Moral Philosophy and Social Action? A John Dewey Award for Interdisciplinary Contributions to Foundational Issues in Occupational Therapy? A Julia Lathrop Award for Political Engagement?

Eleanor Clarke Slagle worked with Adolf Meyer to develop a treatment approach with mentally ill patients known as 'habit training' that was strongly inflected by Pragmatist thought. Philosopher John Dewey and psychologist William James were interested in such issues as the relationships among habit, traditions, environmental challenges, creativity and experimentation, and meaningful contributions by individuals to social change (Dewey 1944, James 1950, 1985). Meyer was intensely interested in the relationship of mental illness to social contexts, viewing it as a 'problem of living' that could be ameliorated by changing the environment. He challenged the dominant biomedical opinion that mental illnesses were caused by incurable lesions and rejected reductionistic views of treatment based on crude behaviourist models of stimulus–response (Lief 1948, Lidz 1966, Breines 1986).

Meyer aimed to offer patients not prescriptions but 'opportunities' to engage in satisfying occupations so they could find their way to an existence no longer dominated by suffering (1922, p. 5). Meyer introduced the 'life chart' as a means of gathering facts to discover relationships between symptoms, pathology and meaningful events in a patient's life (Meyer 1948b; also see Frank 1996). Meyer's views anticipated the 'biopsychosocial' approach in medicine and are validated today by psychoneuroimmunology research, which links health outcomes to lifestyles and daily occupations (Christiansen 2007). Meyer's student, Alexander Leighton, a psychiatrist and a founder of the interdisciplinary Society for Applied Anthropology, later brought Meyer's holistic approach to life history studies in anthropology (Leighton & Leighton 1949; also see Langness & Frank 1981) and to community studies of mental health under conditions of extreme social stress (Leighton 1945, 1959, Leighton et al 1957). Dedicating his book to Adolf Meyer, Leighton (1960) sketched the outlines of a new field that he named social psychiatry.

While working with Adolf Meyer, Eleanor Clarke Slagle attended the Maryland State Conference on Mental Hygiene in 1913. She networked there with Graham Taylor, president of the Chicago School of Civics and Philanthropy, to discuss advancing opportunities for occupational therapy education (Quiroga 1995). This encounter proved productive when Slagle left the Phipps Clinic and returned to Chicago to work for the Occupational Centre of the Illinois Mental Hygiene Society (Breines 1986). Once there, she began to establish her own programmes.

Slagle's lobbying of Taylor apparently paid off: by early 1914 she had resigned her position at the Phipps Clinic to return to Chicago, the hotbed of reform. Back at the Chicago School of Civics and Philanthropy, she gave lectures on occupations. More significantly, under the auspices of the Illinois Society for Mental Hygiene, she started a workshop for the chronically unemployed, called the Experimental Station. Although the programme was organized primarily for patients with mental illness, 'the demand was so great,' Slagle later wrote, 'that all types ... of borderline mental cases and orthopaedic cripples ... were admitted' (Quiroga 1995, p. 46).

The Illinois Mental Hygiene Society sponsored the establishment of the Henry B. Favill Memorial School of Occupations, the first professional school for occupational therapists (Breines 1986). Eleanor Clarke Slagle organized and directed the school from its start in 1915. Its classes were taught at Hull House, where Slagle also resided (Breines 1986). Favill, a physician, had helped to found the Chicago Anti-Tuberculosis Society. There was interest in the Chicago School of Civics and Philanthropy community, starting with its president, Graham Taylor, in extending occupational therapy to tuberculosis patients (Quiroga 1995). Occupational therapy historian Barbara Loomis (1992) writes that the Favill School was 'designed to prepare the students to treat persons with physical or mental illness, soldiers with disabilities, and school-age children with learning disabilities' (p. 36).

But the school's continued existence became tied to the war effort. In March 1917, Slagle, the social worker, met with a group of advocates of occupational therapy in Clifton Springs, New York, including a teacher, a nurse, a psychiatrist, two architects and a secretary, to incorporate the National Society for the Promotion of Occupational Therapy (NSPOT). The purpose was to create a national occupational therapy association so that local and state groups could follow its example. The founders of NSPOT were also aware that the USA was preparing to enter the war in Europe (Quiroga 1995). Many Americans wished to remain neutral, including Jane Addams, who helped to found the Women's International League for Peace and Freedom (Zinn 2003). On 6 April 1917, however, the USA joined its allies – Britain, France and Russia – to fight in the First World War. NSPOT co-founders George Barton, a recovered tuberculosis patient, and Thomas B. Kidner were poised to activate contacts in Canada and the USA to work with people with physical disabilities, as thousands of wounded Allied soldiers already needed rehabilitation (Quiroga 1995). The Hospitals Commission, Canada, invited Slagle twice in 1917 to visit and observe work in Military Hospitals and to make recommendations regarding occupational therapy instruction at Toronto University.

In August 1917, the US Surgeon General established a Division of Orthopedic Surgery in the Medical Department of the Army. Leading orthopaedists Joel Goldthwait and Elliott Brackett argued for expansion of their discipline to include the occupational reconstruction of those wounded in war and the application of similar principles in peacetime (Gritzer & Arluke 1985). Key occupational therapy advocates, apart from the Chicago activists, were closely related by marriage and kinship to the orthopaedists and to the Surgeon General (Frank 1992). Herbert Hall, for example, founder of the 'work cure' who blended Pragmatism with biomechanical principles, was a brother-in-law of the orthopaedist Joel Goldthwait; Hall's occupational therapy programme was established at Devereux Mansion, property owned by his wife's family, the Goldthwaits (Anthony 2005, Reed 2005).The US Surgeon General's endorsement of occupational therapy resulted in the training and deployment of occupational therapy 'reconstruction aides' in the First World War, linking the profession's development to national agendas. In 1918, Eleanor Clarke Slagle conducted and organized the first Red Cross class in occupational therapy, which expanded rapidly. The Surgeon General's office in Washington, DC, invited Slagle to become Consultant in Occupational Therapy and Pre-Vocational Work to the Department of Rehabilitation. She accepted the appointment in December, and visited and reported on 21 hospitals before succumbing to influenza and resigning from that post.

In 1919, Slagle began a year-long stint as President of the National Society for the Promotion of Occupational Therapy. In 1920, the Chicago School of Civics and Philanthropy merged to become the University of Chicago's School of Social Service Administration. The Favill School, which had been part of the Chicago School of Civic and Philanthropy, was closed. Psychiatrist

William Rush Dunton, a co-founder of NSPOT, remarked that prior to the organization of the occupational therapy schools in Boston, Philadelphia and New York, the Favill School had been 'the best place in the USA where instruction in occupational therapy could be secured. Its graduates, who served as aides, were considered the best trained in Army service' (Dunton 1929, p. 77–78, cited in Loomis 1992, p. 36). An alumna of the programme, Geraldine R. Lermit, elaborated on the effect of the armistice on the school's closure:

> When the war was over and the unusual needs created by it had vanished, the need for training seemed to fall off and the Henry B. Favill School proceeded to die a natural death from lack of recruits and like many another worthwhile institution brought to high efficiency by war needs, it passed out of existence early in 1920, shortly after the New York Society of Occupational Therapy had obtained Mrs. Slagle as Executive Secretary.
>
> Lermit, as quoted in Dunton 1929, p. 78–79, and cited in Loomis 1992, p. 36

From 1923 through to her retirement in 1942, Slagle served as Director of Occupational Therapy in the New York State Department of Mental Hygiene, where she amassed a staff of 225. Through most of this period, from 1923 to 1937, Slagle also served as Executive Director of the American Occupational Therapy Association (American Occupational Therapy Association 1967). Slagle has been described as 'an impressive woman who literally built an empire through her belief in occupational therapy and by her political astuteness, achieved control over the Commissioners in New York State to support her programmes' (Cromwell 1977, p. 646).

After the First World War, opportunities for occupational therapists to work with patients beyond the medical phase of rehabilitation were sharply limited when Congress passed the Vocational Rehabilitation Law of 1920 (Gritzer & Arluke 1985). The law addressed a dispute between the US Surgeon General and the Federal Board for Vocational Education, drawing a sharp line between 'medical' and 'vocational' rehabilitation. The occupational therapy profession, now closely allied with medicine, was restricted to the 'medical phase' of restoration of patients in the military and civilian sectors. In 1923, NSPOT changed its name to the American Occupational Therapy Association and invited the American Medical Association (AMA) jointly to accredit occupational therapy schools and oversee AOTA's registration of members (Woodside 1971, Gritzer & Arluke 1985).

As occupational therapy became organized, bureaucratized and subject to the domination of the American medical profession, the linkages to social transformation agendas and contexts shrank. Yet the reform movement did not end, as the career of Julia Lathrop, among many others, shows. In 1912, President William Taft appointed Lathrop as the first head of the newly created US Children's Bureau. Through 1921, as head of the US Children's Bureau, Lathrop directed research into child labour, infant mortality, maternal mortality, juvenile delinquency, mothers' pensions and illegitimacy. The US Children's Bureau, later known as the Department of Maternal and Child Health, remained a last institutional outpost linking occupational therapy with the Hull House reform agenda through the appointment of occupational therapist Wilma West as consultant to the Bureau (Frank 1992). Lathrop herself went on to be president of the Illinois League of Women Voters from 1922 to 1924. She then served as US Commissioner to the Child Welfare Committee of the League of Nations in The Hague from 1924 to 1931 (Addams 2004).

The conservative AMA fought every major health reform proposed in the USA – including public health screenings in schools, private health insurance and health maintenance organizations (Starr 1982). It is no exaggeration to say that the AMA was responsible for stopping every attempt to establish a national health care system in the USA (Starr 1982). Today, the USA stands almost alone among industrialized nations in its choice not to provide health care for all its citizens (Pickstone 1996). Scientific reductionism demanded by medicine forced occupational therapy to reshape its practices and rationale, particularly with the introduction of the rehabilitation paradigm in the Second World War (Kielhofner & Burke 1977). The professional model that the USA exported after the Second World War has had a rehabilitation focus, although other approaches are making inroads, including a widening of the agenda based on occupational science. A shift from rehabilitation's focus solely on function to one on meaningful occupation is appearing in publications by Taiwanese and Japanese occupational scientists educated in the USA at the University of Southern California or having studied with University of Southern California graduates in Asia (see, for example, Lo & Zemke 1996, Chang 2000, in press, Lo & Huang 2000, Minato & Zemke 2004a,b, Lo et al in press).

The profession has remained cautious of politics and involvement in social reform agendas. As historian Estelle Breines comments, the American occupational therapy literature treats Meyer's (1922) paper *The Philosophy of Occupation Therapy* as a foundational text but ignores volumes that he produced from 1890 to 1945. She states: 'While Meyer's article is repeatedly resurrected, assuming a somewhat ritualistic characteristic, his other work is almost never cited by occupational therapists' (Breines 1986, p. 44). One of occupational therapy's most influential theoreticians, Mary Reilly, disavowed any relationship between occupational therapy and the Pragmatist agenda of John Dewey, although her approach, known as Occupational Behaviour, was clearly founded on the legacy of Adolf Meyer, Dewey's friend and colleague (Breines 1986, citing Ruth Levine, personal communication).

Breines notes the anxiety in the USA among scholars and professionals on the Left to dissociate themselves from Marxism and communism during the Cold War (1945–1991). She comments that Dewey's ideas and innovations, which emphasized cooperative approaches, were branded by detractors during that period as 'socialist' or 'pink'. Yet Dewey himself sought to develop democratic and cooperative solutions to industrial struggles. Although influenced by Hegel, Dewey was no Marxist (Westbrook 1991); among Dewey's successors, Sidney Hooks, Reinhold Neihbur and Lionel Trilling turned into Cold Warriors, while only C. Wright Mills approached anything like Marxist critiques of American liberal corporate culture (West 1989). Estelle Breines asks why Slagle 'neglected to incorporate an explicit philosophical foundation' in the educational curriculum (1986, p. 247). Slagle had studied and worked with Addams, Lathrop and Meyer. She must have been fully aware of their affirmation of the leading Pragmatists of their time.

A social transformation model of occupational therapy

In 2004, activists in the profession mobilized to convince the Council of the World Federation of Occupational Therapists (WFOT), meeting in Cape Town, to affirm the profession's commitment to social justice (World Federation of Occupational Therapists 2004). The WFOT Council acknowledged 'the world wide existence of an estimated 600 million people with disabilities, predominantly in (but not limited to) 'developing countries', who with their families and communities are restricted in or denied access to dignified and meaningful participation in daily life'. A position statement on human rights followed (World Federation of Occupational Therapists 2006).

The 2004 WFOT Council position paper on community-based rehabilitation states:

> *Occupational Therapists are developing a critical awareness and understanding about these realities, guided and informed by new notions, such as occupational apartheid, occupational deprivation and occupational justice. Occupational Therapists are committed to advance certain core principles, one of which is the right of all people – including people with disabilities – to develop their capacity and power to construct their own destiny through occupation, which seems congruent with the basic tenets of CBR (Community Based Rehabilitation).*
>
> World Federation of Occupational Therapists 2004 (emphasis added)

To realize this commitment, occupational therapy must enlarge its knowledge base and its partnerships with other professions. A wider set of resources will allow occupational therapy to evolve its own distinctive approach to social issues, population approaches and community development. Professions are distinguished by their unique way of diagnosing problems and treating them (Abbott 1988). Occupational therapy practitioners will need relevant but somewhat distinctive conceptual and theoretical approaches, methods and models of practice and new areas of competency in order to define, classify, diagnose and treat problems in the social sphere (see Chs 1–6). Moving in this direction, Townsend and Wilcock (2004) and Townsend and Whiteford (2005) explore the relationship of the concept of 'occupational justice' to theories of justice in law, philosophy and politics. They lean heavily on the concept of social justice, which is close in origin to economic justice. Thus Elizabeth Townsend and her colleagues try to carve out a distinctive meaning for the concept of 'occupational justice'.

The origin of the term 'social justice' is enlightening. Sklar et al (1998) examine relationships from 1895 to 1933 between American social justice feminists Jane Addams, Florence Kelley and their counterparts in Germany such as Alice Salomon, Minna Cauer and Käthe Schirmacher. These authors note:

> By 1890 'social justice' discourse had entered the vocabulary of a wide range of social activists, including middle-class women reformers. It was a plastic term that could embrace diverse social goals, and applied particularly well to public policies, such as protective labour legislation or widow's pensions. The term gained in ascendancy throughout the decades before World War I because it offered an alternative to charity as the justification for public policies that intervened in the relationships between capital and labor, and signified a redistribution of resources based on fairness rather than pity or fear.

Sklar et al 1998, p. 6

The World Federation of Occupational Therapist's (2004) resolution on community-based rehabilitation recalls the lessons of the progressive era in the USA in highlighting the links between economic disparities, increased risk of chronic illness and disability, and social marginality. These are problems of development – not of the individual organism but of geographical locations and their populations. The USA continues to have uneven development in its cities and rural areas. World system theory addresses the forces that produce particular 'spaces' of uneven development in the North (Chun 2004, Harvey 2006a). The persistence of uneven development in the North was showcased in 2005 by two instances that drew sustained international media attention. In the first case, the failure of the government to build and maintain levees sufficient to protect the mainly poor African American citizens of New Orleans led to the tragedy of hurricane Katrina in August 2006, one of the deadliest and costliest disasters in American history. In the second case, the riots in suburban districts of Paris in October and November 2006 spread throughout the country, leading to an official state of emergency. The violence and destruction of property were triggered by massive unemployment, poverty and social alienation among North Africans.

We turn now, however, to the 'semi-periphery' and 'periphery' where development in global perspective proceeds under policies favourable to multinational corporations. In China, for example, an alarming lack of regulation recapitulates many abuses that the Chicago reformers worked to eradicate in the USA a century ago: child labour, tainted foods and drugs, environmental pollution, and hazardous and inhumane working conditions. The People's Republic of China opened its doors to free trade after the historic meeting in 1972 between President Richard Nixon and Communist Party Chairman Mao Zedong and Prime Minister Zhou En-Lai. We now see a rush to establish free trade with China accompanied by an almost frenzied drive by universities, corporations and professions to stake out institutional footholds there. The rate of growth of the Chinese economy has now outstripped that of Germany, making China the third fastest growing economy in the world at the time of writing.

A spate of investigation reported in the *New York Times* concerns the production and exportation from China to Latin America of toxin-laced cough medicine responsible for the deaths of children in Haiti and Panama in 1997 (Bogdanich 2007, Bogdanich & Hooker 2007). In a related article discussing unregulated business practices in China more broadly, Barboza (2007) notes the 'weak legal system, lax regulations' and a corrupt business culture. He quotes Wenran Jiang, a specialist in China who teaches at the University of Alberta, who comments: 'This is cut-throat market capitalism…But the question has to be asked: is this uniquely Chinese or is there simply a lack of regulation in the market?'. Note that such issues have not been fully resolved in the USA, for example in the food industry, where government enforcement of safeguards put in place during the progressive era is breaking down (Schlosser 2001).

Lack of regulation in economic development correlates with neoliberal policies set by the International Monetary Fund and World Bank as conditions for investment in the periphery and semiperiphery in recent decades (Chun 2004, Harvey 2006a,b). 'Neoliberalism' means that the International Monetary Fund and World Bank will lend money to nations, support private investment and forgive debts if their governments agree to three broad conditions. These include: 1) *privatization* (allowing corporations to profit from the purchase, sale or rights to use natural resources and other assets in the public trust); 2) *austerity* (low taxes on corporations accompanied by reduction of public spending for social programmes); and 3) *trade liberalization* (limited regulation of multinational investors and the conditions related to production and distribution of goods and services).

We note that world system theory and critiques of neoliberalism have emerged on the political Left and been bitterly challenged by economists on the Right. (The term 'neoliberalism' can be confusing. It refers to conservative economic policies and does not map onto common usage of the term 'liberal' in the sense of a Left or centrist political stance.) Neoliberal policies have been fervently advanced by the USA and the UK since the administrations, respectively, of President Ronald Reagan and Prime Minister Margaret Thatcher. Its advocates claim that more and more development will eventually eradicate poverty and improve the quality of life for all. Consequently, privatization has been a key goal of the neoliberal agenda, along with tax incentives to stimulate investments, decreased governmental regulation of business and dismantling of post-Second World War welfare state structures.

Development guided by neoliberal policies produces spectacular bursts of economic growth – sometimes called 'economic miracles' – while creating and widening the gap between rich and poor. Corporations invest in sectors of developing economies that will produce profits for shareholders in the North. This means that essential needs and services from the nation's own standpoint in the South may be overlooked. Environments are not infrequently degraded. So while some local people will benefit disproportionately from the economic growth, critics of neoliberalism argue that the most vulnerable members, who are also the majority, have little control over the changes occurring in their environment and their occupations (Harvey 2006b). Some scholars, including anthropologist Aihwa Ong (2006), however, have begun to examine exceptions to this scenario under neoliberalism in China, Malaysia and Singapore. It is important, then, for occupational therapists to be conversant with local ethnographies of development as well as with broad economic theories.

Cambridge professor Amartya Sen, winner of the 1998 Nobel Prize in Economic Sciences, challenges the narrow premises of neoliberalism in his book *Development as Freedom* (Sen 1999). Cited by numerous occupational scientists, Sen notes that the science of economics originally intended to deal broadly with matters of human value or quality of life, rather than with mere technical concerns to increase profits, as it does today (Watson 2004, Watson & Fourie 2004, Watson & Lagerdien 2004, Kronenberg & Pollard 2005a, Thibeault 2005). Sen argues that the pursuit of wealth alone is a shortsighted goal in international development both morally and practically.

On the moral side, Sen argues that improving living conditions for people defines development and is not something to be 'invested in' after profits are made. On the practical side, he argues that democratic governments also tend to perform better economically, assuming that the government is actually representative. Sen proposes that development is most fully realized when freedom is the goal rather than aggregate growth and profit; consequently, it is important to invest not just in the corporate sector but in social services, education, the environment and overall quality of life so that overall participation is enhanced. Sen is evidently not opposed in principle to private property and profit-making. He simply does not believe that profit alone or aggregate growth is the best measure of successful development, as can be seen in World Bank data cited earlier regarding Latin America. Latin America is among the fastest developing regions in terms of overall economic growth but the elimination of poverty is much slower and the gap between rich and poor is growing wider.

Occupational therapist Hetty Fransen (2005) explains how occupational therapy and development policies meet through community-based rehabilitation. From her vantage at the University of Tunisia, in the 'periphery', Fransen writes:

Discussions on disability often consist of dialectic opposing the individual medical model and the social model. However, not all problems faced by people with disabilities stem from negative social attitudes, nor can impairment be denied as a factor, especially in countries where people don't have access to basic health and education services. The relationship with poverty must be recognized... In its latest definition, community-based rehabilitation is placed within the perspective of inclusive development, with development defined as 'a process by which the members of a society increase their personal and institutional capacities to mobilize and manage resources to produce sustainable and justly distributed improvements in their quality of life consistent with their own aspirations'. Disability has to be re-thought as a development and social issue.

Fransen 2005, p. 172–173

Fransen (2005) cogently bridges social issues and occupational therapy's traditional orientation to helping individuals, noting that 'individually focused rehabilitation' is often still needed. The Pragmatist philosophy of democratic participation that John Dewey and Jane Addams espoused in the progressive era and that supported the Hull House reforms can help to support occupational therapy's renewed engagement in social transformation. Philosopher Cornel West succinctly characterizes Dewey's political vision, which emphasizes transactions between the individual and the social environment: 'For Dewey, the aim of political and social life is the cultural enrichment and moral development of self-begetting individuals and self-regulating communities by means of the release of human powers provoked by novel circumstances and new challenges' (West 1989, p. 103). Dewey based his transactional approach on observations concerning traditional (preindustrial) societies; he developed a laboratory school at the University of Chicago in 1898 to demonstrate this method in education (Dewey 2001; see also DePencier 1967, Schwartz 1992). In this transactional view of the human situation, as recently revisited by occupational scientists Virginia Dickie, Malcolm Cutchin and Ruth Humphry (2006), individuals and their social worlds mutually constitute one another through actions in time. Following Dewey, we would be seriously mistaken to view 'occupation' from the viewpoint solely of individual activity or individual development.

Social transformation in occupational therapy may be represented graphically, using a transactional model (Fig. 7.1). The transactional model posits that individuals who undergo change in their occupational choices, occupation patterns, daily routines, adaptive strategies and so forth, will also introduce some degree of change into their environment. Such changes usually occur quite proximally – within the individual's immediate household – but may also extend to the individual's workplace and other public arenas. Yet overarching changes in the environment are more likely to affect an individual's occupational patterns than the reverse. Such changes are also likely to affect many individuals at once. In the social sciences, the direction and magnitude of such transactions is often discussed in terms of contests between social 'structure' and individual 'agency'.

The life of Diane DeVries, an American woman born in 1950 with severe congenital limb reductions, helps to illustrate these points (Frank 2000). DeVries received state-of-the-art rehabilitation services, including occupational therapy. Later in life, she became an advocate and an activist in the face of discrimination against people with disabilities. Her life provides many examples for occupational therapists to consider, however, regarding the differential impact of individual agency and social structure on her occupational choices and her experience of occupational injustice. Consider the impact in the USA of the Rehabilitation Act of 1973, a law that was fought for by disability rights activists when Diane DeVries was in her twenties and a student in college. Section 504 mandated that all programmes receiving federal funding must be made accessible. As a result, ramps, curb cuts, buses with lifts, universal design toilet stalls, and other features of the built environment support the inclusion of people with disabilities in public places where they were previously excluded because of architectural barriers.

In one swoop, the Rehabilitation Act of 1973 opened opportunities for DeVries's and others' social participation of a magnitude that could not be imagined on an individual by individual basis. The law was not handed down as the gift of a benign and generous government:

129

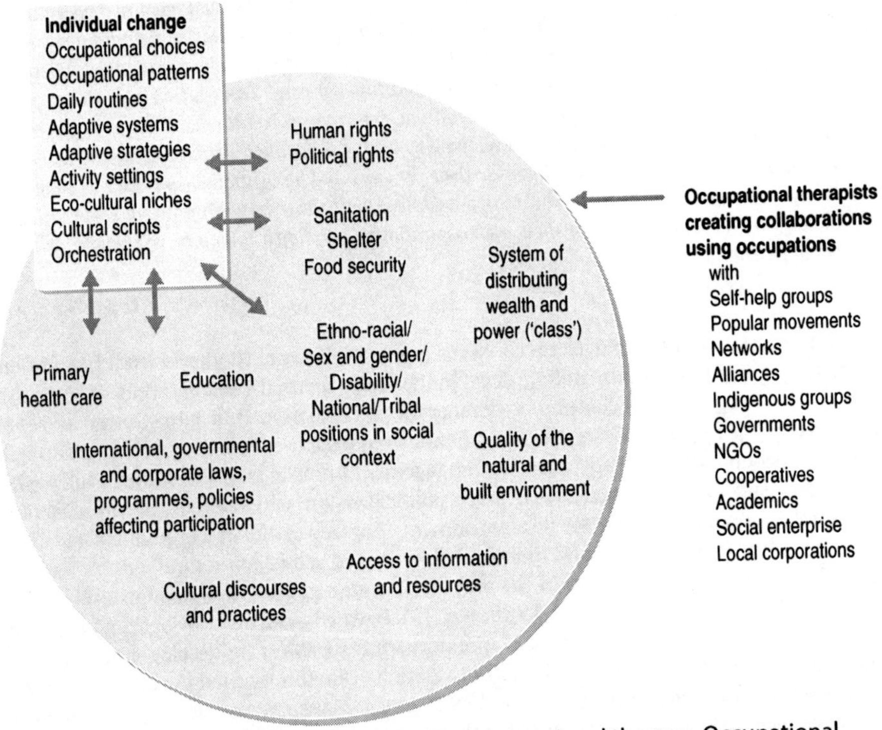

Individual change
Occupational choices
Occupational patterns
Daily routines
Adaptive systems
Adaptive strategies
Activity settings
Eco-cultural niches
Cultural scripts
Orchestration

Human rights
Political rights

Sanitation
Shelter
Food security

System of
distributing
wealth and
power ('class')

**Occupational therapists
creating collaborations
using occupations**
with
Self-help groups
Popular movements
Networks
Alliances
Indigenous groups
Governments
NGOs
Cooperatives
Academics
Social enterprise
Local corporations

Primary
health care

Education

Ethno-racial/
Sex and gender/
Disability/
National/Tribal
positions in social
context

Quality of the
natural and
built environment

International, governmental
and corporate laws,
programmes, policies
affecting participation

Cultural discourses
and practices

Access to information
and resources

Figure 7.1 • A social transformation model of occupational therapy. Occupational therapists collaborate with networks, movements or other associations to promote social participation through engagement in occupations. The transactional view taken from occupational therapy's roots in Pragmatism holds that improved occupational choices for individuals serve, in turn, to develop society. A similar transactional view underpins the 'development as freedom' argument of Nobel Prize-winning economist Amartya Sen.

it resulted from political mobilization by networks of educated individuals with disabilities who founded a social movement to reframe disability by shifting the focus from charity to civil rights (Crewe & Zola 1983, Scotch 2001; see also Charlton 2000). Conversely, in some environments and situations it may not be feasible economically or politically to create such sweeping changes at a given point in history. Consequently, as noted with international efforts to mobilize people with blindness in Tibet and South India, occupational therapists and other workers strive to prepare people with impairments to be maximally mobile and competent where they presently live or choose to live, whether in cities, in mountains or on agricultural flatlands (Tenberken & Kronenberg 2005).

The Social Transformation Model embraces four key principles that should help to guide assessments and practice in actual situations with specific groups and individuals. Occupational therapists who focus on political engagements and social transformation may begin with questions like those below, in italics:

1. **Social environments shape occupational choices.** Factors include human rights; political rights; social status and economic class; access to sanitation, food, water and shelter; access to primary health care; access to education; position based on ethnoracial, gender, age, religious, national or tribal identities; quality of the natural and built environment; and so on.
    Questions for practice: *What are the most important factors in the social environment that limit key occupational choices of the population that I am working with? Has the population*

participated in and agreed with this assessment? What resources within and outside occupational therapy are needed to reconcile professional knowledge with local knowledge in order to effect change?

2. **Individual change and social transformation are transactional.** The relationship between individual occupations and the socially constructed environment is transactional, as discussed in the Pragmatism of John Dewey, Jane Addams and other thinkers and activists in the progressive era. Improvement in one area will have an effect on the other.

   Questions for practice: *What occupational changes for the individual are most likely also to result in social transformation? Which individuals might be engaged to result most effectively in social transformation? What transformations in the social environment are most likely to produce desired changes for the individual's occupational choices?*

3. **The direction and magnitude of effects must be evaluated.** Occupational therapy directed toward social transformation may have a greater impact and more pervasive effects on individuals' occupational choices than interventions focused exclusively on individual change.

   Questions for practice: *How powerful will be the transactional effects if I focus on a particular set of changes or transformations? Can I work at both individual and social change at once? Or, given my professional resources, which is my best choice as where to focus my efforts – on individual changes, social transformation, or both?*

4. **Social transformation requires active collaborations and networks.** Occupational therapy approaches to social transformation require collaboration with active social movements, networks and alliances. Interdisciplinary participation will help to develop a distinctive occupational therapy knowledge base for social transformation, such as in current exchanges between occupational therapists, occupational scientists and anthropologists.

   Questions for practice: *What movements, networks and other groups or organizations are active in the area where I am working? What aims and goals do we share? How can we work together to share insights and expertise? How can I demonstrate how occupational approaches can make our common efforts more effective? Can I collaborate with grantwriters, governments and corporate funders to support my projects? Can we participate in conferences, post information on the Internet, publish in academic journals, make films and write books, and otherwise use media to develop an occupational therapy knowledge base for social transformation?*

Conclusion

The current occupational therapy movement toward political engagement and social transformation recalls the dynamic origins of occupational therapy in the USA prior to the First World War, before the profession was formally organized, bureaucratized and medicalized. The dynamism of those years was characterized by key founders' participation in: 1) social reform movements to gain rights for oppressed and exploited workers; 2) interdisciplinary collaborations across the humanities, social sciences and biomedicine to create new institutions and structures; 3) engagement of academic, business and public sectors under a unifying philosophical approach known as Pragmatism; and 4) transactional efforts to create a more democratic society among diverse classes, ethnic and racial groups by promoting the common good while encouraging individual development.

While recalling these activist roots, we emphatically do not suggest that occupational therapists abandon their hard-won knowledge base, skill sets and traditional legitimacy in biomedicine and rehabilitation sciences. These remain the calling card of the profession and its source of credibility and efficacy. If anything, we anticipate that occupational therapy's work in political and social arenas will continue to grow in tandem with the profession's mainstream. About 50 years ago, occupational therapy theorist Mary Reilly (1962) asserted, 'Occupational therapy can be one of the great ideas of 20th century medicine'. Her prediction may not have come true as she imagined, but 'occupation' is once again emerging as a potent tool for change. In the 21st century, occupational therapy is poised to work toward solutions to problems of living posed by the social and economic conditions of our time.

Acknowledgements

The authors gratefully acknowledge comments by Nick Pollard, Frank Kronenberg, Dikaios Sakellariou, Pamela Block, Erna Blanche, Sharon Kaufman, Brenda Vrkljan, Jessica Marvelle Kramer and Jeffrey S. Reznick.

References

Abbott A 1988 The system of professions: an essay on the division of expert labor. University of Chicago Press, Chicago, IL

Addams J 1930 The second twenty years at Hull-House, September 1909 to September 1929, with a record of growing world consciousness. Macmillan, New York

Addams J 1990 Twenty years at Hull-House (originally published 1910). University of Illinois Press, Urbana, IL

Addams J 2002a The subjective necessity for social settlements (originally published 1893). In: Elshtain J B (ed) The Jane Addams reader. Basic Books, New York: p 14–28

Addams J 2002b The objective value of a social settlement (originally published 1893). In: Elshtain J B (ed) The Jane Addams reader. Basic Books, New York: p 29–45

Addams J 2002c (originally published 1895). The settlement as a factor in the labor movement. In: Elshtain J B (ed) The Jane Addams reader. Basic Books, New York: p 46–61

Addams J 2004 (originally published 1935). My friend, Julia Lathrop. Introduction by Anne Firor Scott. University of Illinois Press, Champaign, IL

American Occupational Therapy Association 1967 American Occupational Therapy Association Then – and Now!. 1917–1967. American Occupational Therapy Association, Washington, DC

American Occupational Therapy Association Commission on Practice, Occupational Therapy Practice Framework, Draft V, August 2000, p 3. (Cited by Department of Occupational Therapy, Colorado State University, Philosophy of the OT Department. Available online at: http://www.ot.cahs.colostate.edu/philosophy.htm)

Anthony S H 2005 Dr Herbert J. Hall: originator of honest work for occupational therapy 1904–23. Occupational Therapy in Health Care 19(3): 3–19

Baer H, Singer M, Susser I 2004 Medical anthropology and the world system, 2nd edn. Praeger, Westport, CT

Barboza D 2007 When fakery turns fatal: good scares raise questions about Chinese entrepreneurs. New York Times 5 June: C1

Barros D, Ghirardi M, Lopes R 2005 Social occupational therapy: a socio-historical perspective. In: Kronenberg F, Simó Algado S, Pollard N (eds) Occupational therapy without borders: learning from the spirit of survivors. Elsevier/Churchill Livingstone, Edinburgh: p 140–151

Beers C 1908 A mind that found itself: an autobiography. Longman, Green, New York

Bogdanich W 2007 FDA traced tainted goods but trail went cold in China. New York Times 17 June: 1

Bogdanich W, Hooker J 2007 From China to Panama, a trail of poisoned medicine. New York Times 6 May: 1

Boris E 1986 Art and labor: Ruskin, Morris and the craftsman ideal in America. Temple University Press, Philadelphia, PA

Breines E 1986 Origins and adaptations: a philosophy of practice. Geri-Rehab, Lebanon, NJ

Cardoso de Oliveira R 2000 Peripheral anthropologies 'versus' central anthropologies. Journal of Latin American Anthropology 4–5: 10–30

Chang L 2000 Illness experience. Journal of the Occupational Therapy Association of the Republic of China 18: 88–89

Chang L in press The representations of biomedical ideology in the experiences of patients in a rehabilitation ward in Taiwan. Journal of the Occupational Therapy Association of the Republic of China 24

Charlton J 2000 Nothing about us without us: disability oppression and empowerment. University of California Press, Berkeley, CA

Christiansen C 2007 Adolf Meyer revisited: connections between lifestyles, resilience and illness. 2006 Ruth Zemke Lecture, Society for the Study of Occupation SSO:USA. Journal of Occupational Science 14(2): 63–76

Chun A 2004 Globalization: critical issues. Berghahn Books, New York

Clark F, Parham D, Carlson M et al 1991 Occupational science: academic innovation in the service of occupational therapy's future. American Journal of Occupational Therapy 45: 300–310

Crewe N, Zola I K 1983 Independent living for physically disabled people: developing, implementing, and evaluating self-help rehabilitation programs. Jossey-Bass, San Francisco, CA

Cromwell F S 1977 Eleanor Clarke Slagle, the leader, the woman. In retrospect on the 60th anniversary of the founding of the AOTA. American Journal of Occupational Therapy 31: 645–648

DePencier I 1967 The history of the laboratory schools: the University of Chicago, 1898–1965. Quadrangle Books, Chicago, IL

Dewey J 1944 Democracy and education: an introduction to the philosophy of education (originally published 1916). Free Press, New York

Dewey J 2001 The school and society and the child and the curriculum. Dover Publications, New York

Diani M, McAdam D 2003 Social movements and networks: relational approaches to collective action. Oxford University Press, Oxford

Dickie V, Cutchin M, Humphry R 2006 Occupation as transactional experience: a critique of individualism in occupational science. Journal of Occupational Science 131: 83–93

Dunton W R Jr 1929 The passing of the Henry B. Favill School. Maryland Psychiatric Quarterly 10: 77–79

Dunton W R Jr 1947 History and development of occupational therapy. In: Willard HB, Spackman CS (eds) Principles of occupational therapy. J B Lippincott, Philadelphia, PA: p 1–9

Frank A G 1967 Capitalism and underdevelopment in Latin America: historical studies of Chile and Brazil. Monthly Review Press, New York

Frank A G 1998 ReORIENT: global economy in the Asian age. University of California Press, Berkeley, CA

Frank G 1992 Opening feminist histories of occupational therapy. American Journal of Occupational Therapy 46: 989–999

Frank G 1996 Life histories in occupational therapy clinical practice. American Journal of Occupational Therapy 50: 251–264

Frank G 2000 Venus on wheels: two decades of dialogue on disability, biography and being female in America. University of California Press, Berkeley, CA

Frank G, Zemke R 2006 What is occupational science and what will it become? Academic and political issues in founding a discipline. Paper presented at the Society for Applied Anthropology and Society for Medical Anthropology Joint Meeting, Vancouver, BC, 28 March–2 April 2006

Frank G, Block P, Zemke R 2008 Introduction. Anthropology, occupational therapy and disability studies: collaborations and prospects. Special theme issue, Practicing Authropology 30(3): 2–5

Frank G, Baum C, Law M (Forthcoming) Occupational therapy in conversation with critical medical anthropology: chronic conditions, health and well-being in global contexts. In: Manderson L, Smith-Morris C (eds) Chronic conditions, fluid states: globalization and the anthropology of illness. Rutgers University Press, New Brunswick, NJ

Fransen H 2005 Challenges for occupational therapy in community-based rehabilitation: occupation in a community approach to handicap in development. In: Kronenberg F, Simó Algado S, Pollard N (eds) Occupational therapy without borders: learning from the spirit of survivors. Elsevier/Churchill Livingstone, Edinburgh: p 166–182

Freire P 1970 Pedagogy of the oppressed. Continuum Books, New York

Galheigo S 2005 Occupational therapy and the social field: clarifying concepts and ideas. In: Kronenberg F, Simó Algado S, Pollard N (eds) Occupational therapy without borders: learning from the spirit of survivors. Elsevier/Churchill Livingstone, Edinburgh: p 87–98

Gordon D 2002 Therapeutics and science in the history of occupational therapy. PhD dissertation, Department of Occupational Science and Occupational Therapy, University of Southern California, Los Angeles, CA

Greenwood D, Levin M 1998 Introduction to action research: social research for social change. Sage, Thousand Oaks, CA

Gritzer G, Arluke A 1985 The making of rehabilitation: a political economy of medical specialization. University of California Press, Berkeley, CA

Gritzer G, Arluke A 1989 The making of rehabilitation: a political economy of medical specialization, 1890–1980. University of California Press, Berkeley, CA

Harvey D 2006a Spaces of global capitalism: towards a theory of uneven geographical development. Verso, London

Harvey D 2006b A brief history of neoliberalism. Oxford University Press, Oxford

Iggers G G 1997 Historiography in the twentieth century: from scientific objectivity to the postmodern challenge. Wesleyan University Press, Middletown, CT

Iwama M 2005 The Kawa model: nature, life flow, and the power of culturally relevant occupational therapy. In: Kronenberg F, Simó Algado S, Pollard N (eds) Occupational therapy without borders: learning from the spirit of survivors. Elsevier/Churchill Livingstone, Edinburgh: p 213–227

James W 1950 The principles of psychology, vols 1–2. Dover, New York

James W 1985 Habit. Occupational Therapy in Mental Health 5: 55–67

Keck M, Sikkink K 1998 Activists beyond borders: advocacy networks in international politics. Cornell University Press, Ithaca, NY

Kielhofner G, Burke J 1977 Occupational therapy after 60 years: an account of changing identity and knowledge. American Journal of Occupational Therapy 31: 675–689

Kondo T 2004 Cultural tensions in occupational therapy practice: considerations from a Japanese vantage point. American Journal of Occupational Therapy 58: 174–184

Kronenberg F, Pollard N 2005a Overcoming occupational apartheid: a preliminary exploration of the political nature of occupational therapy. In: Kronenberg F, Simó Algado S, Pollard N (eds) Occupational therapy without borders: learning from the spirit of survivors. Elsevier/Churchill Livingstone, Edinburgh: p 58–86

Kronenberg F, Pollard N 2005b Introduction. In: Kronenberg F, Simó Algado S, Pollard N (eds) Occupational therapy without borders: learning from the spirit of survivors. Elsevier/Churchill Livingstone, Edinburgh: p 1–13

Kronenberg F, Pollard N 2006 Political dimensions of occupation and the roles of occupational therapy. American Journal of Occupational Therapy 60: 617–625

Kronenberg F, Simó Algado S, Pollard N 2005 Occupational therapy without borders: learning from the spirit of survivors. Elsevier/Churchill Livingstone, Edinburgh

Krotz E 1997 Anthropologies of the South: their rise, their silencing, their characteristics. Critique of Anthropology 173: 237–251

Kuwayama T 2004 Native anthropology: the Japanese challenge to Western academic hegemony. Trans Pacific Press, Melbourne

Langness L L, Frank G 1981 Lives: an anthropological approach to biography. Chandler & Sharp, Novato, CA

Lears T J 1981 No place of grace: antimodernism and the transformation of American culture, 1880–1920. Pantheon Books, New York

Leighton A H 1945 The governing of men: general principles and recommendations based on experience at a Japanese relocation camp. Princeton University Press, Princeton, NJ

Leighton A H 1959 My name is legion: foundations for a theory of man in relation to culture. The Stirling County study of psychiatric disorder and sociocultural environment, vol. 1. Basic Books, New York

Leighton A H 1960 An introduction to social psychiatry. Charles C Thomas, Springfield, IL

Leighton A H, Leighton D 1949 Gregorio, the hand trembler: a psychobiological personality study of a Navaho Indian. Reports of the Ramah Project, No. 1. Peabody Museum of American Archaeology, Cambridge, MA

Leighton A H, Clausen J A, Wilson R N 1957 Explorations in social psychiatry. Basic Books, New York

Levine R E 1986 Historical research: ordering the past to chart our future. Occupational Therapy Journal of Research 65: 259–269

Levine R E 1987 The influence of the Arts and Crafts movement on the professional status of occupational therapy. American Journal of Occupational Therapy 41: 248–253

Lidz T 1966 Adolf Meyer and the development of American psychiatry. American Journal of Psychiatry 123: 320–332

Lief A 1948 Action in Kankakee. In: Lief A (ed) The commonsense psychiatry of Dr Adolf Meyer. McGraw-Hill, New York: p 43–70

Lo J L, Huang S L 2000 Affective experiences during daily occupations: measurement and results. Occupational Therapy International 62: 134–144

Lo J L, Zemke R 1996 The relationship between affective experience during daily occupations and subjective well-being measures. Occupational Therapy in Mental Health 133: 1–21

Lo J L, Lin T W, Chu H et al (in press) Playful tray: adapting Ubicomp and persuasive techniques into play-based occupational therapy for reducing poor eating behavior in young children. Proceedings of Ubicomp

Loomis B 1992 The Henry B. Favill School of Occupations and Eleanor Clarke Slagle. American Journal of Occupational Therapy 46: 34–37

McAdam D, McCarthy J D, Zald M N 1996 Comparative perspectives on social movements: political opportunities, mobilizing structures, and cultural framings. Cambridge University Press, Cambridge

Médecins Sans Frontières 1997 World in crisis: the politics of survival at the end of the 20th century. Routledge, London

Meyer A 1922 The philosophy of occupation therapy. Paper read at the Fifth Annual Meeting of the National Society for the Promotion of Occupational Therapy. Archives of Occupational Therapy 1

Meyer A 1948a (1909) The problem of the state [from The problem of the state in the care of the insane, paper presented at Maryland State Lunacy Commission, Baltimore, MD, 20 January 1909]. In: Lief A 1948 The commonsense psychiatry of Dr Adolf Meyer. McGraw-Hill, New York: p 320–329

Meyer A 1948b (1919) The life-chart [from A paper dedicated to Sir William Osler, in honor of his seventieth birthday, July 12, 1919, by his pupils and coworkers. Contributions to Medical and Biological Research 1(1): 128]. In: Lief A 1948 The commonsense psychiatry of Dr Adolf Meyer. McGraw-Hill, New York: p 418–422

Meyer A 1948c (1935) The mental hygiene movement [from an address, 'The birth and development of the mental-hygiene movement', given at the 25th Anniversary Dinner of the National Committee for Mental Hygiene, New York, 14 November 1934]. In: Lief A 1948 The commonsense psychiatry of Dr Adolf Meyer. McGraw-Hill, New York: p 312–317

Minato M, Zemke R 2004a Occupational choices of persons with schizophrenia living in the community in Japan. Journal of Occupational Science 11: 31–39

Minato M, Zemke R 2004b Time use of people with schizophrenia living in the community. Occupational Therapy International 11: 177–191

Odawara E 2005 Cultural competency in occupational therapy: beyond a cross-cultural view of practice. American Journal of Occupational Therapy 59: 325–334

Ong A 2006 Neoliberalism as exception: mutations in citizenship and sovereignty. Duke University Press, Durham, NC

Ong A, Collier S J 2005 Global assemblages: technology, politics, and ethics as anthropological problems. Blackwell Publishing, Malden, MA

Pickstone J 1996 Medicine, society and the state. In: Porter R (ed) Cambridge illustrated history of medicine. Cambridge University Press, Cambridge: p 304–341

Quiroga V 1995 Occupational therapy. The first 30 years: 1900 to 1930. American Occupational Therapy Association, Bethesda, MD

Reed K L 2005 Dr Hall and the work cure. Occupational Therapy in Health Care 19: 33–50

Reilly M 1962 Occupational therapy can be one of the great ideas of 20th century medicine. American Journal of Occupational Therapy 16: 1–9

Ribeiro G L, Escobar A (eds) 2006 World anthropologies: disciplinary transformations within systems of power. Berg, Oxford

Ruskin J 2007 [Orig. 1850–1853] The stones of Venice. Moyer Bell, Kingston, RI

Saillant F, Genest S 2006 Medical anthropology: regional perspectives and shared concerns. Blackwell, Oxford

Schlosser E 2001 Fast food nation: the dark side of the all-American meal. Harper Perennial, New York

Schwartz K K 1992 Occupational therapy and education: a shared vision. American Journal of Occupational Therapy 46: 12–19

Scotch R 2001 From good will to civil rights: transforming federal disability policy, 2nd edn. Temple University Press, Philadelphia, PA

Sen A 1999 Development as freedom. Anchor Books, New York

Sklar K K 1985 Hull House in the 1890s: a community of women reformers. Signs 10: 658–677

Sklar K K, Schüler A, Strasser S 1998 Social justice feminists in the United States and Germany: a dialogue in documents, 1885–1933. Cornell University Press, Ithaca, NY

Starr P 1982 The social transformation of American medicine: the rise of a sovereign profession. Basic Books, New York

Tarrow S 2005 The new transnational activism. Cambridge University Press, Cambridge

Tenberken S, Kronenberg P 2005 The right to be blind without being disabled. In: Kronenberg F, Simó Algado S, Pollard N (eds) Occupational therapy without borders: learning from the spirit of survivors. Elsevier/Churchill Livingstone, Edinburgh: p 31–39

Thibeault R 2005 Connecting health and social justice: a Lebanese experience. In: Kronenberg F, Simó Algado S, Pollard N (eds) Occupational therapy without borders: learning from the spirit of survivors. Elsevier/Churchill Livingstone, Edinburgh: p 232–244

Townsend E A, Whiteford G 2005 A participatory occupational justice framework: population-based processes of practice. In: Kronenberg F, Simó Algado S, Pollard N (eds) Occupational therapy without borders: learning from the spirit of survivors. Elsevier/Churchill Livingstone, Edinburgh: p 110–126

Townsend E, Wilcock A 2004 Occupational justice. In: Christiansen C, Townsend E (eds) Introduction to occupation: the art and science of living. Prentice Hall, Upper Saddle River, NJ: p 243–273

Wallerstein I 1974 The modern world-system, vol. I: capitalist agriculture and the origins of the European world-economy in the sixteenth century. Academic Press, New York

Wallerstein I 1980 The modern world-system, vol. II: mercantilism and the consolidation of the European world-economy, 1600–1750. Academic Press, New York

Wallerstein I 1989 The modern world-system, vol. III: the second great expansion of the capitalist world-economy, 1730–1840s. Academic Press, San Diego

Wallerstein I 2004 World-systems analysis: an introduction. Duke University Press, Durham, NC

Watson R 2004 A population approach to transformation. In: Watson R, Swartz L (eds) Transformation through occupation. Whurr, London: p 51–65

Watson R, Fourie M 2004 Occupation and occupational therapy. In: Watson R, Swartz L (eds) Transformation through occupation. Whurr, London: p 33–50

Watson R, Lagerdien K 2004 Women empowered through occupation: from deprivation to realized potential. In: Watson R, Swartz L (eds) Transformation through occupation. Whurr, London: p 103–118

Watson R, Swartz L 2004 Transformation through occupation. Whurr, London

Westbrook RB 1991 John Dewey and American democracy. Cornell University Press, New York

West C 1989 The American evasion of philosophy: a genealogy of pragmatism. University of Wisconsin Press, Madison, WI

Wilcock A 2001 A journey from self health to prescription, a history of occupational therapy from the earliest times to the end of the nineteenth century and a source book of writings. College of Occupational Therapists, London

Wilcock A 2002 A journey from prescription to self health, a history of occupational therapy in the United Kingdom during the twentieth century and a source book of archival material. College of Occupational Therapists, London

Wolfensberger W 1975 The origin and nature of our institutional models. Human Policy Press, Syracuse, NY

Wolfensberger W 1996 The principle of normalization in human services. G Allan Roeher, Downsview, ON

Woodside H H 1971 The development of occupational therapy, 1910–1929. American Journal of Occupational Therapy 25: 226–230

World Federation of Occupational Therapists 2004 Position paper on community based rehabilitation. Available online at: http://www.wfot.org/documents.asp?cat=16; accessed 16 July 2007

World Federation of Occupational Therapists 2006 Position statement on human rights. Available online at: http://www.wfot.org/documents.asp?cat=&state=&name=&id=&pagenum=4; accessed 16 July 2007

Yang S, Shek M P, Tsunaka M, Lim H B 2006 Cultural influences on occupational therapy practice in Singapore: a pilot study. Occupational Therapy International 13(3): 176–192

Yerxa E, Clark F, Frank G, Jackson J et al 1990 An introduction to occupational science, a foundation for occupational therapy in the 21st century. Occupational Therapy in Health Care 6(4): 1–18

Yunis M, Jolis A 2003 Banker to the poor: micro-lending and the battle against world poverty (originally published 1997). Public Affairs, New York

Zemke R 2003 Globalization of occupational therapy and occupational science: inspiration or McDonaldization? Keynote address at the Seventh Japanese Occupational Science Seminar, Sapporo, Japan, 22–24 August 2003

Zemke R 2004 Time, space, and the kaleidoscopes of occupation. The 2004 Eleanor Clarke Slagle Lecture. American Journal of Occupational Therapy 58: 608–613

Zemke R, Clark F 1996 Occupational science: the evolving discipline. F A Davis, Philadelphia, PA

Zinn H 2003 A people's history of the United States: 1492–present. HarperCollins, New York

Encouraging student consciousness of the political through community fieldwork

Alison J. Beck, Karin J. Barnes

8

Introduction

With the emergence of interest in politics as a human occupation in the occupational therapy profession, discussion is needed on whether this content should be taught to students in an entry-level programme and, if so, how. Duncan et al (2005) have discussed issues in the development of political literacy through service learning in a South African occupational therapy programme. Wood and colleagues (2005) have described how they uncovered the ethic of occupational justice as a subplot in their curriculum. However, the question remains, how do we include content on political practice in a traditional US occupational therapy curriculum that is already bursting at the seams?

If we take the definition of politics as 'the relationships within a group or organization which allow particular people to have power over others' (Cambridge Dictionaries Online 2006), we already educate our students in the politics of professional, community, health care and educational systems. However, in the USA, content is largely framed within the scope of the traditional medical or public school educational systems of practice (American Occupational Therapy Association 1998). Rarely do we provide educational information about political activities of daily living (pADL) outside of these established communities, nor do we provide opportunities for students outside these accepted areas to be advocates and agents of change within the political arena.

There are several inherent difficulties in the inclusion of content regarding political issues in the curriculum. First, pADLs are about groups and their interactions in larger environments rather than individuals' ability to participate in targeted occupations. Second, we are reluctant to assist students in critiquing how the established medical and public education systems impact people's lives. Third, while traditional occupational therapy educational programmes may advocate for the critiquing of the context of client occupation, the focus is usually on the family, work or school environments. Lastly, for students who may not have developed a political awareness, exploration of the political may be perceived as removed from their future roles as professionals. Thus, learning built on prior experience may require more foundation hours than are available. When teaching students with varied exposure to diverse world views, time is needed to enhance consciousness and without the time they may not be ready to explore these complexities. Yet, political dimensions are present in all basic and instrumental ADLs and significantly impact clients' occupations. The diffuse and complex impact of pADLs challenges the traditional occupational therapy curriculum to incorporate them comprehensively.

Despite obstacles, we are in agreement that it is vital to expose our students to pADL content because of its power to shape their views and actions related to occupation, occupational therapy practice and world awareness. If we do not teach occupational therapy students about pADLs, the profession will be at a disadvantage and our relevance as a community service provider will be challenged. Additionally, if we continue to concentrate on services in isolated occupational therapy settings, without addressing the political component, the relevance and generalization of our efforts will be lost to our clients and their support systems. The continued hegemony of the medical and educational models in everyday occupational therapy practice in the USA means that we need a model that gives us structure and a flow of thought for a global (comprehensive and worldwide) view of practice.

The proposed framework for analysing politics in everyday living, using questions developed by Kronenberg and Pollard (2005) is a conceptual beginning in this endeavour and requires ongoing dialogue about its operationalization into service delivery and education. Therefore, this chapter examines the utility of these pADL questions from the perspective of a professional entry-level Master of Occupational Therapy (MOT) programme at a university in southern USA. A student clinical assignment in which the concepts of the pADL questions were introduced will be described.

Preliminary infusion

The context is a capstone community project course in which second-year students must explore settings that do not employ occupational therapy personnel. Forty hours of immersion in the setting is required. Four students participated in a day centre for people experiencing homelessness and four students participated at a residential facility for children removed from their families. Students were given questions derived from the principles of occupational apartheid and occupational justice (Kronenberg & Pollard 2005) to consider before, during and after their immersion experience. The purpose was to guide the students to examine these environments from an occupational justice perspective and to discover ways to integrate content on pADLs into the curriculum. We will explore the following:

1. What is the efficacy of incorporating the pADL questions into an entry-level MOT student community fieldwork experience?
2. Can questions about the politics of a context be used to assist in the immersion experience so that students begin to recognize the feeling of being 'other' and thus experience the concept of marginalization?
3. How can we assist students to participate as agents of change from the personal level up through to the global level?

We offer our experiences and suggestions to further the discussion on the inclusion of content about political practice in the curriculum. The information presented below arises out of faculty–student discussions, the students' community project papers and their oral presentations of their proposed programmes in their respective settings. The exact pADL questions suggested by Kronenberg and Pollard (2005) were not used but were modified to fit the community assignment of our students.

Question 1: What are the characteristics of the conflict and cooperation situation?

When determining the political nature of a facility and the events within and surrounding it, the initial analysis focuses on 'distinguishable aspects' (Kronenberg & Pollard 2005, p. 71) of the contexts. How comfortable would our students be in participating in and analysing conflict and cooperation in these settings?

We asked our students to describe the context and the events they encountered in the community agencies. They readily identified the occupational injustices of the people receiving services by comparing their occupations to those of typical people. For example, for people receiving services from the day centre for the homeless:

> [they were] barely making it through the day let alone envisioning a retirement plan like people who are not homeless
>
> they wonder where they will sleep tonight, where they will get their next meal
>
> by not having a permanent home these individuals lack an important constancy which could help them in identifying their habitual needs and occupational roles
>
> most feel unworthy of living a decent life because of their addictions or disabilities
>
> [they have a] history of abuse and separation from family support (emotional and financial)
>
> loss of employment to depression to drug abuse to homelessness

At the children's residential facility:

> boys had little or no contact with parents, and they had histories of physical, emotional and sexual abuse
>
> because the group must be with staff at all times, residents must often go along with the majority

The students were able to identify the similarities of conflict and cooperation issues between the two facilities. They could also describe the political relationships between the people and the staff, and themselves and the staff:

> the centre does have rules that have to be followed and if they are not followed they have consequences
>
> by treating all members of the centre with dignity and respect the staff allows its members to make their own decisions regarding attending groups
>
> some staff members shared stories about current clients and their progress... others were quick to inform me of the trouble makers and which ones to handle with caution

It was interesting that, although they could appreciate the complexity of the contexts within which they found themselves, most of the students became overly focused on the conflicts and fewer focused on events indicating cooperation. None of the students was able to articulate the two as interdependent.

Question 2: Who are the actors/occupational beings?

This question asks us to identify the multiple roles of actors as individuals and their relationships within groups and organizations. Their comparative familiarity with assessing individuals, relationships and group behaviours encouraged the students to focus at that level in their exploration of the actors in context:

> the boys live under a constant behaviour management system of two levels
>
> behaviour management controls their participation but their emotional/behavioural problems limit their ability to be 'good'

In the children's facility one student identified that the relationship between staff and residents was not without conflicts:

> the [staff member] stated that residents mainly comply out of fear of repercussions rather than respect
>
> the [staff member] believes that staff must be careful to set boundaries and not get too personal with the residents as they can use things against staff and start rumours, as she says they look for weaknesses because it gives them a sense of control, which she believes is typical of girls, and is even more amplified by the setting

Restrictions were also placed on residents inviting friends over to the residential campus. The friends and their parents are required to go through an interview process and a background check. The child is also required to be chaperoned by a staff member and so the student reported that only one boy had done this:

> 'It's just too much trouble. I don't think anybody would want to go through all that just to hang out. I just sign up for all kinds of activities at school . . . that way I can spend more time with my friends and don't have to be at the cabin all the time.'

Similarly at the day centre for people experiencing homelessness:

> the restrictiveness of the residential facility discouraged participation
>
> the restrictions led to occupational injustices, where participation in occupations was restricted, segregated or underdeveloped . . . many of the restrictions are inevitable
>
> the centre seeks to empower rather than enable philosophy, but disempowering rules, lack of choice and lack of encouragement to make reasoned choices, e.g. people choosing to play Uno rather than to work.

Question 3: How do the actors conduct themselves?

Discerning the motives and reasoning behind the occupational behaviours of the people receiving services was relatively easy for the students. They were able to validate observations through informal interviews and in some events the students could extend this to the staff. Comments interpreted by the students included:

> they feel as if society has labelled them unworthy and they feel segregated from what society allows most to take part in
>
> they are afraid of the pressure associated with living in the 'real world' leading to 'self-sabotage'
>
> schedules for everything which are set by centre staff
>
> no 'loud' behaviour is allowed
>
> lack of staff in day centre to enforce rules so individuals go back into old habits and routines
>
> at the children's facility – staff disempower through behavioural control; boys disempower each other through peer pressure not to behave; school disempowers by not preparing them for the future or assisting them to be on same educational level as peers outside this system

However, the students appeared unaware that they too were actors, and we were not certain that they could articulate what motivated their own occupational behaviours. In a conflict where daycare staff were concerned about the students sitting together rather than interacting with clients in the centre, assumptions and inability to recognize motivations on both sides (students and day centre staff) were not communicated. Cooperation was achieved at least superficially when the students were 'forced' to sit apart but feelings of underappreciation were experienced on both sides that would have needed resolution if the project had continued.

Question 4: What are their means?

Uncovering patterns of power in immediate, local, national and global situations requires an understanding of world views/epistemologies/hegemonic discourses. It originates from an examination of one's own beliefs, which are more easily uncovered through dialogue with others, usually those outside of your comfort circle. With students from variable experiences with this content, were they able to discover power imbalances among the people with whom they interacted? And were the students able to discern those behaviours used in attempts to regain some power but which, in the end, may lead to even further imbalances? They described power imbalances in the following ways:

a simple decision such as planning the daily schedule is decided by the programme director

no participation in meal preparation with inadequate nutrition, no privacy, and schedules for everything set by centre staff

major decisions such as the child's future placement are completed by the case worker. This leaves the child out of the decision making process and causes them to become dependent on others to shape their lives

lack of opportunity of the children to handle and manage their own money

each hour in the schedule is allotted for a specific activity such as game time, leisure and physical activity, but only specific items are allowed and any other activities must be approved

When a homeless client stated that 'I'll kick your boyfriend's ass', did the student see this as a means to regain power lost and to impress her, even though it was ultimately a statement that would cost him power because of its violent nature? Did the student realize her own power in the situation, which might have elicited the client's inappropriate statement?

Question 5: What does the political landscape look like?

Students identified the agency rules but were unable, probably unprepared, to excavate the multiple layers involved in the organizational systems as sources of the conflicts and cooperation. Procedural and financial accountability requirements remained transparent to them. For example, people experiencing homelessness have to sign in upon entering the day centre and sign up for each service they would like to participate in that day (shower, laundry, meal, etc.). Students commented on the restrictiveness of this rule, without exploring why the rule was in place, because of a requirement for receiving federal funding and to provide structure for the staff:

lack of meds making their behaviour unreliable/uncontrollable and therefore making it hard for them to maintain relationships with family, friends and employers; and difficult to make important life choices

Even though students were encouraged to consider the wider influences of state and federal systems, they had difficulty doing so. For example, there was awareness of the occupational injustices caused by people's lack of access to mental health services and medications, without a questioning of the policies and politics perpetuating limited access to care.

At the children's facility, one student noted the poor quality of schooling being offered to the boys in his cabin. The occupational therapy student was pleased that there was cooperation between the local school district and the facility but was concerned that one class included children in all high-school grades and identified the ultimate consequences for the children:

> most have below average academic performance and the most common progression is to jail or the military when they age out of the system

Further encouragement is needed to assist students in examining the relationships behind marginalization and segregation.

Question 6: What is the broader context wherein conflict and cooperation manifest themselves?

We did not have a question for the students in their community project that related to this aspect of political context. Although practitioners through their experiences may be able to expand their analysis to a broader context, can students be expected to do so? If issues of occupational apartheid and occupational justice are calls to action, what changes can students make, and at what level of involvement? What are the restrictions and denials that compromise their future practice and how can they advocate decreasing or removing those limits? We believe that as faculty we currently assist students to advocate for themselves and for their profession. However, we give them few tools with which to help empower people to develop self-advocacy at a grass-roots level.

Discussion

From this first year experience, it appears that community fieldwork, with immersion emphasis on the political, has the potential to expand a student's understanding of the world in which they live and practise. This is a necessary component of an occupational therapy curriculum and it is imperative for educational programmes to incorporate this content so that occupational therapy remains a profession whose practitioners contribute to bringing about change in the lives of all people.

Through our experiences with students in their community fieldwork course we believe that the questions suggested can be easily used to raise consciousness of the political issues in daily life. The pADL questions are focused and yet broad, thus assisting students to explore political issues with the recipients of their services. Applying these questions in settings where marginalization is readily observable leads students to develop confidence in their knowledge of the content. The questions themselves are important in fostering an exploration and understanding of the theories and concepts behind political issues of individuals and systems in people unused to examining activities of daily living in this manner.

However, we suggest that students who have received pADL content integrated throughout the curriculum may have an even richer experience in this capstone course. When pADLs become an accepted part of the evaluation and intervention process in all occupational therapy case studies and community experience reflective assignments, then the transition to more complex real world situations should be facilitated. Partnerships with agencies throughout the world through the use of technologies can expand the students' world views and promote lasting relationships between individuals. Bringing the global into the classroom will also assist in the realization that many issues can also be recognized as occurring locally too. Limitations in access to health care and other power imbalances restricting participation in occupations are present next door as well as across the world.

Assisting students to become agents of change may be the most challenging aspect of raising the consciousness of the political. As faculty, and with our community partners, we need

142

to give the students courage, feelings of injustice for others and confidence that they can make changes. Assessment of the effectiveness of the inclusion of politics in the curriculum will be difficult. Duncan et al suggest looking for the student's 'approach to complex problems and their ability to make sense of political issues such as organizational dynamics, community unrest or culture-bound authority structures' (2005, p. 398). These outcomes may be assessed through student reflective journals, case study discussions and by asking students to develop proposals for occupational therapy services in community settings.

This project has demonstrated that content on politics as occupation can be infused into existing courses in occupational therapy programmes. The use of the pADL questions is a good place to start to foster political consciousness and prepare students to be global practitioners.

Acknowledgements

We would like to thank our MOT students Tanee Jasek, James LeRoux, Monica Obregon, Amee Patel, Kelli Shaner, Patricia Vinton and Sarah Villalobos for their contributions and wish them well for their future practice as politically aware therapists.

References

American Occupational Therapy Association 1998 Standard for an accredited educational programme for the occupational therapist. Available online at: http://www.aota.org/nonmembers/area13/links/LINK31.asp; accessed 31 October 2006

Cambridge Dictionaries Online 2006 Available online at: http://dictionary.cambridge.org/define.asp?key=61275&dict=CALD; accessed 13 October 2006

Duncan M, Buchanan H, Lorenzo T 2005 Politics in occupational therapy education: a South African perspective. In: Kronenberg F, Simó Algado S, Pollard N (eds) Occupational therapy without borders: learning from the spirit of survivors. Elsevier/Churchill Livingstone, Edinburgh: p 390–401

Kronenberg F, Pollard N 2005 Overcoming occupational apartheid: a preliminary exploration of the political nature of occupational therapy. In: Kronenberg F, Simó Algado S, Pollard N (eds) Occupational therapy without borders: learning from the spirit of survivors. Elsevier/Churchill Livingstone, Edinburgh: p 58–86

Wood W, Hooper B, Womack J 2005 Reflections on occupational justice as a subtext of occupation-centered education. In: Kronenberg F, Simó Algado S, Pollard N (eds) Occupational therapy without borders: learning from the spirit of survivors. Elsevier/Churchill Livingstone, Edinburgh: p 378–389

Enacting political activities of daily living in occupational therapy education:
Health Care Disparities in Oregon

Tiffany Boggis

9

Introduction

Students admitted to occupational therapy education programmes arrive on their first day of class eager to learn how to assist individuals with physical or mental disabilities in leading more independent and fulfilling lives. Indeed, this is what they have observed occupational therapists doing in current practice settings. Those entering the occupational therapy profession, however, are often unaware of the larger environmental socioeconomic and political conditions that contribute to disability and the role of the occupational therapist in alleviating these conditions.

Occupational therapy education provides an early opportunity to extend occupational literacy to include issues of occupational justice (Wilcock 1998) and occupational apartheid (Kronenberg & Pollard 2005a). Introducing students to 'ethical, moral and civic principles associated with fairness, empowerment, and equitable access to resources, and the sharing of rights and responsibilities' (Wilcock & Townsend 2000, p. 84) sets the stage for action that addresses issues of disadvantage at an individual, organizational and societal level through hands-on participation. Little has been published about how to implement such a process in overburdened occupational therapy curriculums. The 'political activities of daily living' (pADL) framework (Kronenberg & Pollard 2005a) and dialectical triangle (see Ch. 1) offer a developing model and preliminary tool to use in education.

The purpose of this chapter is to describe one strategy used to develop a politically conscious approach to the education of occupational therapy students. It was designed to encourage students to explore personal and professional values that enable them to envision practice in new contexts that promote occupational health and justice while addressing issues of occupational apartheid associated with health disparities as they acquire skills to facilitate political competency. The successes and challenges in using the pADL framework and dialectical triangle to focus the educational process are discussed.

What does the political landscape look like?

Over the past two decades, empirical studies have presented evidence that medical care contributes relatively little to health when compared with social and societal factors, environmental factors, health behaviours and genetics. Determinants such as socioeconomic status, education, transportation and environmental control have been found to play a more prominent role in health outcomes than medical care alone (McKinlay et al 1989, Institute of Medicine 2003). Unfavourable conditions within this broader environmental context lead to the growing phenomena of health disparity, i.e. differences in the quality of health care or overall rate of disease, disability or death (Carter-Pokras & Baquet 2002) especially for poor, rural and minority populations as compared to the health status of the general population (National Institutes of Health 1999, Eberhardt et al 2001, Hartley 2004, LaVeist 2005).

The World Health Organization has defined health as 'a state of complete physical, mental and social well-being and not merely the absence of disease or infirmity', since 1946 (World Health Organization 1946). Many health-related associations are beginning to notice. The American Medical Association, with its traditional aim to alleviate physical disease or pain, now demonstrates a constructive interest in the non-medical components of health services, including a commitment to eliminate disparities in health care (American Medical Association 2008). With the recently published position statement on community-based rehabilitation, the World Federation of Occupational Therapists (2004) recognizes occupational therapists' engagement in coalitions and strategies with people who experience disabilities to promote equalization of opportunities, social integration and inclusion. In response to the goals outlined in *Healthy People 2010* (United States Department of Health and Human Resources 2005) to 1) increase quality and years of healthy life and 2) eliminate health disparities, the American Occupational Therapy Association (AOTA) conducted a study that concluded 'addressing [health disparities] is no longer an option for AOTA. It is imperative that we do so' (American Occupational Therapy Association 2005b, p. 2). The AOTA statement on health disparities (American Occupational Therapy Association 2006a), updated strategic plan (American Occupational Therapy Association 2006b) and revised occupational therapy educational standards (Accreditation Council for Occupational Therapy Education 2008) that specify actions within multiple contexts to address social issues and prevailing health and welfare needs reflect the seriousness of this conviction.

Clearly, the evolving values of key actors in the political landscape have begun to support a cooperative approach to address health inequities. Yet there remains a discrepancy between what we say we believe and value and what we actually deliver. The disabled community recognizes this: the very population we claim to help accuses us of promoting health disparities by participating exclusively in a health care system that denies access to health and well-being for all populations (French & Swain 2001, Markwalder 2006). We have much to offer our local and global communities in addressing issues of occupational injustice, yet the conflict between reimbursed medical-based care versus unfunded health promotion endeavours results in minimally established services. Because the talk of change does not yet match current practice, occupational therapy students enter their education with limited knowledge of the roles that occupational therapy can play outside traditional medical model systems (see Ch. 3).

How do the actors conduct themselves?

Beyond external evidence and association directives, the need to enact moral and ethical values and beliefs drives some health professionals, including occupational therapists, to address these issues of concern. In a discourse on *Ethics in Practice*, Slater stresses that 'it is ultimately a personal and professional responsibility not only to recognize unethical situations, but also to take action to expose and correct them' (Slater 2005, p. 14). The political will that drives action emerges when our personal aims and motives align with our professional occupational therapy core values and code of ethics (American Occupational Therapy Association 1993, 2005a).

At Pacific University School of Occupational Therapy, 'We envision a world in which our graduates use the skills, knowledge, art, and science of occupational therapy to promote social justice while delivering excellent services to enhance the quality of life of their clients' (Pacific University School of Occupational Therapy 2005). Our vision statement was not a response to any external mandate; rather it emerged from the expressed and subconscious intersection of the personal and professional aims, motives and interests of faculty members (see Ch. 1). Educating students and collaborating with partnering university programmes and community entities enable us to enact our vision through our everyday engagement with our students and the community.

What are our means? The Health Care Disparities in Oregon project

Participating in the Health Care Disparities in Oregon project is the initial means by which we prepare students to serve marginalized populations who experience injustices within our local community while developing occupational literacy in the classroom and beyond. Funded in part by a grant from Learn and Serve America, the project responds to the growing needs in our state and local community while providing primarily our first-year occupational therapy students with an opportunity to take leadership roles as they enact concepts of occupational justice studied in the classroom. In addition to meeting immediate educational goals for occupational therapy students, the overall outcomes of the project are:

* To focus higher education by bringing together faculty, students, staff, citizens and community leaders to address issues of health disparities in Oregon for those of socioeconomic, ethnic and geographical difference
* To support civic education through civic engagement of students in the classroom and in the community
* To build community capacity to address issues through a coalition of sustained partnerships among university schools and departments and between higher education and community organizations.

To focus higher education, the project first offered an Interdisciplinary Health Disparities Seminar that brought together over 65 students and faculty from the four schools of the College of Health Professions at Pacific University. This seminar enabled students and faculty to gain a deeper understanding of the prevalence of health disparities in Oregon, the issues that lead to health disparity, and the complexities involved in identifying and implementing viable solutions to reduce health disparity. Following a discussion by a panel of faculty members and public officials, concurrent small-group breakout sessions provided opportunities to explore four topics in greater depth: 1) the patient–provider relationship, 2) the urban–rural divide in health care, 3) chronic disability and health care and 4) advocacy and the role of the health care professional. Students returned to the large group to share health disparity issues uncovered in the small-group breakout sessions and proposed actions that the health professional could take to address these issues.

The seminar laid the foundational knowledge for occupational therapy students to learn more in the classroom and participate as leaders in the community. Integrated coursework activities required students to expand their understanding of the concepts of occupational justice, occupational apartheid, professional and ethical responsibilities as a health care provider, aspects of cultural competency and the workings of the democratic process. Faculty introduced the pADL framework, described in the textbook *Occupational Therapy Without Borders* (Kronenberg et al 2005), to guide the process for students. The functional application of this framework and its relevance to occupational therapy remained a mystery to most students at this early stage in their education, although students adeptly provided a definition of occupational apartheid and readily recognized how it presents itself in far-off lands through the stories of international contributors in their textbook. They struggled, however, to identify relevant examples within their own lives and communities. Students questioned the usefulness of the pADL framework in guiding daily occupational therapy practice. Clearly, students must gain occupational literacy and political reasoning skills by engaging in a pADL process within their local community to appreciate, recognize and decode conflict and cooperation situations in everyday political situations.

One principle of occupational literacy is that 'everyone is responsible for everything, it is not enough to merely read': occupational literacy is expressed through action (see Ch. 3). Knowles (1990) and Knowles et al (2005) argue that graduate students connect new learning to a known life experience or knowledge base. Adults are practical, focusing on the aspects of learning they perceive most relevant and useful to their future work. Although occupational literacy can provide knowledge, learners require personal experience and participation with social networks in order to synthesize, use and integrate that knowledge (see Ch. 3).

In a contextual service-learning activity, occupational therapy students interviewed stakeholders from multiple community agencies that serve individuals of socioeconomic, ethnic and geographical difference. Four agencies collaborated to identify community members willing to share personal stories. By honing interviewing skills and employing culturally sensitive behaviours within these social networks, students gained an understanding of the unmet needs of Oregonians who experience limited opportunity to engage in occupations that promote health and wellness. The story of Ryan (see Case Study) exemplifies the kind of narrative community members shared. These stories profoundly affected students.

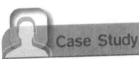 Case Study

The story of Ryan

Ryan is an 18-year-old Native American teenager who grew up on rural reservation lands with his siblings and his mother, who was addicted to both alcohol and gambling. Older siblings, who would often take him along to house parties where he experienced situations of violence, drugs and alcohol abuse, supervised Ryan. Ryan's mother was not working and often spent the family's money at the casino, the only leisure occupation offered on the reservation. This often left the family in desperate circumstances. At one point the food situation in Ryan's family was so dire that Ryan's mother killed the family dog to feed to her children.

Many miles away from his rural reservation, Ryan is thriving at the urban Native American school that he now attends. He does well in classes, participates in sports and mentors other teenagers. When asked if he would ever return to his reservation he is resolute in his refusal. Ryan reflected on how isolated he felt at the reservation. He thinks about his family and wonders why no one seemed to notice the gravity of their situation. No services existed at the reservation or nearby to help his mother with her alcoholism and gambling or to support his brothers and sisters and prevent the dangerous situations they experienced. Currently the entire family is separated from each other and Ryan is the only member of the family engaging in occupations that support his health and well-being.

Adapted with permission from: Ford K, Waring L, Boggis T 2007 Living on the edge: the hidden voices of health disparities. OT Practice Magazine 12: 20. © 2007 American Occupational Therapy Association.

Hearing narratives first-hand creates a real-life context that allows students to relate their learning and knowledge acquired in the classroom to practice, as evidenced by students' reflections on the experience.

> *I drive to work, to school and back again. I don't see how others live. This helped me to see what others in situations different from myself experience. This is important because OTs work with everybody.*

Occupational therapy student

> *I come from a rural area and health disparity is a norm for that population. The [interviewees'] stories are pretty tragic to hear. Knowing that I am going to be in this profession and knowing the skills of the profession... it means a lot to me to know that I have a chance to make a difference.*

Occupational therapy student

The interview experience provides a context for students to reflect on their own 3-P Archaeology (i.e. dialectical triangle). The initial aim of the student may have been simply to 'get through' the interview assignment, yet student feedback evidenced an engagement in the process that fostered a transformation that aligned personal and professional motives and interests: students responded to the call for action as responsible professionals and participating citizens, marking their entrance into the political dimension of practice.

> *I thought I would just go out and get the information and bring it back for the assignment. But [Ryan] really wanted to tell me his story. It was more like getting to know each other as humans rather than an interview. He just let it all out... and it made my jaw drop! He wanted me to [share] his story so that it might help his family and community. So I went to the state legislature and it was pretty powerful.*

Occupational therapy student

> *Putting a face to the situation, getting that one-to-one experience of the interview, puts it in perspective. It came right back to my doorstep... that [health disparity] is not just something for 'others' to figure out. I can do something about it too.*

Occupational therapy student

Students developed beginning research skills to transcribe and analyse interview data, and then identified major themes to address to reduce health disparities. Analysis of the themes fostered self-discovery of the relationship between the domains of occupational therapy and health disparities. For example, students recognized how a lack of access to resources, one of the research themes that emerged, negatively affected participation in health-promoting self-care, social and leisure occupations, as illustrated in the story of Ryan. They gained skill to 'critically read and interpret occupation' (see Ch. 3) that offers a way to democratic participation and is a prerequisite if democracy is to enable social change and occupational justice through civil participation. Engagement in this political reasoning process prepared students for a visit to the state capital, giving them opportunity to realize two goals of the pADL process: 1) to enable people-centred empowerment and 2) to encourage occupational justice (Kronenberg & Pollard 2005a, p. 71).

With these goals in mind, occupational therapy students, faculty and community stakeholders accompanied 20 low-income Latina women from our local community on a trip to our state capital to learn how state-elected officials are addressing health care disparities and to deepen participants' understanding of the legislative process. Students and community members demonstrated leadership and civic responsibility in the democratic process by sharing the effects of health disparity on their own lives or the lives of those who experience it. By telling their stories, students and community members were able to challenge the dominant and normative social and cultural forces that contribute to occupational injustices (Galvin 2005). Student representatives asked provocative questions of legislators that sparked dialogue about specific issues related to health disparity. Engaging in the occupational literacy process located the questions that supported students in identifying the need for change and enabled them to share responsibility with marginalized members of our community by facilitating greater social participation (see Ch. 3). Some public policy players stated that our presence in the Capitol that day was one of the most significant political actions seen in recent times and that it would inform health policy in Oregon.

What is the broader context wherein conflict and cooperation manifest themselves?

For the final health disparities project activity, students became leading political actors to help organize a community Health Disparities Forum as their means to educate and spark discussion among key community stakeholders using a Microsoft PowerPoint presentation to outline the health disparity themes they discovered and presenting the real-life stories gained through their interviews to illustrate each theme. Students suggested actions to address issues related to each of the themes at an individual, community and state level. The forum culminated in an animated, passionate dialogue among participants that included students, faculty, community stakeholders and public officials.

The community dialogue revealed the complexity involved in implementing some of the solutions students offered and heightened students' awareness of the multiple conflicting situations in the broader economic, political and cultural contexts of health disparity. Although no one challenged the idealist goals of students to lower heath care costs, subsidize preventive health clinics, provide universal health coverage and expand services in rural areas, the dialogue exposed the conflicting motives and priorities of taxpayers, government officials and stakeholders who operate within the current system of care. One audience member stated that current priorities misdirect valuable human, material and financial resources toward the war in Iraq. A public official noted that change would not occur until we found the financial will and means to support change. A lobbyist pointedly asked students: 'In an environment of limited financial resources would you support universal health insurance to meet basic and preventative needs if it meant that occupational therapy services would no longer be covered?'. Although action steps remained elusive, the forum served to establish a social network for future cooperative endeavours to alleviate health disparity.

Educational outcomes and the pADL process

Through personal interaction with community members of socioeconomic, ethnic and geographical difference, students deepened their knowledge and tested their ability to explore the effects that health disparity has on the lived experiences of those less fortunate than themselves. Student reflections on the process illustrate that engagement in civic education in the classroom and service-learning in the community profoundly affected their attitudes about the values of lifelong citizenship and service to promote access to health care and health-promoting occupations for the common good. Analysing their collected data and sharing their findings with public officials at the state capital, students developed the social, cultural and analytical skills necessary to participate effectively in the American democratic system to address health policy issues. In addition, first-year students honed their knowledge and skills in interviewing, leadership, oral presentation, cultural competency, research and ethical practice – skills that will serve them well as they continue their occupational therapy education.

Despite lack of an intimate textbook understanding of the pADL process, students began to recognize and analyse previously unnoticed effects of the confluence of factors that inform complex public health issues such as health disparities. Participating in the pADL process, students set out on their journeys toward the occupational literacy that will enable them to make informed choices about their social participation and emerge as leading actors in the broader political landscape (see Ch. 3).

Students demonstrated a heightened awareness and understanding of the political nature of how people participate in daily life by actively pursuing opportunities to use their political reasoning skills to enact pADLs in both their personal lives and in their budding professional role. For example, students independently organized themselves to contribute to a fund-raising event for the benefit of the Oregon Public Broadcasting (OPB) service. The self-identified student leader of the event sent an e-mail that reflects this personal and professional growth: 'I just wanted to send out a big THANK YOU to the volunteers for OPB! They stuck with the commitment and represented the School of Occupational Therapy with professionalism and in the process exercised their pADLs!'.

Goals revisited

In addition to supporting the civic education of students, the School of Occupational Therapy at Pacific University brought together key members of our College of Health Professions and support services to focus higher education on the issue of health disparities and developed partnerships with local organizations and community members to build community capacity. Increased capacity for action set the stage for a university-wide collaboration: the Human Health, Human Dignity: Setting the Oregon Standard project, led by the Pacific Institute for Ethics and Social Responsibility. Students and faculty across university departments engaged in a dialogue about current health policy by participating in university-wide seminars. An ensuing town hall event, open to the public, built on situations of conflict and cooperation uncovered by seminar participants. Occupationally literate students demonstrate skills and feel empowered to make choices about how to facilitate change that enables others to respond to issues of those in need.

Many occupational therapy students voluntarily participated in these seminars and some students chose to facilitate seminars, a role most often assumed by a faculty member. Participation at this level indicates the intersection of students' personal and professional and political aims, motives and interests, and demonstrates a level of occupational literacy and political competency.

Future directions

Participation in these activities as first-year students sets the stage for them as third-year students to learn further how to empower others. Two courses encourage students to pursue occupational justice issues: one designed to promote visionary occupational therapy programme development and the other to enact innovative practice. The pADL framework and dialectical triangle will be useful tools for students as they reflect on prior experiences and project forward to imagine and analyse feasible visionary practice options.

Just as the occupational therapy process guides intervention with individual clients, the pADL process guides intervention for action within local and global systems. The key principles of pADL are: 'think globally, act locally; nothing changes if nothing is done to change; the aim is not to obtain the goals but the processes above all; and there is no public ethic without a personal ethic' (Kronenberg & Pollard 2005b, p. 5). Embodiment of these principles guides us as we strive to promote occupational justice by facilitating collaborative community partnerships to alleviate health disparities.

References

Accreditation Council for Occupational Therapy Education 2008 Accreditation standards for a master's-degree-level educational program for the occupational therapist. Available online at: http://www.aotoa.org/Educate/Accredit/StandardsReview.aspx; accessed 13 February 2008

American Medical Association 2008 Commission to end health care disparities. Available online at: http://www.ama-assn.org/ama/pub/category/12809.html; accessed 29 March 2008

American Occupational Therapy Association 1993 Core values and attitudes of occupational therapy practice. American Journal of Occupational Therapy 47: 1085–1086

American Occupational Therapy Association 2005a Occupational therapy code of ethics. American Journal of Occupational Therapy 59: 639–642

American Occupational Therapy Association 2005b AOTA Board Task Force on Health Disparities. Report to board of directors. American Occupational Therapy Association. Bethesda, MD

American Occupational Therapy Association 2006a AOTA's statement on health disparities. American Journal of Occupational Therapy 60: 697

American Occupational Therapy Association 2006b AOTA strategic goals and objectives 2006–2009. Available online at: http://www.aota.org/members/area6/links/link03.asp?PLACE=/members/area6/links/link03.asp; accessed 24 November 2006

Carter-Pokras O, Baquet C 2002 What is a 'health disparity'? Public Health Report 117: 426–434

Eberhardt M S, Ingram D D, Makuc D M et al 2001 Urban and rural health chartbook. National Center for Health Statistics, Hyattsville, MD

French S, Swain J 2001 The relationship between disabled people and health and welfare professionals. In: Albrecht G L, Seelman K D, Bury M (eds) Handbook of disability studies. Sage, Thousand Oaks, CA: p 734–753

Galvin R D 2005 Researching the disabled identity: contextualizing the identity of transformation which accompany the onset of impairment. Sociology of Health and Illness 27: 393–413

Hartley D 2004 Rural health disparities, population health, and rural culture. American Journal of Public Health 94: 1675–1678

Institute of Medicine 2003 Unequal treatment: confronting racial and ethnic disparities in healthcare. National Academies Press, Washington, DC. Available online at: http://www.nap.edu/catalog/10260.html; accessed 24 November 2006

Knowles M S 1990 The adult learner: a neglected species, 4th edn. Gulf Publishing Company, Houston, TX

Knowles M S, Holton E F, Swanson R A 2005 The adult learner: the definitive classic in adult education and human resource development, 6th edn. Elsevier, London

Kronenberg F, Pollard N 2005a Overcoming occupational apartheid, a preliminary exploration of the political nature of occupational therapy. In: Kronenberg F, Simó Algado S, Pollard N (eds) Occupational therapy without borders: learning from the spirit of survivors. Elsevier/Churchill Livingstone, Edinburgh: p 58–86

Kronenberg F, Pollard N 2005b Introduction, a beginning. In: Kronenberg F, Simó Algado S, Pollard N (eds) Occupational therapy without borders: learning from the spirit of survivors. Elsevier/Churchill Livingstone, Edinburgh: p 113

Kronenberg F, Simó Algado S, Pollard N 2005 Occupational therapy without borders: learning from the spirit of survivors. Elsevier/Churchill Livingstone, Edinburgh

LaVeist T A 2005 Minority populations and health: an introduction to health disparities in the United States. Jossey-Bass, San Francisco, CA

Markwalder A 2006 A call to action: a guide for managed care plans serving Californians with disabilities. Disability Rights Advocates. Available online at: http://www.dralegal.org/publications/call_to_action.php; accessed 24 November 2006

McKinlay J B, McKinlay S, Beaglehole R 1989 Review of the evidence concerning the impact of medical measures on the recent morbidity and mortality in the United States. International Journal of Health Services 19: 181–208

National Institutes of Health 1999 NIH strategic plan to reduce and eliminate health disparities, fiscal years 2000–2006. Department of Health and Human Services, Washington, DC. Available online at: http://obssr.od.nih.gov/Content/Strategic_Planning/Health_Disparities/HealthDisp.htm; accessed 27 September 2006

Pacific University School of Occupational Therapy 2005 Occupational therapy vision statement. Pacific University School of Occupational Therapy, Hillsboro, OR

Slater D Y 2005 Ethics in practice. OT Practice Magazine October 17: 13–15

United States Department of Health and Human Resources 2005 Healthy People 2010. Available online at: http://www.healthypeople.gov/document/; accessed 7 January 2006

Wilcock A 1998 An occupational perspective of health. Slack, Thorofare, NJ

Wilcock A, Townsend E 2000 Occupational terminology interactive dialogue. Journal of Occupational Science 7: 84–86

World Federation of Occupational Therapists 2004 Position paper on community based rehabilitation (CBR). Available online at: http://www.wfot.org.au/documents.asp?cat=16; accessed 28 October 2006

World Health Organization 1946 Preamble to the Constitution as adopted by the International Health Conference, New York, 19 June–22 July 1946; signed on 22 July 1946 by the representatives of 61 States (Official Records of the World Health Organization, no. 2, p 100). Available online at: http://www.searo.who.int/EN/Section898/Section1441.htm; accessed 5 July 2007

Individual blame or systemic failure? Re-evaluating occupational disengagement in an Indigenous community

Tamar Paluch, Shana Boltin,
Linsey Howie

Our connection

Australia is a country of vast distances and untamed wilderness. Lying just below the Tropic of Capricorn, the Cape York Peninsula covers 150 000 square kilometres at the northern tip of Australia. With landscapes of rainforest in the southeast, wetlands in the west and dry scrubland in between, Cape York is one of the most pristine areas of our country. It is home to 15 000 people – mainly Indigenous Australians – spread across 17 communities. In the wet season (December– April) access is limited to sea or air, as the roads are washed out. Delivery of fresh fruits, vegetables and milk is via the weekly barge. Weipa, the Cape's port and hub, lies 800 km north-west of Cairns, the northernmost main city of Queensland. One of the world's most lucrative and largest bauxite mining operations is situated at Weipa, providing the region's main source of employment.

It was here that our thoughts on Indigenous disadvantage were developed during a final-year fieldwork placement for the Bachelor of Occupational Therapy at La Trobe University, Melbourne. Our narrative reflects views developed through living and working with this remote Indigenous community, in-depth discussion with key personnel and community members, and observations of and engagement in daily routines and occupations. In preparing for our work with remote Indigenous communities we were struck by the paucity of literature regarding allied health work in these settings. Furthermore, the biomedical focus of our undergraduate studies largely neglected the application of occupational therapy with diverse social groups and non-traditional settings. Our commitment to community development and social justice was both a motivating factor and a guiding principle to our 10-week placement.

The stories of Indigenous people around the world too often share common threads. A history of dispossession, victimization and genocide has left a devastating legacy of disempowerment, disenfranchisement and marginalization. Disproportionately high unemployment and incarceration rates, unchecked substance abuse, epidemic levels of violence and suicide, poor educational achievement, devastating health outcomes and deep poverty are all part of their experience. So too are the often misguided and ill-informed responses of governments to ameliorate the complex problems that beleaguer these communities (Baum 2002).

Australia remains one of the few countries that has failed to deliver a treaty or formal recognition of past injustices against its Indigenous population (Ring & Firman 1998). Fundamentally a treaty (Brennan 2003) involves recognition of Aboriginal Australians' traditional cultural rites and rituals spanning thousands of years, and their relationship to the land. More so, a treaty demands recognition of the systemic injustices that were initiated with European settlement and continue to this day (Brennan 2003). 'It is clear that land and reconciliation are as central to improving indigenous health status as are adequate infrastructure and healthcare services' (Baum 2002, p. 253). In the late 1990s, statistics indicated that mortality rates of Indigenous Australians were comparable to those of the New Zealand Maori in the early 1970s (Ring & Firman 1998). The improved health outcomes of the Indigenous populations of the USA, Canada and New Zealand have been attributed, in part, to the establishment of various treaties and agreements (Ring & Firman 1998, Brennan 2004). Failure meaningfully to recognize the traumatic history of European settlement and its enduring legacy for Indigenous Australians will continue to be a real obstacle to securing improved health and social status for this population.

The 1967 constitutional referendum was a defining moment for the lives of Indigenous Australians (Pearson 2002). The referendum afforded official recognition of the Indigenous population by the Federal Government and granted parliamentary representation, inclusion in the national census and access to social security. Entitlement to equal pay for labour was also enshrined in this referendum. Shortly after the referendum granted Indigenous Australians equal rights, the entitlement to equal pay resulted in widespread retrenchment and unemployment. Faced with a large population who had lost their homes and their jobs, the Federal Government responded with welfare payments. The potential benefits of equal citizenship were undermined by these events and to a large extent cemented Indigenous Australia's exclusion from the mainstream workforce and economy.

Social welfare is vital to supporting the humanitarian rights of disadvantaged community members (Baum 2002). However, the Indigenous experience of welfare over the past 30 years has been predominantly negative. The 'passive welfare system' (Pearson 2000), as it has been termed, delivers unconditional monetary and housing benefits to all unemployed adults. In doing so it locks its recipients into a welfare system that does not offer real employment opportunity or self-determination.

The effectiveness of the welfare system has been questioned primarily by the Cape York Institute, a think tank that aims to develop Indigenous social and economic policies. The Institute's strategy involves the establishment of social and business enterprises in order to create real opportunities for community and economic development (Cape York Institute for Policy and Leadership 2006). Noel Pearson, director of the Institute, is a prominent Indigenous lawyer and advocate who has taken a leading role in the historical struggle for land rights and self-determination. In recent years Pearson's focus has been on reforming the current passive welfare system, which he claims fuels the alcohol or 'grog' epidemic that exists in the Aboriginal communities. By breaking down the passive welfare system, Pearson (2000) believes that the rights of Indigenous Australians to take responsibility for their own lives will be reinstated.

In August 2005 we began our placement in one of these Indigenous enterprise facilities endorsed by Pearson. Within the enterprise, a work-readiness programme sought to provide Indigenous young adults with the chance to enter the workplace with appropriate skills for maintaining employment, as well as an awareness of their workers' rights. From the outset we were aware that we would not be working in a traditional health care facility with occupational therapy support. While it is now widely acknowledged that health lies beyond the mere absence of disease (World Health Organization 1986), the Indigenous understanding of health has much to offer in furthering understanding of this notion: 'Aboriginal health is not just the physical well being of an individual but... the social, emotional and cultural well being of the whole community. It is a whole-of-life view and includes the cyclical concept of life-death-life' (National Aboriginal Health Strategy Working Party 1989).

In addition to reframing our perceptions of health, the conventional parameters of occupational therapy practice were also challenged. The impact of bureaucratic processes, geographical location and culture (see Ch. 4) changed the need for, and the viability of, strict timelines, tangible and measurable outcomes and individual-focused interventions (for further discussion of the dichotomy between Indigenous and Western concepts of time see Yalmambirra 2000). Finding ourselves outside the traditional framework of occupational therapy practice required us thoroughly to re-examine the profession's role and the potential contributions that we could make in the time available to us. As a consequence of this, we made a significant shift from active therapist to participant observer. Initially this move took us well and truly out of our comfort zone, leaving us rather uncertain of the 9 weeks ahead of us. However, over time this obstacle evolved into an unexpected opportunity. Taking on the participant observer role was essential to gaining the trust and respect of the employees. This role allowed us to be immersed in the environment and experience of the work setting, and supported us to get to know the other employees. It also gave us the opportunity to develop a deeper understanding of the power of the environment to impact on the occupational engagement of communities and individuals.

Given the widespread nature of occupational dysfunction and social disadvantage within the Cape York community, we were interested in exploring the link between these two factors. This demanded a broader understanding of the environment as a prime determinant of the potential for occupational engagement and participation. Our knowledge of the concepts proposed by Townsend and Wilcock (2004) on occupational justice, and Kronenberg et al's (2005) contribution to the political realm of occupational therapy practice, lent support to, and inspired us to reconsider the centrality of, the political and historical dimensions of environment and how these are manifest in practice.

The application of a political activities of daily living (pADL) framework (Kronenberg & Pollard 2005; see Ch. 1) as a means of addressing the political context of occupational injustice is proposed by Kronenberg et al (2005). One shortcoming, which hindered our use of the pADL tool, was our own lack of exposure to the broader understanding of health that it advocates (see Ch. 8). Having used this tool at an earlier stage would have enriched our learning and comprehension of the political complexities of Indigenous health. However, we arrived at this understanding through the creation of our own model, which emerged over time through an organic process of observation and reflection. Only after this did the pADL framework start to make a lot more sense to us.

We developed the 'model for understanding occupational injustice in a marginalized population' (Fig. 10.1) not as a practical tool, rather as a way of articulating the multilayered nature of occupational dysfunction evident in Cape York. In doing so, it has supported the identification and conceptualization of the potential impact of chronic unemployment and welfare dependence on the health and well-being of this community.

This model represents a merging of Kielhofner's (2002) Model of Human Occupation and the passive welfare paradigm discussed by Noel Pearson (2000). The model was influenced by Richard Trudgen (2000) who, in his book *Why Warriors Lie Down and Die*, writes 'Welfare leads to a level of dependence that is crippling and creates... loss of roles, loss of mastery and hopelessness... this translates into destructive social behaviour – neglect of responsibility, drug abuse, violence, self-abuse, homicide, incest and suicide' (Trudgen 2000, p. 8). These sentiments were echoed by local community members, one of whom stated simply: 'No ownership, no sense of achievement, no real jobs' (personal communication 2005; see Chs 4, 5).

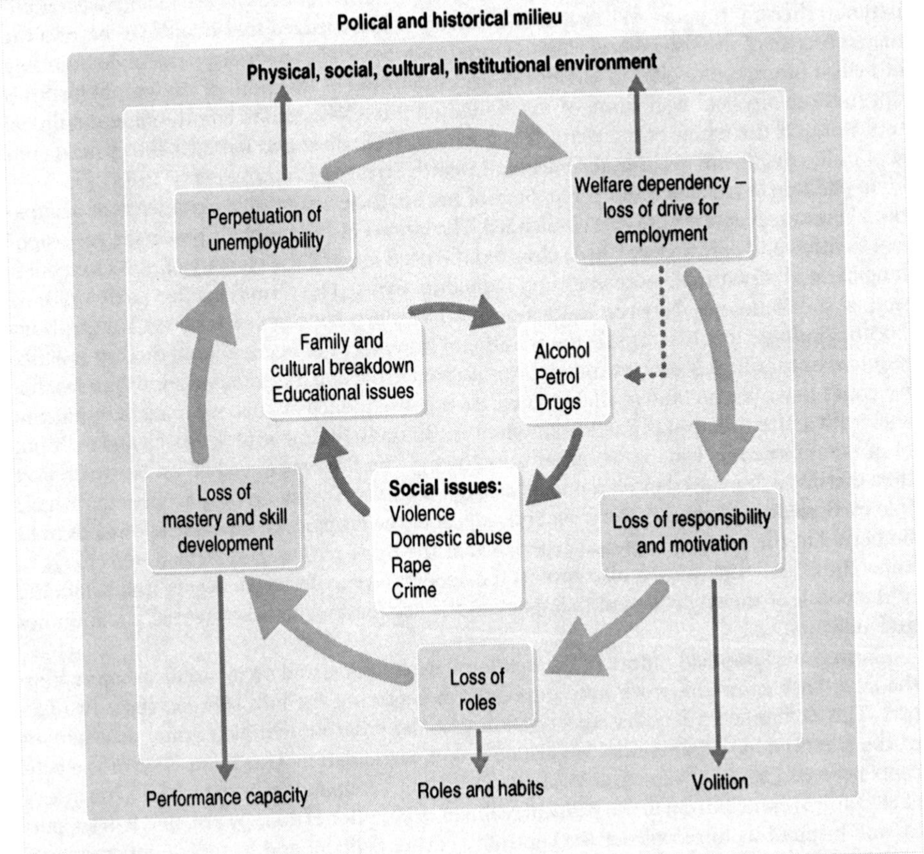

Polical and historical milieu

Physical, social, cultural, institutional environment

Perpetuation of unemployability

Welfare dependency – loss of drive for employment

Family and cultural breakdown Educational issues

Alcohol Petrol Drugs

Loss of mastery and skill development

Social issues:
Violence
Domestic abuse
Rape
Crime

Loss of responsibility and motivation

Loss of roles

Performance capacity   Roles and habits   Volition

Figure 10.1 • The model for understanding occupational injustice in a marginalized community.

During our placement in Cape York we observed the deeply entrenched consequences of historical dispossession and subsequent social and economic marginalization (see Chs 19, 20). This is illustrated by the inner circle of our model. It reflects the assertion that passive welfare dependence is a significant contributor to the increase in drug and alcohol abuse, which fuels a destructive cycle of domestic, psychological, physical and sexual violence, incest and crime, ultimately resulting in the breakdown of familial, cultural and educational values and structures (Pearson 2000). The human experience of these realities is expressed through a sense of disempowerment, hopelessness, boredom and lack of inspiration.

The outer circle of the model depicts these components as the psychological and occupational effects of welfare dependency. An entrenched culture of chronic unemployment and welfare handouts leads to a loss of self-responsibility. This in turn impacts on the roles that individuals adopt and their opportunity to acquire new skills, all of which perpetuate the unemployment cycle. The young adults with whom we worked were reluctant to believe in their capabilities for success and achievement, yet were clearly frustrated by the lack of such opportunities. Not only had they constantly met with systemic obstacles in their attempts to gain or maintain employment, they also had very few people from whom to learn that success and achievement were possible in the first place.

Each aspect of the outer circle correlates to a facet of the Model of Human Occupation (Kielhofner 2002). The loss of responsibility and motivation to pursue employment is linked to volition; the loss of roles and structure is linked to roles and habits; and the loss of mastery and skill development is linked to diminished performance capacity.

Both the Model of Human Occupation (Kielhofner 2002) and the Canadian Model of Occupational Performance (Canadian Association of Occupational Therapists 2002) – the two primary models employed by occupational therapists in practice in Australia – identify the conventional notions of the environment as physical, social, cultural and institutional. In this context, they are clearly implicated in the perpetuation of welfare dependence and long-term unemployment. However, it is the political and historical environments that serve as an incubator for these interactions.

The Australian government has been criticized for the poor infrastructure and service delivery in rural and remote areas in general, and for Indigenous communities in particular (Baum 2002). This criticism is congruent with Whiteford's (2004) discussion of locational disadvantage as an integral element in considering the impact of people's physical environment on their health and well-being. Understanding the physical environment in terms of locational disadvantage provides insight into the relationship between the geographically remote nature of Indigenous communities and the perpetuation of antisocial and undesirable occupations. According to Whiteford (2004), geographic isolation is a significant player in occupational opportunity. Firstly, social isolation results in the limited availability of occupational role models and opportunity to observe, explore and experience positive social behaviours. Secondly, limited access to educational, employment and leisure resources results in restricted occupational opportunities for community members. Overall the range of viable productive and leisure occupations is limited. This in turn hampers any prospect for change, as little or no ability or incentive to move beyond this paradigm exists.

Social environmental factors can be seen in terms of the wider social setting and those relevant to the Indigenous community. The former refers to the struggle to confront and overcome negative stereotypes and racist attacks on the streets and in the workplace, which are too often inflamed by the electronic and print media. For example, a local primary school experienced the parents of Caucasian pupils wanting to separate the children into Indigenous and non-Indigenous classes because they believed their children were at risk of being disadvantaged academically. Attitudes such as these continue to impact on the psyche of Indigenous individuals and communities and exacerbate feelings of exclusion and marginality (Baum 2002). Social pressures within the Indigenous community are also an important factor in this environment. Pressure placed on individuals not to challenge the community norms, for example by pursuing a life away from the home town (Neill 2002, Bennett 2005), is not uncommon. For example, family members are often discouraged from pursuing careers or educational opportunities beyond the level of parents or siblings. Furthermore, the 'tall poppy syndrome' (Bennett 2005) is common – where a certain community member is successful, their success is not always welcomed or supported by the family.

The cultural environment becomes all the more relevant when working with a population that is characterized by strong cultural traditions and values. This has implications for the delivery of person- and community-centred practice. In order to ensure that this fundamental tenet is upheld, Indigenous beliefs and practices, including the Indigenous definition of health, must be embraced. When such factors are not taken into consideration, organizations risk providing inappropriate services that further isolate individuals and reinforce feelings of cultural alienation. For instance, it is widely known that the experience of service delivery to Indigenous communities has been characterized by racism and discrimination for many years (Henry et al 2004; see also Chs 4, 19, 20).

Issues of service delivery extend into the institutional environment, which is defined by Egan and Townsend (2005, p. 206) as 'the administrative rules, both implicit and explicit, which govern how things are done'. Noel Pearson (2000) writes of an 'explosion in the number and variety of Indigenous organizations in the region' (p. 44). This development results in a 'confusing mess of structures in competition, if not in conflict, over access to resources and

159

representation' (Pearson 2000, p. 44). The lack of coordination between services and organizations results in wasted and sometimes misused resources. Aboriginal-controlled health services and enterprises are a promising means of empowering and engaging communities, but unfortunately widespread mismanagement and vested interests of unscrupulous providers undermine the real potential of these services (Baum 2005).

Our appraisal of the conventional environmental disablers of occupational engagement invariably led us back to a consideration of the overarching impact of the political and historical milieu. Our experience in Cape York was a gateway into conceptualizing the occupational impact of chronic unemployment for remote Indigenous communities in particular. However, we wonder whether a similar appraisal can shed light on other marginalized populations that are socially and economically excluded from mainstream society? Such population groups include people with mental illness, people with physical disabilities, refugees and migrant groups.

The complexity of health and well-being in socially disadvantaged communities requires reflective, socially informed and socially active occupational therapists. The challenge to us is to engage with and honour the events that have shaped the current experiences of the communities that we serve. This demands a greater knowledge of, and sensitivity to, the events of the world around us. It also requires us to integrate an awareness of contemporary issues into our own professional practice and in our encounters with individuals and communities.

Fundamental to this is a paradigm shift that challenges the traditional biomedical approach of occupational therapy practice. A political perspective on occupational engagement supports this by moving beyond individual culpability (as advocated by the biomedical model), which invariably deepens the marginalization and prejudice that these communities experience. An established political discourse compels us to confront the relationship between health and the political, structural and systemic factors that support or hinder occupational opportunity (see Chs 1, 2, 7–9).

Acknowledgements

The authors gratefully acknowledge the assistance of Indigenous Enterprise Partnerships for facilitating our placement in Cape York. Special thanks to the enterprise director and staff for their guidance and support throughout our placement.

References

Baum F 2002 The new public health. Oxford University Press, Melbourne, Victoria

Bennett J 2005 Indigenous entrepreneurship, social capital and tourism enterprise development: lessons from Cape York. Unpublished Thesis, La Trobe University

Brennan S 2003 The Treaty Project Issues Paper No.1: Why treaty and why this project? S Brennan, Sydney, New South Wales. Available online at: http://www.gtcentre.unsw.edu.au/Publications/docs/treatyPapers/Issues_Paper1.pdf: accessed 22 October 2007

Brennan S 2004 The Treaty Project Issues Paper No.4: Could a treaty make a practical difference in people's lives? The question of health and wellbeing. S Brennan, Sydney, New South Wales. Available online at: http://www.gtcentre.unsw.edu.au/Publications/docs/treatyPapers/Issues_Paper1.pdf: accessed 22 October 2007

Canadian Association of Occupational Therapists 2002 Enabling occupation: an occupational therapy perspective, revised edn. CAOT Publications ACE, Ottawa, Ontario

Cape York Institute for Policy and Leadership 2006 About the Cape York Institute. Available online at: http://www.cyi.org.au/about.aspx: accessed 22 October 2007

Egan M, Townsend E 2005 Countering disability-related marginalization using three Canadian models. In: Kronenberg F, Simó Algado S, Pollard N (eds) Occupational therapy without borders: learning from the spirit of survivors. Elsevier/Churchill Livingstone, Edinburgh: p 197–212

Henry B R, Houston S, Mooney G H 2004 Institutional racism in Australian healthcare: a plea for decency. Medical Journal of Australia 180: 517–520

Kielhofner G 2002 Model of human occupation: theory and application, 3rd edn. Lippincott Williams & Wilkins, Baltimore, MD

Kronenberg F, Pollard N 2005 Overcoming occupational apartheid – a preliminary exploration of the political nature of occupational therapy. In: Kronenberg F, Simó Algado S, Pollard N (eds) Occupational therapy without borders: learning from the spirit of survivors. Elsevier/Churchill Livingstone, Edinburgh: p 58–86

Kronenberg F, Simó Algado S, Pollard N (eds) 2005 Occupational therapy without borders: learning from the spirit of survivors. Elsevier/ Churchill Livingstone, Edinburgh

National Aboriginal Health Strategy Working Party 1989 A National Aboriginal Health Strategy. Department of Aboriginal Affairs, Canberra

Neill R 2002 White out: How politics is killing black Australia. Allen & Unwin, Sydney, New South Wales

Pearson N 2000 Our right to take responsibility. Noel Pearson & Associates, Cairns, Queensland

Pearson N 2002 Passive welfare and social enterprise. Available online at: http://www.isx.

org.au/resources /speeches/1020214184_ 31770.html: accessed 22 October 2007

Ring I T, Firman D 1998 Reducing indigenous mortality in Australia: lessons from other countries. Medical Journal of Australia 168: 528–529, 532–533

Townsend E, Wilcock A 2004 Occupational justice. In: Christiansen C, Townsend E (eds) Introduction to occupation: the art and science of living. Prentice Hall, Thorofare, NJ: p 243–273

Trudgen R 2000 Djambatj mala – why warriors lie down and die. Aboriginal Resource & Development Services, Darwin, Northern Territory

Whiteford G 2004 When people cannot participate: occupational deprivation. In: Christiansen C, Townsend E (eds) Introduction to occupation: the art and science of living. Prentice Hall, Thorofare, NJ: p 221–242

World Health Organization 1986 Ottawa charter for health promotion: 1st international conference on health promotion. Available online at: http://www.who.int/hpr/NPH/docs/: accessed 22 October 2007

Yalmambirra 2000 Black time...white time: my time...your time. Journal of Occupational Science 7: 133–137

Political practice in occupational therapy in Georgia:

'challenging change' through social action

11

Maria Kapanadze, Medea Despotashvili,
Nino Skhirtladze

Why has my star of destiny faded away?
Why am I travelling alone?
No father, no mother, no-one with me
I lie in the street, on my own.
Well brought up, warmly dressed,
Why am I on the street?
I have sinned greatly before God,
I deserve it.

Zura Kanashvili, 'I have sinned'.

The rationale

About 5000 children in Georgia live and work on the street (Save the Children 2004). They represent a vulnerable social group with a very specific background and needs. Street children encounter particular barriers and problems, which are mostly related to the lack of basic essentials, educational and vocational opportunities. These deficits detrimentally affect their quality of life and exclude them from social participation. Holistic rehabilitation programmes for street children are based upon egalitarian principles and are vital to increasing their participation in community life (see Ch. 21).

Governmental and non-governmental organizations acknowledge the importance of resolving this issue at micro, meso and macro levels. The holistic approach derives from a wide understanding of health promotion. It aims for a better understanding of existing programmes and services, and especially of children's needs within an overall context. The occupational therapy perspective may introduce a client-centred approach (within the psychosocial frame of reference) in the needs assessment of street children and three-level analysis (i.e. macro, meso and micro) of their context (see Chs 1, 2). At all levels, a genuinely child-centred approach is needed if children are to be taken seriously and involved in research, programme design and implementation (Van Beers 1996).

Getting started

The small pilot project was carried out through the collaboration of three occupational therapy students (MK, MD, NS) and the Children's Social Adaptation Centre, a government organization working with street children. The project was realized in September–October 2005, in connection with an education module coordinated by the European Network of Occupational Therapy in Higher Education: 'Occupational Therapy with Street Children and Refugees'. It was an initial step in the process of exploring the occupational therapy role with street children in Georgia. Hence, the programme recognized the importance of the participatory strategies used in community-based rehabilitation and their applications in local contexts (Kronenberg 2003).

Social vulnerability is a significant indicator of service provision quality levels. Programmes are often directed towards poverty reduction and establishing basic socioeconomic responsibilities but lack adaptive strategies for the inclusion, facilitation and education of relevant actors. Therefore the project had to demonstrate its ability to accommodate these issues through cycles of participatory action research, including the identification of issues, initial planning and cycles of action, reflection and modification. An understanding of the political dimension of everyday practice is very important both for professional development and in determining the relevance of occupational therapy in promoting social change.

Two main directions in needs assessment were developed in parallel with the progress of the project: 1) negotiations within the interdisciplinary team and 2) the facilitation of the children's group by incorporating elements of expressive therapy, forum (and interactive) theatre techniques and communication skills training.

'Acting out'

Over the period of a month a group of adolescents (gathered on voluntary basis) who were living at the centre worked on the material for and planned a photo-exhibition. The participants also wanted to share their paintings and poems with the public. The whole process of planning and organization of the exhibition was led by the young people. The baseline for occupational therapy intervention was the provision of an enriched context for the children to express themselves and show their initiative and creativity through meaningful occupations. The project created an occupational space that appeared to offer an experience of success for the young people living at the centre and an opportunity to express themselves to an audience (i.e. guests who were invited to the exhibition).

> *Challenges to change:*
> *I look at the exhibition and my eyes are full with tears*
> *I have no idea what will happen to me...*
> *I perceive the beautiful colours in which poetry is written.*
> *I live the poetry.*
> *I love my motherland.*
>
> Anri

The project (which consisted of failures and disappointments, along with success and joy, like every process in life) showed us a different and unique experiential perspective of the rehabilitation process. The most important facets of occupational therapy engagement were:

- a focus on the process of 'doing', which created opportunities for expression of participants' potential without the need to correct mistakes
- the establishment of trust between the participants

Reflections:

Establishing trust with children had to be the first step for further development. The setting of our first meeting was very symbolic. All the children were sitting on the stage and they brought three chairs for us and placed them on the opposite side, facing them. The setting was chosen spontaneously. I observed the changing relationship and the increasing trust between the children and our selves from one meeting to the next. I noticed that my trust towards the children was increasing as much as I saw changes in them.

Nino

Children set up several 'tests' for us. In the most significant of these they took our bags and ran playfully from the room – but through that playfulness we could read a question in their eyes: 'Am I just a street child to you, how much do you trust me?' As our mobile phones rang they ran to bring them to us.

The children had free access to the camera and other materials, despite warnings from the staff to keep our belongings locked in a separate room from them. It made us especially proud of them.

Medea

- The process was led by participants – participation in the exhibition was voluntary, the group was open and decisions about exhibition content and organization details were made by the young people
- Being open to challenge the professional boundaries through 'continuous professional learning through action': integrating sociocultural and political knowledge and skills with creativity

Reflections:

It does not really matter whether you realize your plans or not, the important thing is to change plans to the authentic needs of internal and external situations.

Nino

- Establishing effective partnering within the working group, interdisciplinary team and the wider circle of society

Reflections:

Our unique personal histories from different professional backgrounds and with different tempos promoted a deep understanding of the nuances of the process and facilitated the compatibility of the group.

Maria

The people who were invited to our photo exhibition still call us and share their impressions. Even people who weren't there have learned about it and ask about further plans. I would say that the challenge was not just about the change but also discovery.

Medea

- Being sensitive to personal values

Reflections:

The whole process of our work pushed me to make new discoveries in the children, in people I worked with and in myself.

Medea

Working on the pilot project was not an ordinary assignment; I felt that this experience of studying occupational therapy opened a door onto real life.

Nino

A space for reflection

How such occupational engagements become operational in the sense of a political practice (see Ch. 1) of daily living is a major point for reflection that is important to consider when trying to effect 'best practices'. Thinking from a global perspective in a world of diverse attitudes, ethics and dilemmas, we are obliged to question the service we are providing and ask whether we are sustaining the long-term environmental and systemic conditions that continue to deprive people of meaningful occupations. How can we accommodate the negative aspects of the actors involved? Where is the basis for empowerment and/or the means for humanity in what we do? Our pilot experience suggests the following occupational therapy points regarding relevant political practice at the organizational level with street children:

- General: practitioners should investigate, understand and 'advocate' their own role when addressing occupational apartheid (see Ch. 4), show the relevance of their own role to the other multidisciplinary members and search for ways to enable effective partnering between all stakeholders
- Specific: enable street children to be active participants in building their own future (to strengthen their capacities and talents, and avoid pitfalls), developing public awareness and knowledge on everyday issues of street children, through local actions and the promotion and facilitation of 'healthy' attitudes.

The experience we have gained makes us feel ourselves responsible (*response-able*) for the continuation and further development of occupational therapy practice in the field. It is in line with the idea that 'once we have seen over the border and experienced whatever lies there we are not then able to "not see" and "not-experience" what we have seen and experienced' (Kronenberg & Pollard 2005, p. 2).

References

Van Beers H 1996 A plea for a child-centred approach in research with street children. Childhood 3: 195–201

Kronenberg F 2003 Position paper on community based rehabilitation for the International Consultation on Reviewing CBR. WFOT – CBR Project Team. Organized by the World Health Organization (WHO) in collaboration with other United Nations Agencies, NGOs and DPOs, and hosted by the Government of Finland, Helsinki, Finland. Available online at: http://www.wfot. org/office_files/CBRposition%20Final%20CM 2004%281%29.pdf; accessed 23 October 2007

Kronenberg F, Pollard N 2005 A beginning... In: Kronenberg F, Simó Algado S, Pollard N (eds) Occupational therapy without borders: learning from the spirit of survivors. Elsevier Churchill Livingstone, Edinburgh: p 1–13

Save the Children 2004 OCHA Situation Report Georgia for October 2004. Available online at: http://iys.cidi.org/humanitarian//hsr/04b/ ixl114.html; accessed 22 October 2007

When the therapist met the evangelists:
a story of the enablement of an inner-city community

*Julie Coleman with Jeff
and Vanessa Kirby*

12

This is the story of Connect Befriending Scheme – a project that works because it effectively empowers and enables some vulnerable and lonely people living in an impoverished inner-city area of Sheffield, UK. This is not an occupational therapy project but work developed by Anglican Church-funded community workers, otherwise known as Church Army evangelists. It is discussed in this book because the project was encountered by the author, an occupational therapist, and she felt right at home. As one of the volunteer befrienders I began to see parallels between the approach used by Connect and the principles of community-based rehabilitation as explored by Sakellariou and Pollard (2006) and Kronenberg et al (2005) (see also Chs 15, 16). What follows is a description of the project and a discussion of what makes it relevant to this book.

Connect Befriending Scheme is based in the political ward of Burngreave, a multicultural inner-city community 1 mile north of Sheffield city centre in the UK. It is the second poorest ward in Sheffield (Hanson 2003). Some 42% of the population of Burngreave is made up of black and ethnic minority groups (National Health Service 2004).

Because it is poor it is also rich and diverse. I like it because people are really friendly, welcoming and tolerant. It's the place I choose to live and I am proud of it. There are some who cannot see the richness here and only see the poverty, the crime and are fearful of the mix of cultures.

Connect Befriending Scheme is a simple idea. Its aims to do something small, to link vulnerable and isolated people living in this community with volunteers and share friendship. This need was identified by the community itself via a survey that was conducted by the local Anglican minister Martyn Snow (Advisory Group for Christchurch Pitsmoor 2002).

Funding was found to employ two community workers, Jeff and Vanessa Kirby, to set up the project in January 2004. Their first task was to invest 5 months of their time networking and engaging in research in the local area and visiting a similar befriending scheme in another city.

The Kirbys got to know people, found out how the neighbourhood worked, and made connections. They ran stalls at community events and publicized the project in the local community magazine. They visited as many of the community organizations as they could to look for potential volunteers and build links with groups and individuals who might be in touch with people who could benefit from a befriender. They listened respectfully, paying close attention to the detail of every relationship with each group and each person. In responding to people's concerns they were clear about the mission of Connect but prepared to be vulnerable. This approach enabled them to establish a visibility and credibility in the neighbourhood with many different groups.

By July 2004 Connect was able to recruit its first volunteer befrienders. These were local people from a range of ages and backgrounds, reflecting the ethnic diversity of the area. Befrienders were given a training programme, designed by the community workers to enhance and promote connectedness. Supported with expenses for travel and childcare, it involved a commitment to 1.5 hours a week for 6 weeks and was compulsory, as were criminal record checks.

The training programme aimed to harness and increase volunteers' awareness of their own skills in relating to others, focusing on listening, and personal boundaries. It was fun and creative, using role play, with a strong social element to the training with time for refreshments and chat. Jeff and Vanessa also spent time with the befrienders to assess their strengths and attributes. The programme acknowledged that people volunteer not only out of a desire to help but also out of their own needs. We all are vulnerable and, through the befriending training, people developed their own skills and found friendship and practical help from other befrienders.

The befriending relationship is one in which the friend and befriender give and receive emotional support and share precious time together. The relationship offers both friend and befriender the space to mature socially (Argyle & Henderson 1990), a reciprocity that is not generally possible within service user–service provider relationships.

Many of the first referrals came from the community nurse team with whom links were made during the networking stage of the project. They included the frail elderly, recovering drug users, people with learning difficulties and people with mental health needs. Each person was visited by the community workers and carefully assessed to ensure the person's needs were within the capacity of a volunteer. The volunteers were then matched with the people referred to the scheme (they became known as 'friends'). The first meeting would be facilitated by Jeff or Vanessa, or sometimes the referrer.

The scheme has been running since October 2004. The befriender/friend has a minimum of an hour's contact per week. The relationship is monitored by formal supervision of the volunteer every 6 weeks, depending on the needs of individual volunteers. The befriender is encouraged to keep a record of visits.

An integral part of the project is Connect Coffee. This monthly meeting for friends, befrienders and referrers has a multifaceted purpose. Referrers and potential referrers make up many of the invited speakers, thus promoting the project in the community and encouraging referrals. It is also a chance for informal supervision of the befrienders as it acts as a drop-in and point of contact. It also facilitates and strengthens the network of befrienders and provides a neutral venue for befrienders and friends to meet. In addition the project has used small grants from local regeneration funds to fund events such as a Christmas meal and a boat trip for the befrienders, and a shopping trip for friends and their befrienders.

Between 2004 and 2006 four rounds of training took place, producing 22 trained volunteers. Of 46 people who have been referred, 16 are currently being befriended and six people are on a waiting list to be matched with a befriender. More importantly, a community has been given an infrastructure to better serve its more vulnerable members.

Connect is in the process of becoming something that is owned by the people involved with it. It is not 'Jeff and Vanessa's project'. There is a subtle distinction here, one that is difficult to measure, which concerns how people are treated, how something feels, how much attention has been paid to details; it is about an attitude, an orientation. The giving, receiving and empowerment that have occurred make it community-based rehabilitation. Something small has been created that is collaborative, sustainable and promotes interdependence (Sakellariou & Pollard 2006). The next stage in the project's development is to hand it back to the community. Currently it is being coordinated by Karen Skidmore who is curate of Christchurch Pitsmoor. Jeff and Vanessa have formally said goodbye to the scheme, although they continue to live and work in the area on other Church Army projects. Information about their new projects can be found on the website of one of their supporting churches (St Barnabas 2006).

So what has this got to do with occupational therapy?

If you were to ask Jeff and Vanessa to talk about why they did this work you would get a rationale containing a discussion about Jesus's concern for the marginalized and oppressed and the Isaiah agenda as discussed in Raymond Fung's book, *The Isaiah Vision: An Ecumenical Strategy for Congregational Evangelism* (Fung 1992).

If an occupational therapist was coordinating this project the rationale would need to be just as clear and involve a discussion about the prevention of occupational apartheid (see Ch. 4) and social exclusion, coupled with reference to the current political will for health promotion activities at grass-roots level (Department of Health 2006). For example, an 80-year-old woman (who doesn't know her neighbours and who has no living family) stopped her daily calls to the community nurse team as the befriender addressed her need for social contact. When the befriender was ill, the calls started again.

In her address to the World Federation of Occupational Therapists, Marilyn Pattison urges occupational therapists to move beyond the traditional boundaries of the profession and to become innovative entrepreneurs. She argues that this does not mean a move away from the core skills, rather it involves using those skills in more sophisticated and effective ways (Pattison 2006, p. 167).

Occupational therapists may have something to learn from this particular style of entrepreneurial evangelism. Indeed, like occupational therapy, evangelists have struggled to communicate the power of their approach and risk discrimination because of a perceived oversimplification of their realm of concern (see Ch. 16). As Pattison (2006) points out, occupational therapists do not simply provide crafts for people. It could equally be said that evangelists do not merely shout at people on street corners.

References

Advisory Group for Christchurch Pitsmoor 2002 Three year development plan for Christ Church Pitsmoor. Available online at: http://www.christchurchpitsmoor.com: accessed 22 October 2007

Argyle M, Henderson M 1990 The anatomy of relationships. Chapter 4, Friendship. Penguin Books, London

Department of Health 2006 Our health, our care, our say: making it happen. Available online at: http://www.dh.gov.uk/: accessed 22 October 2007

Fung R 1992 The Isaiah vision: an ecumenical strategy for congregational evangelism. Risk Book Series, no. 52. WCC Publications, Geneva

Hanson R 2003 Richard Hanson photography. Available online at: http://www.hansonphoto.co.uk/html/pitsmoor.html: accessed 22 October 2007

Kronenberg F, Fransen H, Pollard N 2005 The WFOT position paper on community-based rehabilitation: a call upon the profession to engage with people affected by occupational apartheid. WFOT Bulletin 51: 5–13

National Health Service 2004 Sheffield NHS website. Burngreave neighbourhood profile. Available online at: http://www.sheffield.nhs.uk/healthdata/resources/nopctburngreave34.pdf: accessed 22 October 2007

Pattison M 2006 OT – outstanding talent: an entrepreneurial approach to practice. Australian Occupational Therapy Journal 53: 166–172

Sakellariou D, Pollard N 2006 Rehabilitation: in the community or with the community. British Journal of Occupational Therapy 69(12): 562–567

St Barnabas 2006 Website of St Barnabas Church Linthorpe and Ayresome. Available online at: http://www.st-barnabas.net/Mission/Kirbys/kirbys.html: accessed 22 October 2007

The Sleaford MACA group

13

Catherine McNulty

MACA is a community creative arts group based in Sleaford, a small market town in Lincolnshire. The group meets in a church hall one afternoon a month to share skills, talents and to have fun. MACA makes links with the local community whenever possible through events such as art exhibitions, concerts and specific project work. Group members are usually connected with the local community mental health services. The group has its origins in the thinking and personal experience of Catherine McNulty, an occupational therapist working for Lincolnshire Partnership NHS Foundation Trust mental health services.

Beginnings

My asters came second. That was the start of it. The seeds of my thinking were from a personal experience of entering some flowers I had grown and nurtured from a packet of seeds in the local village garden and craft show. It is surprising how some life experiences can have a significant meaning and impact on future events. Only with reflection and deeper analysis can the evidence be uncovered (Schon 1983).

Growing up in a family with seven siblings in a small market town, I felt my roots were very working class. When I married at 18 and moved into a small village, I seemed to be on the outside of what I thought was a fairly middle-class culture. The emphasis here is on my own perception and related lack of confidence (see Chs 5, 14). With a young family of three sons I met with other young mothers but I often felt out of my social depth, whatever that was or is. It seems much less important these days, if it is important at all. After returning to full-time employment and having the opportunity to train as an occupational therapist, my attitudes started to change.

My thoughts and feelings about being an outsider in my local culture also changed. I think these had shackled me, to a degree. Through the experiences of employment and education my self-confidence has grown, I am much less concerned about class difference and my place within it. I think this is related to gains in self-worth and confidence.

This is an interesting concept, given the work I now do as an occupational therapist working in the community mental health service. People who have mental health needs very often also have difficulty with low self-esteem and self-confidence. Just working on these areas alone can be helpful in promoting mental health. Stigmatized by having mental health problems, people often feel separate and different from their local culture (Department of Health 1999, College of Occupational Therapists 2007).

In the late summer of 1998 I decided to enter the local village craft and produce show. I had never done this before as I thought it was something that only well-to-do folk did. I entered some flowers I had grown from seed and nurtured to full bloom, and also a christening gown I had made for the baptism of my younger sister's first baby.

My asters came second in their class and the christening gown got a first in one of the sewing class groups. I was given two certificates and overheard people's comments, particularly about the christening gown. It was a real confidence booster, and I also felt accepted and more part of the culture of the village I lived in. I had qualified as an occupational therapist a year or so earlier and reflecting upon my own experience I thought there was some mileage here for my work with people who had mental health needs. Making a link with my local community through creativity helped me to feel I belonged more, and I felt good about that.

The MACA group

I was working as an occupational therapist in mental health services. For part of my week I was based at a small rehabilitation unit at the Beaconfield site in Grantham. Along with the rehabilitation unit there was an acute unit, a base for the community mental health team and day services.

Many of the people I worked with had difficulty with motivation. Following my achievements in the village show, I thought about having a similar 'craft and produce event' for the Beaconfield site. The event was held during the autumn. Grantham is a rural market town and, from a local cultural perspective, the timing would link with the harvest festival period.

Over the weeks prior to the event it was great to see people talking about it and getting their stuff ready. Ten residents lived at the rehabilitation unit at the time and everyone was involved in some way. It was a real team effort. Staff members helped to support and encourage people, and on the actual day the whole unit was involved. The event was open to all the other units and services on the Beaconfield site and there were many entries.

The event had been planned to enable people of all abilities to contribute to it. There were categories for creative writing and poetry, artwork, craftwork, flower and foliage arrangements and home baking, with tasting to find the best. The unit was bursting at the seams. The judging took place just as it had done for me, with the exhibition closed while the judges looked carefully at all the entries before making their decisions. The award ceremony took place after lunch. The certificates were proudly accepted. There were smiles and applause and a speech from the judges on how difficult their task had been. Everyone who entered had a reward in some way.

The day was everything I thought it would be, and more. A follow-up art exhibition was arranged in the town centre, using an empty shop in the shopping precinct. It lasted a whole month and was reported in the local paper. It was an opportunity for social inclusion, putting these talented artists on the local map, and was the first of many art exhibitions we held, making links with the local community through creativity.

A second event was staged in a local church the following summer, an afternoon concert and art exhibition of Music And Creative Activities (which gave rise to the name of the MACA group). The performers were people who used the mental health services and staff from various teams. The venue had wonderful acoustics and a very supportive group of parishioners who provided refreshments for the audience.

The church was packed out. After weeks of practice and preparation the concert went perfectly. People smiled with their achievements, confidence and enjoyment, again the result of team effort. I learned many things about the power of group work on this scale and the potential of human beings who have a common goal, working together.

We took the art exhibition from the concert to display in the local library. This was the beginning of a really positive relationship with the library and the first of many exhibitions held there. Poetry books we had produced were placed on the shelves for people to read. What was being achieved might be described today in terms of policy buzz words like social inclusion and citizenship. We were engaging with the local community in ways that hadn't been done before and it felt good.

Both events were very successful. Observing people proudly bringing their entries for the craft and produce event, and then receiving their certificates and praise from their peers, being part of the concert preparation seeing the courage and pleasure people gained, I had felt really moved. There was something tangible and very different happening. It seemed that participants in both events had gained confidence and self-esteem. Being involved and engaged in these creative arts projects had a profound effect on their motivation. They were a celebration of 'doing, being and becoming' (Wilcock 1998, p. 248).

In autumn 1999 we started to meet regularly to harness some of the energy, the potential healing power of creativity, and to continue building links with the local community. We became known as the MACA group, taken from the title of our first afternoon concert. The group moved to Sleaford in 2002, where my work as an occupational therapist is based with the local community mental health team. Over all the years (1999–2007) I have been involved with MACA, it has been consistently well attended, which indicates the importance it has for its members.

The MACA group's relaxed nature is an important factor in providing opportunities in multiple layers of various occupational roles and 'small achievable tasks' (Cracknell 1995, p. 343) for those involved. Group members come forward to take on responsibilities, from making sure there are sufficient resources for drinks and actually putting the kettle on through to making suggestions for projects on which the group can work or be involved. People have opportunities to develop confidence, try out new things, write poetry and songs. There is always plenty of encouragement around and group members have become volunteers for the group.

Some comments from group members about the benefits of coming to the MACA group:

- I can see and play instruments and that gets me out, so I can meet people
- Enjoy the group, gives me a reason to come out, which is important
- I enjoy singing and playing guitar
- A place where everyone can express ideas in a creative way, either in music, art poetry or theatrical way, hope that it maintains its relaxed and friendly atmosphere
- Enjoyable, meet people, like music
- Uplifting, inspirational
- Good way of socializing, getting together and having great fun, no inhibitions, sometimes you can go somewhere and meet people you feel strange and different from the rest, unsure, but here you can mix and enjoy yourself
- A unique creative environment for people of all abilities to take part in creative activities, either in a group or individually, it is an open and accepting place for people to grow in confidence
- Laid back, somewhere you can gather your wits and meet others
- It's all right here
- When I come to this group it's the closest I am to my old self.

It can be difficult, and therefore important, for people with complex mental health needs to gain a sense of enjoyment (Emerson et al 1998), and these developments describe what Csikszentmihalyi (1992, 1997) calls 'flow', in which the exchange and interaction is unconscious and spontaneous. We are just a bunch of people making music and doing creative arts, but skill in this area is always unique. When people are involved in MACA group projects their mental health needs become less significant to them and people take risks in getting involved in things. Individuals come forward to volunteer for doing things that they identify strongly with. Doing things 'as an artist' has helped individuals to overcome anxiety. Ideas put forward by individuals are the backbone of the project and are supported. For example, one member suggested we could do a gig in a pub, so we did. It was a great success. Another suggestion was to publish a book of poetry. The book was published in partnership with the print shop at a local prison.

This is refreshing and energizing to be part of, but the MACA group also has a political significance. These initiatives, which came out of the group, were opportunities to facilitate forms of social inclusion (Department of Health 2004, College of Occupational Therapists 2007: see Ch. 14). Others are that it is set within the local community, renting out a church hall. The name is known locally within the church communities and the local art scene. Further links have developed with the local arts council and a creative landscape project known as 'The Nettles Project'. MACA was actually invited to perform for two consecutive years in the 'Sleaford Live' music festival, which meant we had a slot in the festival programme, a booklet sent out to thousands of local addresses. Being visible in the local community is a means of demonstrating social inclusion. Both performances had an audience of 30 to 40 people, which is a fair achievement for a midweek afternoon concert in a small market town. This was a real experience, real audience and real applause. When the group meets and we talk about these tangible achievements the creative energy and value of citizenship is truly apparent and more ideas come forward.

In September 2006 the group celebrated going solo, functioning outside of mental health services. The group has elected a committee and adopted a constitution. Although folks are still growing into their roles there are some volunteers who help and support the group. However, in the current climate of health service debt and the marketplace agenda of hospital trusts, there is a need to show the evidence base and the worth of this group. The basis for occupational therapy input to MACA could change and without this input or other sufficiently robust support it may begin to flag and even close. There is a need to identify clearly 'what that something is' that is provided by occupational therapy. Perhaps it is the occupational thinking, the way I have personally approached things and the opportunities I see from the occupational focus, using this in partnerships and linking in with the local community to build social capital. People are social animals by nature and if isolated become alienated, as Putnam's (2000) picture of the decline of social capital suggests. A fair and just society works to meet our human needs through our interdependence, the result of humanity engaging in occupations.

There is room to grow with this project, and opportunity for a research project, but to do this it needs more resources and time. Until then, here are some of MACA's achievements.

- Appearing at the first National Institute of Mental Health in England East Midlands Conference at Nottingham University
- Recording a CD
- Publishing a poetry book
- Taking part in the 'Sleaford Live' music festivals
- Appearance at the Hearing Voices Conference in Sleaford
- Photography for Lincolnshire Partnership NHS Foundation Trust
- Guest appearance at the Support Treatment in Early Psychosis Conference at the Bentley Hotel in Lincoln.

References

College of Occupational Therapists 2007 Recovering ordinary lives: the strategy for occupational therapy in mental health services 2007–2017. College of Occupational Therapists, London

Cracknell E 1995 A small, achievable task. British Journal of Occupational Therapy 58: 343–344

Csikszentmihalyi M 1992 The psychology of happiness. Rider, London

Csikszentmihalyi M 1997 Living well: the psychology of everyday life. Weidenfeld & Nicholson, London

Department of Health 1999 National service framework for mental health. Available online at: http://www.dh.gov.uk; accessed 22 October 2007

Department of Health 2004 Choosing health: making healthier choices easier. Stationery Office, London. Available online at: http://www.dh.gov.uk/en/Publicationsandstatistics/Publications/PublicationsPolicyandGuidance/DH_4094550; accessed 22 October 2007

Emerson H, Cook J, Polatajko H, Segal R 1998 Enjoyment experiences as described by persons with schizophrenia: a qualitative study. Canadian Journal of Occupational Therapy 65: 183–192

Putnam R 2000 Bowling alone: the collapse and revival of American community. Simon & Schuster, London

Schon D 1983 The reflective practitioner. New York, Basic Books

Wilcock A 1998 Doing, being, becoming. Canadian Journal of Occupational Therapy 65: 248–257

The Transatlantic Fed:
from individual stories of disability to collective action

14

Brendan Abel, Melodie Clarke,
Stephen Parks

> *Since all men are 'political beings,' all are also legislators... Every man, in as much as he is active, i.e. living, contributes to modifying the social environment in which he develops (to modifying certain of its characteristics or preserving others); in other words, he tends to establish 'norms,' rules of living or behaviour. One's circle of activity may be greater or smaller, one's awareness of one's own perceptions may be greater or smaller; furthermore, the representation to power may be greater or smaller, and will be put into practice to a greater or lesser extent in its normative systemic expression by the 'represented'.*

Antonio Gramsci 1971, p. 265

At the outset, we should note that none of us is an occupational therapist. In taking on the work described below, we were probably more animated by the idea of exploring our role as 'political beings' within a university community. More than therapists, we saw ourselves as would-be legislators attempting to ameliorate or modify what we felt to be the obstacles facing those from a working-class background at an exclusive United States campus. This focus on our identity as part of a collective working-class community gradually shaped a collaborative writing project that interacted with policy debates around disability and education. Before that story can be told, however, some background is necessary.

The Transatlantic Fed is a partnership between the Federation of Worker Writers and Community Publishers (FWWCP) and the Writing Program, Syracuse University. At the outset, the Transatlantic Fed was a listserv discussion group bringing together a Syracuse University Civic Writing class and FWWCP members charged with the task of addressing a seemingly straightforward question: Does the working class in Great Britain and the USA share similar experiences? This was not an innocent question to ask in the context of Syracuse University, an educational institution where university fees can average over $40 000 a year and where, not surprisingly, the number of working-class students is relatively small. Indeed, Parks developed the connection with the FWWCP as a means to provide working-class students at Syracuse University with an entry point into a tradition of writing and analysing working-class experience for the knowledge and insights it can provide. An additional goal for Parks was also to provide a forum for more privileged students to learn about the reality of working-class life.

Within a class of approximately 20 students, the Transatlantic Fed project attracted six students, all from working-class backgrounds, half of whom also faced issues of physical or mental disability. The online conversation with the FWWCP soon focused on the intersection of class, education and disability. As might be expected, the initial stories were personal, individual and focused on the discrimination the participants faced daily. Eric Davidson wrote: 'I don't know what it's like in the USA, but in the UK there is a lot of prejudice against Survivors – we are seen as incapable, socially inept, self-obsessed, boring, incapable of self-expression . . . right down the list to smelly.'

This sharing of individual stories, however, soon led to larger questions of what actions could possibly be taken. For instance, in a response to a participant writing about her illness, Anne wrote:

> It was interesting to read of your illness. I suffer from systemic lupus erythematosus . . . basically my body is allergic to itself and this is manifested in short-term memory recall, which I find very frustrating. At present I'm fighting to get my working hours put back on to the 09.00–17.00 basis and have presented both therapist and doctor's lines – to no avail sometimes, so maybe we could do something on these lines.

The question of 'what to do' echoed throughout the posts and called forth the role of potential legislators within each participant. Before moving on to the actions taken by the group, however, it is worth spending a moment discussing Gramsci's (1971) conception of legislators.

A fundamental tenet of this idea is the belief that we are always already participating in collective aspects of public life. Even our most immediate or personal actions work to reaffirm or to resist normative systemic expression. For instance, the sheer act of the students bringing working-class experience and writing into an institution that could be viewed as structured against such opportunities was a legislative moment – it affected in a small way who could speak and what could be said. More broadly, it could be argued that such work was an attempt to enact an emerging collective belief among participants that such personal issues needed to be systemically represented within the legislative framework of the university. For Gramsci (1971), then, the initial work of legislators is to elaborate this emergent collective sensibility across the locations where one has legislative authority, moving to create spaces where a new definition of normative representation and behaviour exists. Later, the work becomes that of further articulating those spaces within the system, ultimately creating a new 'governance' structure in a way that has affinities with de Certeau's (1984) concepts of tactics and strategies.

Within the context of using personal writing about class/disability as a means to alter the 'normative representations' and governance structures of a variety of institutions, the work of the Transatlantic Fed began to take on more meaning. The writing produced became an attempt to enact a collective role as legislators to affect local change within discussions occurring at Syracuse University and the FWWCP (see also Chs 3, 6). To track these changes at Syracuse University, we want to examine the particular trajectory of one participant, Melodie Clarke, whose work is chosen not for its individual merits but for how it speaks to the collective effort of the Transatlantic Fed.

As with many of the Transatlantic Fed members, Clarke's initial posts to the group focused on the particulars of her situation:

> Our discussions about class, education and disability made me become interested about what is being done on our campus to address these issues. I had a wonderful experience with a particular event that I would like to share with you.
>
> At Syracuse University they're doing a program called Writing on the Wall. In this program they are having 130 concrete blocks painted with symbols or words that symbolize oppression. They can be painted by students and Faculty . . . I painted a block with the word disability and a small flower. They had us fill out a card explaining why you chose the word that you did or what the symbol you used meant. I wrote that people don't see me, they see the disability and don't look past that to see me. I feel like I have to prove myself to become visible again.

I've been thinking about this subject for a couple of days now. I am using a walker (I'm being weaned off of it to using a cane) and wear braces on both hands. I feel that when I meet people they look at my disabilities and don't look farther to see me as a person. I am a person beyond the disabilities. I have dreams, feelings and aspirations like everyone else. I feel that people are putting me in a box and it gets harder and harder to push or break my way through.

It even goes on at the University level, where just because you have a ramp on the outside of a building does not make it handicap-accessible. I get so frustrated at times because I can't get downstairs to the Bursar's Office or upstairs to Financial Aid. I also get frustrated by people who treat me like I'm not there or they have prejudged me based on my appearance or disability. Frustration eventually turns into depression and sadness. I keep pushing against the box wall to get people to see me for who I am, not my disability, not my disease (sarcoidosis), not because they feel sorry for me and not treating me really different from every other student.

In response, Nick Pollard wrote back stating:

The other day I took several masters students to meet some people I occasionally work with in a centre for people with early onset of dementia, an unrelated condition but also one which is not sufficiently recognized and often not diagnosed early enough for people to be enabled to make choices for themselves about managing their own lives. One of the service users there was a local politician and has been instrumental in getting the day centre set up in a way that favours what the service users want to do. He advised my students – OT managers in the health service: 'What you want to do is get some service users together and take them with you to argue for resources. You're professionals, and you'll get fobbed off. Service users can say things that are a bit naughty and make the arguments, they haven't got anyone paying their wages. Let them do the talking.' His other maxims, following this, were 'keep battling on', and 'only fight battles you can win'.

Out of such interchanges, the idea emerged of participants developing a performance piece that could be used in a variety of contexts to highlight how typical discussion of the 'Syracuse University student' denied the reality of working-class existence. Within weeks, Abel had coordinated efforts to turn the writings of the Transatlantic Fed into a short performance piece that was read in front of Writing Program faculty and students at an end of year 'celebration of writing'. (To read the full performance piece, see www.transatlanticfed.blogspot.com.) With their stories of the difficulties in receiving equal educational access faced by working-class, disabled students stood in stark contrast to other humorous student pieces focusing on rides on yachts. The effect of the presentation on the student population was clear, however. When a new course focused specifically on working-class identity linked to the Transatlantic Fed was offered, it immediately filled with Writing Program students; a later course also filled within 2 weeks.

To return to Gramsci, the Syracuse University Transatlantic Fed members had found a seam within the Syracuse University curriculum that allowed topics of working-class identity and disability to become part of the offerings of an academic department. Within their limited power as 'professor' or 'student' legislators, changes had occurred into what would count as the 'normative representation' of what counted as acceptable academic study within our institution. Here connections could be made to Gramsci's conception of the intellectual: 'All men are intellectuals, but not all men have in society the function of intellectuals' (1971, p. 9). By drawing on the heritage of the FWWCP, students were using an alternative tradition by which to claim the role of intellectual within the confines of the Syracuse University classroom. It was student interest that allowed, for instance, a second Transatlantic Fed-focused writing course to be taught. Also, by the end of the second Transatlantic Fed class, when it became clear that traditional sources of university funding would be unable to continue the partnership with the FWWCP, Syracuse University student members of the Transatlantic Fed formed into a student group, accessing funding from student activities fees to support continued dialogue and partnership among working-class students in Syracuse University and FWWCP members.

While Clarke certainly participated in such work, there are other ways to map out her writing on to an attempt to alter the framework in which disability conversations occurred on campus. In one of her original posts, Clarke discussed what she perceived as the dissonance between public avowals of disability access and the actual physical layout of the campus. Throughout her time in the set of classes that made up the Transatlantic Fed project, Clarke took pictures documenting this contradiction. As the second class ended, Clarke worked with fellow students to create an online map where students could follow the daily hurdles she faced in navigating the campus. (As noted above, Clarke often makes use of a walker with wheels.) These pictures are then further contextualized by photos showing the economic and educational class divide between Syracuse University and the city of Syracuse. (For the initial writing by Clarke that helped to generate this project, use the web link at the end of the chapter.) Recognizing the need to allow others to participate, this online map can be amended and added to by those who visit the site. Finally, Transatlantic Fed members are working to take many of the images produced by Clarke and sponsor a gallery showing in the Syracuse University student centre. This event, to be sponsored by student and faculty disability organizations, will hopefully begin a larger discussion about issues of normality and class privilege with the university administration.

One way to conclude the Transatlantic Fed's legislative role at Syracuse University would be frame it around a final piece of writing done by Clarke, a piece performed at a community reading, featuring Syracuse University students, FWWCP members and Syracuse residents:

Silent no more
Once upon a time
I endured in silence
Told by others
'Stay silent'
'Don't talk'
'Shush'
'Shut up'
'Don't you dare cry'
'I don't want to hear it'
Silence was ingrained
Into my life
My personality
By endless repetition
As I grew older
I still found it hard
To talk freely
To share my ideas
My dreams
My ambitions
I found writing
Helped to free
What was locked
Deep inside
Waiting to be set free
My heart
My mind
My soul
No longer
Will I stay silent

Letting others
Decide whether I can
Have a say or not
I am in charge
Of my voice
Of my heart
I am no longer
Willing to be
Pushed into invisibility
Which is where
Silence leads to
For if we don't speak
We fade slowly
Into the background
We become forgotten
Like a half
Remembered dream
I am silent no more
My voice will be heard
Sometimes above the
Roars of the crowd
For I am silent
No More!

Before the Transatlantic Fed, the life of this poem would have been relatively easy to predict. Written for class, the poem might have been shared with other students, discussed as a personal statement of triumph, its metaphors or line structure discussed. It would have been seen, that is, as a personal narrative. Within the context of the Transatlantic Fed, however, the poem takes on, à la Gramsci, legislative intent. The poem is part of a larger effort to alter what is taught within the university and what voices are listened to within those university classrooms. Coupled with a student group, the poem intersects with larger issues of gaining the funds to enable self-representation and working-class collaboration. Finally, when placed within the context of gallery showings, the poem becomes a means by which to leverage the previous work of the FWWCP into ongoing collective efforts to make Syracuse University a more accessible and responsive campus to those with disabilities. In this way, Clarke's story becomes a vehicle to understanding the collective work necessary to alter Syracuse University's 'governance structure'.

But what about the FWWCP? Here the larger collective goals can be represented by following the efforts of Brendan Abel. The previous work demonstrated the ability of the Transatlantic Fed to use personal histories to produce collective (if limited) change within an institution. The FWWCP offered a different context for such work. First, the FWWCP has a long history of work with both personal narrative and issues of disability. One of its members, Survivors Poetry, has been producing writing and advocating on such issues for more than a decade. Within this environment, the Transatlantic Fed's work worked to organize and actualize in writing a more latent discussion – the goals of education. That is, since its conception, the FWWCP had been producing writing that focused on working-class experiences of education – marginalization, lack of resources and curricular bias (i.e. developing an occupational literacy; see Ch. 3, see also Ch. 5). As noted by Abel in his work producing the Transatlantic Fed performance piece, participants in the Transatlantic Fed had taken up this history, producing personal stories documenting their own educational experiences (see Ch. 1):

I was one of the 'scruffs'. I was pushed aside, left at the back, not included in discussions,
etc. in class. If I put my hand up to ask a question one certain teacher would give me a
withering look and tell me to put my hand down! When I did get to ask a question I was

usually told, 'Because I said so!' or 'Don't be stupid, girl!' I wasn't the only one, there were quite a few of us. So that kind of thing (class divide – no pun intended!) certainly did impinge on my education.

Even in the state-run (catholic-run) schools there were class divides also. I know I was one of the poorest ones, so I was the scruff, the thicko, the stupid one, whose parents couldn't afford the correct school uniform, I was poor, so, therefore I was stupid, etc., etc. [Even the school's head mistress], a nun, told me so quite often, usually when she was giving me 'six of the best' (a good whacking with a long cane on each of my hands).

Pat Smart

The strange thing is, somehow, I didn't realize that there would be so much of a class difference between me and other college students...age, yes, but not class.

I have to pass up on many opportunities here on campus because I either don't have the time, because I have to work so much, or else I don't have the money. For example, I simply cannot take an unpaid internship. I can't volunteer my time to anything. I simply must be paid, because I have no other source of income.

Joan DeArtemis

When performed at Syracuse University, the script produced a set of work around disability. When read at the FWWCP Festival of Writing in 2006, the same script produced an intense discussion of what should be the FWWCP's vision of educational equity. At a workshop the following day, formulated by Abel, Transatlantic Fed members, along with FWWCP participants, made use of their legislative roles and created the following educational manifesto, entitled *The Republic of Letters II*, positioning it as a sequel to Morley and Worpole's (1982) seminal publication on the goals of the FWWCP:

1. Education should teach a global humanity (not the humanities) based on an alternative sense of history and where cooperative values and restorative justice are primary.
2. Education should take place in a safe environment free from traditional social/economic biases with self-respect for each other as individuals as well as members of different classes, heritages and sexualities.
3. All educators must move from subconsciously teaching students to be a Westernized version of 'them' to teaching the essential equality among all individuals and cultures.
4. The conceptual equality taught to students must also be manifested in equal funding and equal access to well maintained school facilities.
5. To base an educational system on any other values [than these] accepts a fundamental inequity in society and acceptance that not all human potential will be fulfilled.

Coordinated by Abel, the work of the Transatlantic Fed has now turned to working collaboratively with members of Syracuse University, the city of Syracuse and the FWWCP member groups to produce a publication that will make clear the meaning and action to be taken in response to this educational manifesto – a publication that will no doubt begin in the personal and ultimately record case studies where collective working-class efforts have produced such change.

As stated at the outset, none of us is an occupational therapist. We would argue, however, that a project such as the Transatlantic Fed can demonstrate the importance of using writing to highlight the individual's collective identity as a latent community 'legislator' and to recognize the ability of collective action by such legislators to affect what counts as 'normative representation' within an institution or organization. Too often, we would argue, what goes for 'normal' is a restrictive and exclusionary concept and set of occupational practices – normal, that is, works both to deny resources to working-class communities and to deny the existence of those whose abilities do not fit into common definitions of normal (see Chs 1, 6, 13).

What should be the contours of this new normality? Perhaps listening and recording the voices of those most excluded from the current paradigm can provide an answer.

Acknowledgements

Submitted by Brendan Abel, Melodie Clarke and Steve Parks on behalf of the original Transatlantic Fed members: Lynn Ashburner (UK), Dave Chambers (UK), Eric Davidson (UK), Joan DeArtemis (USA), Tim Diggles (UK), Ann Lambie (UK), Rosie Lugosi (UK), Cathy Nicles (USA), Candra McKenzie (USA), Steve Oakley (UK), Nick Pollard (UK), Pat Smart (UK).

Further resources

For more detail on these experiences, see www.transatlanticfed.blogspot.com.

References

De Certeau M 1984 The practice of everyday life (trans SF Rendall). University of California Press, Berkeley, CA

Gramsci A 1971 Selections from the prison notebooks (trans/ed Q Hoare, G Smith). International Publishers, New York

Morley D, Worpole K 1982 The republic of letters. Comedia/MPG, London

Working with refugees and asylum seekers:
challenging occupational apartheid

15

Richard Davies

This paper is a personal commentary on the issues facing asylum seekers and refugees following their arrival in the UK. The national and local population of this group is described, followed by comments on the core qualities that make occupational therapists well situated to deal with the complexities associated with this work. The personal skills of listening and empathy are discussed, along with the appropriateness of occupation as a therapeutic medium. Finally the concept of occupational apartheid is discussed, as experienced by this group of clients with reference to their exclusion from particular occupations through their nationality and status in society.

The day service I work in serves a population of people aged 16 and upwards who are experiencing mental health problems in a major city in the north of England. Based in an economically disadvantaged area of the city, the area is culturally diverse and has long been home for people from a variety of ethnic origins. The day service has for some time attempted to engage creatively with hard to reach communities in its locality who have not accessed secondary services for a variety of reasons, not least of all the stigma associated in many communities with mental illness.

In response to this problem the day service has sourced community funds to appoint two workers, one Pakistani woman and one Yemeni man, to work with their respective lingual communities to improve mental health care provision in non-traditional settings. Called 'emotional wellbeing workers' to avoid the stigma often associated with mental health issues, the concept of *sukhoon*, meaning relief or inner peace in Urdu and Arabic, forms the focus of their interventions with their communities. They often work in community centres to identify individuals not currently accessing the health care system. This may be followed up by offering individual and group work in culturally appropriate ways. In this way they aim to engage meaningfully with the issues that people face in their respective Urdu- and Arabic-speaking communities.

Through this work and a wide range of other contacts the day service has been able to uncover previously unmet mental health needs. Consequently an increasing number of asylum seekers and refugees with occupational needs are being introduced into the service.

The local and national picture for asylum seekers and refugees

During recent years the numbers of asylum seekers coming to the UK increased from 26 205 asylum applications received by the UK Home Office in 1990 to a peak of 84 130 asylum applications in 2002 (Peach & Henson 2005). This figure fell dramatically to 25 710 in 2005 following a range of changes introduced by the UK government to reduce the number of asylum applications made by foreign nationals entering the country (Heath et al 2006).

The point of arrival for most asylum seekers is London and the ports on the south-east coast. This raised concerns about the pressures being placed on local services in these areas and the government responded by introducing a dispersal system in an attempt to relocate asylum seekers more equitably across a greater number of host cities. The system obliged asylum seekers to move to northern UK cities in order to continue receiving accommodation and support.

A specific terminology is used in the UK to describe those at various stages of the asylum system. A person whose asylum application has been successful and who has been offered indefinite leave to remain is described as a refugee. In 2005 only 7% of initial decisions granted refugee status, although a further 24% were allowed appeal or discretionary leave. Someone who has fled persecution and has applied for asylum but whose application is still being processed is described as an asylum seeker. For those whose asylum claim has been rejected the term 'failed asylum seeker' is most usually applied, although 'denied asylum seeker' and 'unsuccessful asylum seeker' may also be used. For the purpose of this piece the term 'denied asylum seeker' will be used, as the location of the marginalization is identified as systematic, that is within the structure of the asylum process rather than within the pathological agency of the individual.

The largest groups of asylum seekers in the city where the day service is based are Iranians, Iraqis, Somalis, Yemenis, Congolese and Afghans. In March 2005 the National Asylum Support Service, the part of the Home Office that offers support and accommodation to asylum seekers, supported 1450 asylum seekers from 56 different nationalities in the city. This probably underestimates the true number of asylum seekers in the city; many new arrivals may be supported by their family and friends who are already resident there. This is a common pattern of migration, where people often move along patterns initiated by 'bridgehead communities' who facilitate the settlement of other people from the same region to their host region.

In addition to this, a significant number of denied asylum seekers have not been successful in their application and have exhausted all rights of appeal. This population is not supported by the government and does not show up in National Asylum Support Service figures. A local asylum seeker charity estimates this population at around 1000 people who are receiving no help from the state and rely solely on support from friends and charities.

Asylum seekers and refugees have been located in many areas around the city and the ethnically diverse area where the day service is located was identified as one of a number of appropriate locations for refugees and asylum seekers to be relocated into. This places the day service at the centre of a large population of occupationally disadvantaged individuals who have difficulty accessing traditional routes to social inclusion.

Working with individual experience

Whiteford (2004) details the experiences of Maria, a Bosnian woman, as a refugee in Australia and highlights the challenges she faced as she sought to engage in occupations in order to recreate a life in a new country with her two young daughters. Difficulties included:

- isolation through lack of language competence
- reduced opportunities to participate in leisure and work because of language difficulties and financial status

* difficulties in maintaining a habitual routine in an unfamiliar environment
* loss of family for practical and emotional support
* loss of sense of 'connectedness' to others in the community because of a contrast between the social and physical environment of the country of origin and the host country.

The difficulties encountered by Maria are familiar to the client population I work with in the UK. Similarly, some of the occupationally focused interventions she identifies are familiar. 'Facilitating community and social participation through the use of pre-existing structures and facilities' (Whiteford 2004, p. 196) is possible by linking people into a diverse range of activities, from groups offering community walking programmes or community vegetable gardening to a local employment project for refugees.

Additionally the bureaucracy of the asylum system impacts upon the occupational life of the asylum seeker, as Helen Claire Smith (2005, p. 474) has identified: 'Asylum, and the long wait for approval, is a dehumanizing process forcing people into an apathetic and passive position. Occupationally speaking it is a disaster. Individuals are not permitted to work and often find it difficult to integrate into an unwelcoming society.' An additional irony is that much of this population has skills that the economy needs. A spokesperson from a non-governmental organization, the National Institute of Adult Continuing Education (2001, p. 1) has commented: 'asylum seekers may have skills, qualifications and qualities which are needed in the UK and in the local economy'.

Smith (2005) sees her role as working with the drive and abilities of individuals who have demonstrated great resilience and resourcefulness in seeking a better life. However, she has identified one important structural barrier for refugees in that the government places restrictions on those individuals' occupational activity.

Currently asylum seekers in the UK are denied access to paid work, which in itself would be an important therapeutic tool in developing feelings of self-worth and promoting good mental health within the asylum seeker community. In a briefing paper, the Refugee Council (2007, p. 6–7) states: '[B]eing able to get a job opens up many more opportunities. There is potential to meet a wider range of people and experience different working environments... It will help lift people out of poverty, gain greater self respect and help regenerate their neighbourhoods. It is what asylum seekers want.'

How is it possible for a therapist to maintain a positive outlook in the face of such bureaucratic intransigence when people are prevented from working? In short, it makes the job more difficult but not impossible. As Smith says:

Start by remembering that many of the issues that we face when helping refugees are not really new to us. It is easy to see all the differences and forget what is common to us all. Use your everyday helping skills: listening, demonstrating respect and seeing the client as an individual with a unique identity and aspirations. Our clients are searching for empathy more than an answer to their complex problems and needs.

Smith 2005, p. 475

In this I am reminded of a recent discussion I had in my car with a client I shall call Patrice. He is deeply traumatized by events in Africa where he was a teacher and a peaceful member of a political group who opposed the government. His trauma began 4 years ago when government soldiers forced their way in to his home and arrested him in front of his pregnant wife. They took him to a prison where he was tortured and sentenced to death. He managed to escape and fled to the UK but does not know whether his wife and child are still alive. His first asylum application has failed and at the time of writing he is appealing the decision.

When I first met Patrice he was deeply traumatized by this experience coupled with the trauma of his subsequent flight from his country of origin and the treatment he has received from the bureaucratic machinations of the asylum system. He was silent or mumbled monosyllables, eyes and head averted downwards, shaking and rocking backwards and forwards in his chair. Over the weeks and months he became engaged in occupations and made friends and relationships with people attending the day service.

In the car, Patrice told me he was 'happy' when I saw him because I listened to him. 'Some people they don't listen, but you listen.' I was struck by the simplicity of the thing that he found valuable about our work together. Although the aims of my intervention with Patrice focused on his occupations, it was easy to forget the importance of developing occupational building blocks through the simple act of being respectful.

At the day service, Patrice has worked with us to increase his occupational participation through gardening, walking groups and volunteer opportunities within the grounds of the building. Certainly we have discussed his symptoms and how activity can reduce the frequency, intensity and duration of his fragmented intrusive thoughts, and how he sleeps better at night after exercise. However, he talks about gardening as important to him in other ways. He says his world is fragmented and shattered (Medical Foundation for the Care of Victims of Torture 2006), he does not know whether his wife and child are alive or indeed if his child was ever born. He lives with the uncertainty every day that he may be deported back to what he sees in his mind as a repeat of the incarceration, torture and death sentence he has endured already.

Patrice's experiences are splintered, fragmented and disorganized as he goes through a daily round of confused and frightening thoughts that intensify, particularly during the night. Patrice is, however, afforded some relief by the regular activity of allotment gardening that is carried out in partnership with a local organic growing project. He told me how important the activity is to him as it introduces a sense of order into his life through the natural rhythms of the activity. These include the regular meetings he has with people he can trust, looking forward to and anticipating the enjoyment he expects to experience as a result of being with them. He describes the orderliness of the growing process: the systematic planning of crops, sowing seed and then cultivating the crop – lining plants out in rows and ordered beds, followed by harvest and eating the resulting produce. All of this is in contrast to the turmoil he has come to expect as a daily experience. The activity enables him to feel a sense of order in at least one part of his life and he can relate the activity to when he grew crops at home, in happier times.

In this observation I am reminded of Ann Wilcock's description of 'doing, being and becoming' (1998, p. 248). While doing the activity he is reflecting and understanding how the vegetable garden is meeting his needs for order and his sense of being. It is a process in which he feels he is becoming a different person.

Approaching structural boundaries

Prior to July 2002, asylum seekers who had been waiting for longer than 6 months for their appeals were allowed to apply for permission to work. The government revoked this right for two reasons. First, they claimed that asylum decisions were being processed within the 6-month window, and second, they felt that the system could be abused by people whose sole aim was to gain employment in the UK job market (Refugee Council 2007).

In relation to the first claim, the reality for many people is that, even when an initial decision is received relatively quickly, subsequent legal processes may take longer than the time frame quoted by the Home Office (Refugee Council 2007).

No evidence exists that the second claim is the case and Bloch, referring to Home Office research, states that denying permission to work to asylum seekers persists 'despite the absence of any evidence that access to welfare benefits or employment are significant "pull"' factors influencing the decisions of asylum seekers (Bloch 2004, p. 9).

Patrice and others like him are experiencing occupational apartheid (Kronenberg & Pollard 2005; see Ch. 4) imposed upon them by their status as asylum seekers. Although he is forced to accept £38 per week, 30% less than the minimum the government say a single person should live on, he is unable to work legally to improve his living conditions. Clearly, living in poverty will substantially increase an individual's chance of suffering poor health and will contribute to making pre-existing conditions worse, as well as contributing to new conditions of ill-health. However the occupational injustice of this system needs to be addressed as well as the clinical considerations.

A report commissioned by Refugee Action (Dumper et al 2006) researched the experiences of denied asylum seekers and revealed that most people interviewed who talked about work stated that they did not want to work simply for more money but emphasized work as a means to support themselves for reasons of dignity, pride, independence and self-esteem. This clearly involves a role for occupational therapy in engaging individuals in work to improve their health and well-being. 'Dignity, as created through the opportunity to interact with the world in a meaningful way through living diverse occupational lives, not just those focused on material gain' (Whiteford 2000, p. 204).

Unfortunately an already complex situation is made more difficult when attempting to address the needs of denied asylum seekers. For those whose asylum claim and subsequent appeal has been denied, access to food and housing support is available under section 4 of the Asylum and Immigration Act 2004. However, in order to access this support, denied asylum seekers must agree to return to their country of origin.

Many denied asylum seekers are unable to return home; for example, without travel documents a country may not accept that the individual is a national of their country, particularly if they have a dissident history. Many asylum seekers feel that a return to their country of origin is unacceptable as a safe route to return may be unavailable to them and to acquiesce to going back would in effect be signing their own death warrant. Many people claim that their asylum application has been processed unjustly. The experience of Patrice, outlined above, is just one example of many.

A letter to *The Times* newspaper in 2005 from the Right Reverend Dr John Sentamu, Archbishop of York, and seven Church of England Bishops began the 'Living Ghosts' campaign. This aims to improve living conditions for denied asylum seekers through restoring the right to paid work or receipt of benefits until the time of removal. In the letter they stated:

> [I]t is inhuman and unacceptable that some people seeking asylum are left homeless and destitute by government policies... As a society we have international and legal responsibilities to welcome those fleeing adversity from other parts of the world and provide social security. But the threat of destitution is being used as a way of pressuring refused asylum seekers to leave the country.

The government reject the claim that their policies make people destitute. Immigration Minister Tony McNulty stated: 'It is apparent that many unsuccessful asylum seekers who have exhausted all rights of appeal choose not to access support from central government. Instead, we hear that they are destitute or living on food parcels' (*The Guardian*, 9 January 2006).

Whichever way you view it, the reality for many people is that their already meagre financial and social support is taken away. Amnesty International commissioned a report entitled *Down and Out in London*, which details the conditions destitute denied asylum seekers live in. Government policies again are challenged as the report suggests that the 'very aim of the Home Office policy is to make rejected asylum seekers destitute to force them to go home' (Amnesty International 2006, p. 6).

Money is withdrawn for food, shelter and anything else we would expect in order to live in dignity. Many people sleep rough on the streets or on a friend's floor. Being denied government support, asylum seekers are refused health care unless that person can pay impossibly high bills, which may be many thousands of pounds. Examples are numerous from across the range of health services. The Refugee Council describe how they have worked with 17 women denied access to maternity care. One woman, whom they named C:

> gave birth in hospital, and her baby was admitted to the special care unit after birth. C was invoiced £3024 in maternity costs, an amount she was wholly unable to pay. She then refused to attend follow up checks with her baby because of her fear of the debt collectors, and that the hospital would use the appointment as a way to deport her.

Kelly & Stevenson 2006, p. 11.

There are exceptions for free emergency care, for example detention under the mental health act or life-threatening care upon admission to an accident and emergency (A&E) unit. This has led to some dire situations. One Arab man with bowel cancer was admitted to A&E with uncontrolled bleeding. He was scheduled for an operation once the bleeding had stopped. However, he was discovered to be a denied asylum seeker and was informed that the operation he needed had been cancelled as he could not settle the bill for many thousands of pounds. He was asked instead to present himself to A&E again 'when his condition deteriorates' (Kelly & Stevenson 2006, p. 12).

This places a dilemma in front of the health care professional who can see the needs of a potential patient but is prevented from working with that individual because of the denied asylum seeker's status in society. Not only does it involve a risk of disciplinary action for the worker but also places the client at risk of being pursued with a bill potentially for thousands of pounds. The Refugee Council has identified instances where clients have received letters from hospital trusts demanding payment for care. One example reads 'failure to respond to this letter will result in this matter being transferred to [debt collection agency], who will take all necessary steps including litigation to recover this debt' (Kelly & Stevenson 2006, p. 15). Mistakes can also occur. I have experience of one client who was billed for an investigation into a suspected heart condition, despite his asylum claim still being at the appeal stage.

Common sense suggests that these bills cannot be paid when the person in receipt of the health care is destitute. However, for someone fleeing from a country where officialdom is seen as oppressive, the fear of debt can only add to the mental ill-health of an individual (Kelly & Stevenson 2006). The first principle of medical ethics and professional codes of conduct, *primum non nocere* – 'first, do no harm' – appears to be particularly relevant to this issue.

So what can be done? Whiteford (2004) describes four responses to addressing the longer-term needs of refugees from an occupational perspective as researcher, advocate, educator and lobbyist. With regard to the first of these, a growing body of research is beginning to emerge. In the UK Helen Claire Smith is particularly involved in researching and reporting on refugee issues (2005).

At the day service, advocacy for denied asylum seekers is developed by forming alliances with those they are in touch with in the community. Prevented from offering help to denied asylum seekers directly, we seek to assist in ways that support those groups that are not under the same legal restraints as ourselves. This includes offering mental health support and advice to workers from local churches or community organizations who are working with this group of people. The first thing to acknowledge to those we work with is that we do not know all the answers but we may be able to work together to identify ways of working with the community that can help to reduce the occupational deprivation that people may be experiencing and to enable people to live more fulfilling occupational lives. We offer a community space to local community groups with a health focus to meet; this is free of charge and can be accessed by refugees or asylum seeker groups, destitute or not.

Education through mental health awareness training for community workers is a valuable way of supporting those who are able to offer support directly to denied asylum seekers. Church groups, outreach workers and cultural projects have received training in our local geographical area. As part of that process, ongoing supervision from the day service team to support individual community workers and volunteers is valuable for the development of strong community links.

Lobbying decision-makers is both a personal duty and a societal responsibility (see Chs 1, 4). Influencing policy at a local level may appear trivial but, by acting locally and thinking globally, real change can be achieved if enough people are prepared to take action. Joining Amnesty International and the Refugee Council's Just Fair campaign are ways in which individuals can make a real difference to people's lives through submitting correspondence to key players in the decision-making processes.

Conclusion

When working with asylum seekers and refugees it is of course paramount to work with the spirit of the individual, which has enabled them to overcome privations most of us will never have to endure (Smith 2005). This chapter has offered some examples of how the day service I work at has begun to engage more meaningfully with this client group through awareness of these external constraints, which are political in their origin and implementation. Within these constraints there are opportunities to work meaningfully with asylum seekers' and refugees' aspirations. We can begin to dismantle the occupational deprivation experienced by our clients through engaging in appropriate occupational forms. This may be through assisting with orienting to a new environment or reintroducing valued roles into daily activity. Where marginalization is the result of systematic exclusion from services we can work with those who are able to help by supporting the supporters. Most of all we can help by listening closely to those who have the greatest expertise in this complex area and who demonstrate the greatest strength of all, the clients themselves.

References

Amnesty International 2006 Down and out in London: the road to destitution for rejected asylum seekers. Amnesty International. London. Available online at: http://www.amnesty.org.uk/uploads/documents/doc_17382.pdf; accessed 19 October 2007

Bloch A, 2004 Making it work. Asylum and migration. Working paper 2. Institute for Public Policy Research, London

Dumper H, Hutton C, Lukes S 2006 The destitution trap: research into destitution among refused asylum seekers in the UK. Refugee Action Report. Amnesty International, London. Available online at: http://www.amnesty.org.uk/uploads/documents/doc_17360.pdf; accessed 19 October 2007

Heath T, Jeffries R, Pearce S 2006 Asylum statistics United Kingdom 2005. Available online at: http://www.homeoffice.gov.uk/rds/pdfs06/hosb1406.pdf; accessed 26 November 2006

Kelly N, Stevenson J 2006 First do no harm: denying healthcare to people whose asylum claims have failed. Refugee Council Report. Refugee Council, London. Available online at: http://www.refugeecouncil.org.uk/policy/position/2006/healthcare.htm; accessed 13 February 2008

Kronenberg F, Pollard N 2005 Overcoming occupational apartheid, a preliminary exploration of the political nature of occupational therapy. In: Kronenberg F, Simó Algado S, Pollard N (eds) Occupational therapy without borders: learning from the spirit of survivors. Elsevier Churchill Livingstone, Edinburgh: p 58–86

Medical Foundation for the Care of Victims of Torture 2006 Suicide in asylum seekers and refugees. Medical Foundation for the Care of Victims of Torture. London. Available online at: http://www.torturecare.org.uk/files/brief29.rtf; accessed 30 November 2006

National Institute of Adult Continuing Education 2001 Asylum seekers and adult learning: dispelling the myths. NIACE, Leicester. Available online at: http://www.niace.org.uk/projects/Asylum; accessed 19 October 2007

Peach E, Henson R 2005 ICAR statistics paper. Key statistics about asylum seeker arrivals in the UK. Information Centre about Asylum and Refugees in the UK, London. Available online at http://www.icar.org.uk/download.php?id=76; accessed 26 November 2006

Refugee Council 2007 Briefing paper: Social exclusion, refugee integration, and the right to work for asylum seekers. Refugee Council, London. Available online at: http://www.refugeecouncil.org.uk/NR/rdonlyres/6F10BF62-B164-4D81-BA34-CE85797AB857/0/RightToWorkJuly2007.pdf; accessed 29 October 2007

Sentamu J 2005 Letter. The Times 3 December

Smith H C 2005 Feel the fear and do it anyway: meeting the occupational needs of refugees and people seeking asylum. British Journal of Occupational Therapy 68: 474–476

Whiteford G 2000 Occupational deprivation: global challenge in the new millennium. British Journal of Occupational Therapy 63: 200–204

Whiteford G 2004 Occupational issues of refugees. In: Molineux M (ed) Occupation for occupational therapists. Blackwell, Oxford: p 183–199

Wilcock A 1998 Reflections on doing, being and becoming. Canadian Journal of Occupational Therapy 65: 248–256

Illustrating occupational needs of refugees

16

Clarissa Wilson

> *It isn't for the moment that you are struck that you need courage, but for the long uphill climb back to sanity and faith and security.*
>
> Anne Morrow Lindbergh

No one chooses to be a refugee (Office of the High Commissioner for Human Rights 2007). Refugees are ordinary people with long stories (Fine 1991). Escaping danger is the first of many challenges. To survive, they must navigate a new culture, language, set of life skills and, sometimes, occupational deprivation (Whiteford 2005). Amid occupational chaos, refugees adapt to lost life roles, new life roles and drastically changed life roles (Driver & Beltran 1998). Consider Nada's story:

> *Nada escapes after her husband was killed. She arrives in a crowded refugee camp and still has flashbacks to the dangerous journey. Daily camp existence is precarious. The perpetual limbo of not knowing, not being able to influence when it ends is grinding. The disabling effects of occupational deprivation while being 'warehoused' for 12 years accumulate. Her child can't remember anything else. Once finally safe in a settlement country, she has new roles as a head of house, language student and money manager. She has lost roles in community, family and religious activities. She has drastically changed roles as a provider of food, health and parenting.*

Refugees are not inherently disabled or diseased (Schwartzman et al 2006). Nada will intuitively press on towards occupational performance and well-being (Wilcock 1993, Lentin 2002). Yet healing and community reintegration may stall with mounting occupational problems. Personal and occupational problems (e.g. trauma and new life skills) are likely to be compounded and perhaps overshadowed by environmental problems (e.g. politics of poverty, restrictive visas, cultural accessibility of services, community discrimination, etc.) (Whiteford 2000, Drexler 2005). Nada soon finds herself trapped and treading water in an occupational void of disruption, dysfunction and deprivation. These occupational problems perpetuate 'refugee-ism' long past the initial trauma, haunting and undermining her recovery.

Perhaps settled refugees or church groups could help. Perhaps professionals such as trauma counsellors could help. But what happens when the primary issues are occupational in nature (Yerxa 1993)? What happens when community and professional intuition is not enough? When navigating the variables to create and enable occupational opportunities is so complex that the helping community and professionals are equally stuck?

Occupational therapists have long enabled life skills for new life roles through redesigning and recycling occupations after lost life roles. Occupational therapists have long been facilitating the person, occupation and environment to promote occupational performance and well-being (Polatajko 2001). Our mandate of creating and enabling occupational opportunities is not limited to disability or disease (Gray 1998). Our profession exists to enable occupationally well people and occupationally just societies (Kronenberg et al 2005). Occupational Opportunities for Refugees and Asylum Seekers (OOFRAS) exists to help our profession uphold its mandate with refugees (Smith 2005).

Illustrating occupational opportunities for refugees and asylum seekers

Never doubt that a small group of thoughtful, committed citizens can change the world; indeed, it's the only thing that ever has.

Margaret Mead

Following Gail Whiteford's paper on the occupational deprivation of refugees and asylum seekers at the 2003 OT Australia conference in Melbourne, I asked: 'How has the profession responded to these occupational needs?'. Other than individual, isolated and ad hoc initiatives, there was no visible professional response. Questions are political, always personal and quite possibly costly (Peavey 1997). You pay the price of responding to something you may prefer to un-know, or you pay the price of bearing your personal and professional incongruence.

So, I wrote a position paper outlining occupation as a human right, even for refugees (Wilson 2003). Vigorous conversations ensued. I was told that the profession did have an obligation to respond but was 'not ready'. In all likelihood, it would not respond even if the Department of Immigration directly asked for occupational therapists.

Follow-up conversations with occupational therapists refined these impressions. Occupational therapists felt overwhelmed – what can one therapist do? Some felt lost – where and how to begin? Others felt unprepared – what do I need to know? And they felt alone – where can I go for support? So OOFRAS was born to inspire, empower and equip occupational therapists for refugee initiatives.

OOFRAS is an extraordinary community comprised of ordinary occupational therapists and students. It is not a product, a process, a programme, or a place – but a people. We work together to see the occupational needs of refugees and asylum seekers addressed. OOFRAS is visible as the sum of a global infrastructure and local initiatives. Globally, the collaborative operates through the website (Occupational Opportunities for Refugees and Asylum Seekers 2007). Local networks, refugee initiatives and OOFRAS groups emerge according to local interest, intention, availability, skill and experience.

The coordination team is comprised of five Australian occupational therapists who voluntarily serve and lead the collaborative: Sally Datson, Jessica Leggatt, Crissy Hubbard, Linda Rylands and Clarissa Wilson. There are no official resources, assets or funding. Our resources are relationships. Our assets are divine synergy and the willingness to give things a go. Our funding is of the 'just enough, just in time' variety. We set things like the website, scholarship, printed resources, fundraising and student projects in motion, trusting that the funding will somehow follow. And it has.

OOFRAS focuses on capacity building within two domains: individual occupational therapists and the occupational therapy profession. Our 'inspire, empower, equip, initiate' anthem guides how we provide ideas, knowledge, skills and initiative opportunities to individuals at different stages of readiness. Our 'research, education, capacity building, systemic advocacy, direct services' anthem guides initiatives to build a robust field of practice to support individual action (Wilson 2006).

We started with a clear idea of where we wanted to go, but had no idea about how to get there. We started with raw enthusiasm, but no more than naive political intuition. But that's OK (Bornstein 2004). Where would the world be if no one did anything till they knew what they were doing (Sloane 1976)?

Illustrating political engagement

Nobody made a greater mistake than he who did nothing because he could only do a little.

Edmund Burke

Like other grand notions, 'politics' sounds ethereal, sophisticated and almost glamorous. Who, me? No, not for the likes of the ordinary, the mundane, the practical, the plebs like me with bills to pay (Griffin 2001).

This vague, self-limiting notion is merely a murky fog obscuring the dazzling power and responsibility we each possess (Thibeault 2006). However, sentiments about dazzling power are feeble, futile and bordering on the fictitious until power can be experientially discovered, lived, tested and known (Dees et al 2002).

OOFRAS is an opportunity to experience vicariously, then to live, test and know the gravity of and delight in our power. We know any dream we can accomplish on our own is tragically small. So politics is inseparable from community. The allure of a handful of painfully ordinary occupational therapists becoming politically charged can arouse others to the stunning power of their personal choices in ordinary situations. This process is confronting and anything but ordinary.

A sample of past OOFRAS initiatives demonstrate that there are many grooves. If you can't find one, you have permission to make one! These initiatives apply for political engagement in most areas. Examples include:

* Social initiatives like BBQs with refugees, refugee church, multicultural festivals
* Writing initiatives like position papers, newsletters and website pages
* Catalyst initiatives like calling for others to join OOFRAS groups and listserves
* Research initiatives like conducting an occupational needs analysis, survey of local services to understand gaps in funding and services
* Network initiatives like conference workshops, posters, papers, resources and display tables
* Educational initiatives like guest lectures, coordinating student fieldwork and projects
* Professional development initiatives like transcultural mental health, legal system, trauma recovery training
* Resource development initiatives like brochures, fact sheets, booklets and orientation packs
* Mentoring initiatives like offering to support an individual or to be an ally to a local OOFRAS group
* Fundraising initiatives like doing a T-shirt rally in your own area or hosting an event
* Supporting initiatives like buying a T-shirt or forwarding on information to others.

You get the idea – there are many opportunities to participate!

Participation sparks self-perpetuating momentum and synergy (Townsend 1999). In the past, we generated initiatives, now we also respond to and with initiatives of others by speaking at occupational therapy lectures and multidisciplinary panels, invitations to explore occupational therapy roles in refugee transition schools or writing media releases. We also see evidence of changed lives changing lives when practising therapists who encountered OOFRAS for a student project reconnect later to get politically engaged at another level.

The cost of *not* investing in community and doing ad hoc, grass-roots refugee initiatives is evidenced by lack of political impact, coordination, efficient support and representation.

So here is your invitation. We invite occupational therapists to consider three simple steps: find an opportunity that suits, find local synergy and find a way to invest your experience back into the community. Talk with other OOFRAS therapists, browse the 'what can I do' web pages for opportunity ideas. The coordination team can help get the word out so you can find local synergy. The essence is to do *something* and to do it *together*.

So be assured, politics is not otherworldly, its implications are so very tangible. It's not limited to the sophisticates, it's for anyone who cares enough to ask: 'How could this work?'. It's not glamorous, it's gritty, tedious and costly. It isn't enshrined in lofty pontifications, it's situated in the practicalities and logistics of action. It's not for the complacent, it usually requires personal changes to how we invest time and energy. While we would welcome companions for the OOFRAS journey, it would be even more exciting to see all types of therapist together embracing the political as personal – right where they are at. To commend occupational opportunity as a human right, we need to cherish it through the mundane political happenings all around us.

Resources to get you started

Refugee focus

United Nations High Commissioner for Refugees (UNHCR): www.unhcr.org

European Council on Refugees and Exiles (ECRE): www.ecre.org

Refugees International: www.refugeesinternational.org

Harvard Program in Refugee Trauma: www.hprt-cambridge.org/index.html

Researchers for Asylum Seekers: http://www.ras.unimelb.edu.au/

Amnesty International: www.amnesty.org

Occupational focus

Occupational Opportunities for Refugees and Asylum Seekers (OOFRAS): www.oofras.com

Occupational Therapy International Outreach Network (OTION): www.wfot.org

Kronenberg F, Simó Algado S, Pollard N (eds) 2005 Occupational therapy without borders: learning from the spirit of survivors. Elsevier/Churchill Livingstone, Edinburgh

References

Bornstein D 2004 How to change the world: social entrepreneurs and the power of new ideas. Oxford University Press, New York

Dees J, Emerson J, Economy P 2002 Strategic tools for social entrepreneurs: enhancing the performance of your enterprising nonprofit. John Wiley, Chichester

Drexler M 2005 Health disparities and the body politic. Harvard School of Public Health, Boston, MA. Available online at: http://www.hsph.harvard.edu/disparities/book; accessed 16 February 2007

Driver C, Beltran R 1998 Impact of refugee trauma on children's occupational role as school students. Australian Occupational Therapy Journal 45: 23–38

Fine S 1991 Eleanor Clarke Slagle Lecture: Resilience and human adaptability; who rises above adversity? American Occupational Therapy Journal 45: 493–503

Gray J 1998 Putting occupation into practice: occupational as ends, occupation as means. American Journal of Occupational Therapy 52: 354–364

Griffin S 2001 Occupational therapy and the concept of power: a review of the literature. Australian Occupational Therapy Journal 48: 24–34

Kronenberg F, Simó Algado S, Pollard N 2005 Occupational therapy without borders: learning from the spirit of survivors. Elsevier/Churchill Livingstone, Edinburgh

Lentin P 2002 The human spirit and occupation: surviving and creating a life. Journal of Occupational Science 9: 143–152

Occupational Opportunities for Refugees and Asylum Seekers 2007 Website. Available online at: http://www.oofras.com; accessed 16 February 2007

Office of the High Commissioner for Human Rights 2007 Human rights and refugees: fact sheet 20. Office of the High Commissioner for Human Rights, United Nations, Geneva. Available online at: http://www.unhchr.ch/html/menu6/2/fs20.htm; accessed 16 February 2007

Peavey F 1997 Strategic questioning: an approach to creating personal and social change. Jobs Research Trust, New Plymouth, Taranaki, New Zealand. Available online at: http://www.jobsletter.org.nz/pdf/stratq97.pdf; accessed 16 February 2007

Polatajko H 2001 The evolution of our occupational perspective: the journey from diversion through therapeutic use to enablement. Canadian Journal of Occupational Therapy 68: 203–207

Schwartzman A, Atler K, Borg B, Schwartzman R 2006 Fueling the engines: a role for occupational therapists in promoting healthy life transitions. Occupational Therapy in Health Care 20: 39–59

Sloane J 1976 Sylvia Docker Lecture: After the pioneers. Australian Occupational Therapy Journal 23: 7–19

Smith H 2005 'Feel the fear and do it anyway': meeting the occupational needs of refugees and people seeking asylum. British Journal of Occupational Therapy 68: 474–476

Thibeault R 2006 Globalisation, universities and the future of occupational therapy: dispatches for the majority world. Australian Occupational Therapy Journal 53: 159–165

Townsend E 1999 Enabling occupation in the 21st century: making good intentions a reality. Australian Occupational Therapy Journal 46: 147–159

Whiteford G 2000 Occupational deprivation: global challenge in the new millennium. British Journal of Occupational Therapy 63: 200–204

Whiteford G 2005 Understanding the occupational deprivation of refugees: a case study from Kosovo. Canadian Journal of Occupational Therapy 77: 78–88

Wilcock A 1993 A theory for the human need for occupation. Journal of Occupational Science Australia 1: 17–24

Wilson C 2003 Position statement and challenge to occupational therapists. OOFRAS, Kenmore, Queensland. Available online at: http://www.oofras.com/index.php?snap_cms/displayTemplate&t=editable/About_Us; accessed 16 February 2007

Wilson C 2006 The idiOTs guide to working with refugees. Clarissa Wilson, Melbourne, Victoria

Yerxa E 1993 Occupational science: a new source of power for participants in occupational therapy. Occupational Science Australia 1: 3–10

Reflections on working with south Sudanese refugees in settlement and capacity building in regional Australia

17

Andrina Mitchell

This chapter uses the experiences of an occupational therapist working with Sudanese refugees as a case study illustrating how occupational therapy skills can be used in the settlement process on both an individual level and in capacity building with whole communities. The following is an overview of the two diverse roles that the therapist played, a description of the specific refugee community and a discussion of the challenges faced concerning:

- acculturation
- intercultural awareness
- the barriers to engagement
- professional self-care and burnout.

Roles

The occupational therapist was employed by local government in two separate roles. Firstly, she acted as a case manager for newly arrived refugee entrants for the first 6 months after arrival. Through this federally funded programme, entrants arrived under the Special Humanitarian Program, meaning that the refugee entrants had been sponsored by Sudanese family or friends already settled in Australia. Generally, the new arrivals lived with their sponsor for the first 3–6 months to adjust and to pay back the debts incurred in the immigration process.

Settlement issues and living skills were addressed jointly by the Special Humanitarian Program sponsors and case manager. Typically, sponsors saw it as their responsibility to orientate the new arrivals to Australian culture; however, this created some problems as their level of understanding was not always as comprehensive as they believed it to be. Areas of priority in this role included access to services (health, education, children's services and financial assistance), securing housing, the provision of a culturally appropriate household goods package and undertaking relevant life skills training (tenancy, budgeting, public transport, etc.). Secondly, through state government funding, the occupational therapist was employed as a community consultant as part of a pilot project which sought to build the capacity of emerging refugee communities. The outcomes of this position were to:

- enhance refugee community self-determination and governance skills through mentoring/training
- develop the leadership capacity of women and youth

- empower the community to support new arrivals in settlement
- become financially self-sustaining through engaging mentors to support them in applying for/managing grants and setting up community enterprises.

The key performance indicators (KPIs) of both programmes were specific in outcomes, time lines, brokerage funds management and reporting requirements.

In addition to these tasks, roles also involved:

- instigating and facilitating monthly case coordination meetings with the relevant key service providers. Issues around privacy, confidentiality and informed consent with clients had to be resolved. These meetings were essential for peer support, identifying and addressing gaps in service delivery, and allowing for strategic future planning with joint funding applications
- developing, implementing and supervising a volunteer training programme
- advocating for the refugee community at a local level, for example with real estate agents, who went from reluctant participants to eventually become champions of the programme
- assisting the Sudanese community to advocate for themselves and to become cultural consultants around programme development, particularly in relation to children's services and legal issues
- lobbying, in conjunction with service providers and the Sudanese community, for changes to the current funding arrangements around service provision.

The refugee community and the local community

The local south Sudanese refugee community was diverse, made up of about 90 to 95 individuals, with more than half of them less than 12 years old. The ethnic mix was made up of five main tribes (Azande, Chollo, Nuer, Nuba and Dinka), with a roughly equal mix of Christians and Muslims. Originally, 11 Sudanese families chose to relocate from the state's capital city to this regional town of 30 000 people. All had been in Australia for 2–3 years, spoke functional English, had car licences and were ready for work. Of the original families, eight remained after 18 months. They, in turn, sponsored another 11 families, couples and individuals. Developing language proficiency was the main focus of this group's initial settlement period.

In addition to the core Sudanese community, there were also about 10 to 20 transient members, mostly youth, who worked at the local abattoir when they could and then disappeared back to the city for months on end. These individuals were harder to engage with, as they were relatively disconnected from the larger Sudanese community, generally ignoring the elders and demonstrating their own set of values, beliefs and behaviours. Their occasional antisocial behaviour was strongly disapproved of by the Sudanese community as it went against their cultural norms and was particularly detrimental to their reputation.

It should be noted that the host township was extraordinarily homogeneous as a group before the Sudanese arrived, with 97% coming from a Christian, English or Irish background – 1% Aboriginal, 2% European and Asian backgrounds (Department of Sustainability and Environment 2001).

Acculturation

Acculturation is a predictable settlement process that migrants and refugees move through where contact is made, cultural values are compared and the new culture is totally or partially accepted or rejected (Fig. 17.1). In true acculturation, both cultures are changed as a result of the interaction.

In regard to refugee health, better outcomes are seen in those who become integrated or assimilated into the new culture (Plavsic 2002). Turner (2003) reinforces the importance of acknowledging this process by stating that 'the question of utmost importance to the health

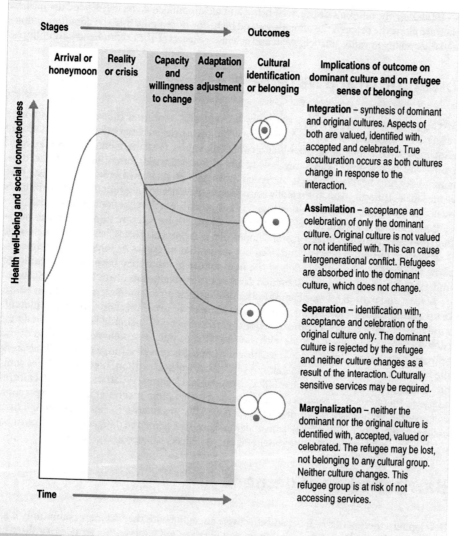

Figure 17.1 Stages, outcomes and implications of the acculturation process.
Source: adapted from Berry et al 1986, as cited in Culhane 2004.

worker here is "where is the client in the acculturation continuum/journey?"'. Typically, the new arrival will pass from initial optimism and hope to a crisis, often brought on through difficulties with language, finances or not understanding the new culture. At this point, depending upon their capacity and willingness to change or adapt, the refugee will take one of four paths, becoming integrated, assimilated, separated or marginalized (Berry 1998, cited in Culhane 2004).

Factors that influence these divergent paths include:

* the level of choice in the migration process
* ease of language acquisition
* feelings of belongingness
* cultural similarities and understanding
* occupational opportunities
* prior experiences of torture and trauma
* openness to change
* experiences of acceptance or discrimination in the new culture.

Ultimately, the refugee's health, well-being and social connectedness will depend upon where they are along the process, the acceptance and inclusion of diversity into the dominant culture and their ability to value, participate in and celebrate aspects of the original and new cultures.

Intercultural awareness

Working with refugees requires a degree of intercultural awareness that results from honest reflection of the therapist's own culture and a willingness to learn about other cultures. Cultural contemplation can include an examination of beliefs, values, customs, technology, gender roles, spirituality, taboos, world views, mythology and attitudes towards family, independence, time, community and health. Through increased awareness of their own culture, therapists may reduce their ethnocentrism, the usually unconscious tendency to judge another culture by one's own, usually with the presupposition that one's own culture is the superior or correct one.

Both the host and refugee cultures can experience ethnocentrism; interactions are therefore most effective when intercultural competence is reciprocal. This is generally seen at stage 3 of the acculturation process and does not mean that migrants or refugees should necessarily take on the values and beliefs of the new culture but that they have the opportunity to understand the new cultural system and draw realistic conclusions about how to navigate it.

Respect and trust in refugee communities take time for professionals to earn but can be lost in an instant through an unintended cultural blunder. To avoid this and assist with intercultural awareness, a range of cultural advisors is recommended. It should be remembered that each of these individuals will come with their own issues, agendas, prejudices, allegiances and refugee experiences. Therefore, it is worthwhile having access to a range of individuals from the represented tribes, religions, ages and genders. A word of caution, however: refugee communities, like all communities, have hidden agendas and factions. When working with cultural advisors, therapists can inadvertently get entangled in these machinations. Transparency, documentation, honesty, accountability and neutrality are essential – but, even then, it may not be enough to save them from 'smear' campaigns. Any perceived danger to a subgroup can result in the gatekeepers shutting the threat out – silenced, isolated and powerless.

Barriers to engagement

Developing a therapeutic rapport and effectively engaging with the Sudanese community is an ongoing challenge. Five of the most significant barriers and intervention strategies utilized by the occupational therapist are described in Table 17.1 to illustrate the issues.

How occupational therapists can take care of themselves to avoid burnout

Working with refugees is hard work emotionally, particularly when the programme is a new one and the infrastructure is still being developed. The experience of burnout occurs because of high work demands and limited resources, support, acknowledgement and time. Generally there is also a perceived lack of control to change the situation and unrealistic expectations. 'As a worker, one is exposed to trauma vicariously and affected by it … characteristically, there is a constant tension between over-involvement and under-involvement' (Kaplan 1998, p. 131).

The involvement continuum swings from over-involvement to under-involvement. Over-involvement is characterized by the crusader approach, having weak boundaries, taking work home, accepting excessive responsibility and being overly accommodating. Under-involvement, at the other extreme, is demonstrated by cynicism, minimizing contact with and blaming the clients, and generally being inflexible and uncooperative (Kaplan 1998).

Table 17.1 • Barriers to engagement and intervention strategies

Issue	Barriers to engagement	Intervention strategies
Language and literacy	New arrivals' lack of proficiency in host country's dominant language, English	Work in partnership with language school
	Refugee literacy levels varied ranging from university graduates to those with limited, interrupted or no education	Support with volunteers, childcare and transport arrangements for increased access to English lessons
	Lack of qualified interpreters within 2 hours' travel. Reliance on telephone interpreters. Refugees using friends and children as interpreters	Support base-level interpreter training of local refugees to get qualified
	Lack of translated information on services	Arrange staff professional development on working with qualified interpreters, rather than using children/friends
		Instigate a local Sudanese community radio programme for information dissemination and cultural education in first language.
		Development of newsletter in Arabic – to be created in weekly computer class
		Development of translated settlement information hub – hard-copy and online
		Development of bilingual booklet and DVD re access to children's services
	Misunderstandings between workers and clients due to language barriers	Work with cultural interpreter
		Learning basic Arabic words for welcome, hello, goodbye, thank you and 'my name is…'
		Using culturally respectful terms such as Uncle, Aunt, Grandma and Grandpa
		Active listening
Effects of torture and trauma	Lack of trust in services – particularly in government-funded programmes	Explain role clearly and repeat often
		Ensure that all publicity and media coverage has explicit permission of the refugees, as there have been cases of family and friends back home being punished in retribution for refugee activities in Australia
	Frequent missed appointments, due to lack of perceived importance, the effects of torture and trauma, and because appointments are not common in Sudan: people are used to attending services only when needed and waiting on-site until it is their turn	Allow time for missed appointments, arrange home visits or attend group meetings where the community meets and conduct appointment informally. Contact them on mobile phone to remind them just prior to appointment.

(Continued)

Table 17.1 • Barriers to engagement and intervention strategies—Cont'd

Issue	Barriers to engagement	Intervention strategies
	Generally, the community does not accept that depression exists as an illness – marked cultural stigma around mental illness. No framework to understand counselling services, elders actively blocking community access to the service as it's 'not the way we do it'	Encouraging the whole refugee community to attend general parenting, health and well-being workshops where mental health issues are raised in a non-threatening manner Develop rapport and allow time
	Ongoing traumatizing of refugees through torture and trauma of family and friends home in Sudan and in camps. Approximately once a month, a friend or relative of someone in the community went missing or died, resulting in the entire local community entering a mourning period for between a week and a month, disrupting work, home and student roles and further harming their mental health	KPIs need to be flexible enough to accommodate the inevitable delays that they cause Work in partnership to raise awareness of effects of torture and trauma with other service providers, including schools, police, childcare and health providers Accept the validity of Sudanese counselling practices, i.e. a group of elders listens to issues and tells the person what they must do to fix it. Likewise, accept that Sudanese mourning rituals are significant, meaningful practices and occupations. Time should be allowed for them
	Clients demonstrating symptoms of post-traumatic stress disorder, depression, anxiety and anger	Work with the Victorian Foundation for Survivors of Torture Recovery goals to restore: • safety, reduce fear and anxiety • attachments and connections • identity, meaning and purpose • dignity and value (Kaplan 1998)
Conflict resolution skills	As with any community group, interpersonal conflicts, factions and alliances existed	Acknowledge factions, request representatives for all meetings but always work with whole community Formation of interfaith women's choir Mediate between refugee subgroup and service partners to address issues of disengagement
	Cultural norm of walking away from issue rather than dealing with it, e.g. not returning to a service instead of addressing issue through feedback Expectation that if one member of the community had an issue with a service provider, the whole community would be obliged to boycott the service or face being ostracized	Develop and encourage use of feedback and complaints systems within children's services Role model effective conflict resolution skills within group

Table 17.1 ● Barriers to engagement and intervention strategies—Cont'd

Issue	Barriers to engagement	Intervention strategies
	Norm of men to control women and children through 'disciplining' them	Support of attendance at parenting courses where negotiation skills with children are learned
		Education sessions on legal issues in Australia re children's and women's rights to safety
	Lack of experience of individuals taking on leadership roles, delegation, or responsibility for decision-making	Facilitate leadership workshops
		Encourage leaders to join other community groups to learn how they function and manage conflict effectively
	Lack of skill development in governance skills and inclusive communication and decision-making processes	Work with training organizations involved with the refugees to include communication, conflict resolution, assertion and negotiation training as part of their coursework
Intercultural attitudinal conflict with regard to inclusiveness and equal rights	Occupational therapists' KPIs did not take into account cultural norms, such as women and youth not being allowed or encouraged to take on leadership roles	Youth leadership training done through conference attendance of Sudanese youth across Australia
		Women's leadership course facilitated by discussing motherhood role and extending it into basic leadership principles
	Occupational therapists' KPIs demanded inclusiveness of all members of the community; however, this was not a cultural norm – subgroups repeatedly blocked from information and governance processes	Explain and encourage inclusive behaviour addressing exclusions based on tribe, age, sex and religion within community regarding decision-making. Arrange childcare and transport for increased access for women and isolated subgroups to community strategic planning sessions and Annual General Meeting. Direct invitations to all members
	Australian legislation re equal rights for women, independent financial support for women and teenagers, allowing family units to break down and ensuing loss of status/power experienced by men	Reinforce equal rights issues and legislation
Intercultural attitudinal conflict regarding time	Making people wait can be a sign of status for Sudanese elders	Decide on an acceptable amount of time to wait, and then leave. Explain if possible. Make sure that there is something else to do whilst waiting.

(Continued)

203

Table 17.1 Barriers to engagement and intervention strategies—Cont'd

Issue	Barriers to engagement	Intervention strategies
	Local Sudanese have had limited experience of appointment systems. Culturally, the norm is to arrive at a service when it is needed and just wait in turn	Set up a monthly clinic with onsite interpreters, for maternal child health nurses instead of using an appointment system Offer home visits or meeting at other places, such as English class. Make appointments for out of hours times, nights and weekends
	Difficult to get agreement from the whole community in time to put in grant applications, etc. as the decision-making process is fraught with conflicting opinions and poor conflict management skills	Allow plenty of time for grant applications etc. and prepare to miss the deadline – apply again next year Encourage learning from consequences of actions/ inaction, and ensure understanding of what they can get out of the grant, etc.

To protect against burnout and over/under-involvement occupational therapists should:

- ensure stronger peer support, effective and regular supervision and debriefing as often as needed
- keep firm boundaries with clients and time (i.e. not taking work home)
- pace oneself and remember the 'big picture'
- take time off to recharge
- practise reflection on purpose, expectations and effectiveness
- practise a form of expression to release emotions
- acknowledge and celebrate achievements.

204

Conclusion

This chapter used the experiences of an occupational therapist working in rural Victoria, Australia to explore issues around the acculturation process in the settlement and capacity building of Sudanese refugees. The occupational therapy profession has valuable contributions to make in this area because of the profession's ability to work on an individual level with skill development, adaptation and accommodation, and on a community level effecting change through advocacy, lobbying and strategic policy and programme planning. A number of barriers to engagement with this community have been identified and the strategies used by the occupational therapist have been described. Because of the complexities of this work, however, it is acknowledged that occupational therapists working in this sector may also require:

- additional specialist skills (e.g. working with interpreters)
- access to a wider knowledge base (e.g. the effects of torture and trauma and health issues specific to different ethnic groups)
- considerable professional experience in case management, vocational rehabilitation, mental health, family-based therapy, community health and/or community development programmes.

Alternatively, they should be well positioned in a diverse multiskilled team and be connected into an extensive professional network with refugee-specific expertise. Effective management, supervision and debriefing should also be available to ensure quality service provision and to prevent therapist 'burnout'.

References

Berry J W, Trimble J, Olmeda E 1986 The assessment of acculturation. In: Lonner W J, Berry J W (eds) Field methods in cross-cultural research. Sage, London: p 82–104

Culhane S 2004 An intercultural model: acculturation attitudes in second language acquisition. Electronic Journal of Foreign Language Teaching 1: 50–61. Available online at: http://e-flt.nus.edu.sg/v1n12004/culhane. pdf; accessed 15 October 2007

Department of Sustainability and Environment 2001 Know your area. Department of Infrastructure, Melbourne, Victoria. Available online at: http://www.doi.vic.gov. au/Doi/knowyour.nsf/webPageSummaries/ LGA-Warrnambool+(C)-Ethnicity#2001 Countryofbirthlga; accessed 15 October 2007

Kaplan I 1998 Rebuilding shattered lives. Victorian Foundation for Survivors of Torture. Brunswick, Victoria. Available online at: http:// www.foundationhouse.org.au/pub_rebuilding_ 2.htm; accessed 15 October 2007

Plavsic M 2002 Acculturation. South East European Refugee Assistance Network. Available online at: http://www.see-ran.org/expanded/ ?id=00123; accessed 15 October 2007

Turner G 2003 Transcultural health education for multicultural Australia: culture or acculturation? MMHA's Synergy magazine 3 Mental Health Workforce development. Multicultural Mental Health Australia. Paramatta, New South Wales. Available online at: http://www.mmha.org.au/mmha-products/ synergy/2003_No3/InMyOpinion1/; accessed 15 October 2007

Forging partnerships to address health-related needs:

targeting embedded rural communities in the horseracing industry

Karin J. Opacich, Shannon Lizer,
Peggy Goetsch

Context and population of interest

The term 'invisible populations' describes groups of people who may not be mapped or counted by conventional strategies and whose health-related needs may be consequently overlooked or underestimated. Among such populations are 'embedded rural communities' associated with the horseracing industry in Illinois and nearly 150 racetracks across the USA. These communities can most accurately be characterized as rural in lifestyle, engaging in typically rural occupations but geographically situated in urban and suburban locations accessible to horseracing customers.

The 2005 American Horse Council census reports that over 383 000 people are employed in the racing industry (American Horse Council 2005) with thousands more working in other equine-related endeavours. A cohort of that workforce, thousands of people who actually take care of the horses, live on or near US racetracks and can be considered members of *back-stretch* communities. (The backstretch is the portion of the racetrack farthest from the grand-stand and nearest the stabling area. Backstretch workers maintain the stables and care for the horses, and they usually live on or near the racetrack.) Because the work is associated with assigned racing dates or time-limited 'meets', the workers migrate from track to track, some remaining at one or two work sites in the state and others travelling across state lines. In Illinois and most other racing venues, a large proportion of the workers migrate from rural towns and primitive farms in Mexico, Guatemala and Ecuador where economic conditions are very harsh and opportunities are severely limited. The jobs they assume in the racing industry may entail similar agricultural work, e.g. tending livestock, maintaining stables and caring for equipment. It is not uncommon for entire worker communities to emanate from particu-lar towns or regions, indicative of a growing phenomenon called *chain migration* (Marotta & Garcia 2003).

Bateson (1996) described women's occupations as 'enfolded', and occupations and occupational roles for this population are similarly intertwined. They live in the same environment where they work, where they recreate, where they raise their children and where they worship. Their inclusion in this community is contingent upon their ability to perform a job even as they age. Occupational choices are limited to those that are both culturally acceptable and available in a limited and rather idiosyncratic context. While the lifestyle of backstretch workers might seem unattractive to most, it does afford steady work, marginal housing, education for their children and a semblance of community. Much like the military, the backstretch tends to accommodate a broad spectrum of personalities, behaviours and abilities, making it possible for some who might not succeed in a broader social context to live acceptably.

A large proportion of the workforce, by virtue of low socioeconomic status, limited education, immigration status, race and ethnicity, and access to social resources, is vulnerable to disparities in health and health care (Clancy & Chesley 2003, Murdock et al 2003, Health Resources and Services Administration 2004, Mokdad et al 2004). While the scientific literature discretely addresses issues associated with agricultural workers and safety (Purschwitz 2003, Frank et al 2004), migrant worker health (Hansen & Donohoe 2003, Villarejo 2003) and the perils of horse-related activity (Press et al 1995, Waller et al 2000, Abu-Zidan & Rao 2003), there is little available that addresses the combined impact of these content areas and informs this industry about the unique health needs of its workforce, and none specific to the backstretch population (see also Chs 4, 5).

Unlike typical employers, which sponsor health programmes, racetracks are structured to host trainers and their operations, who, in turn, employ other horsemen. Trainers are required to pay for workers' compensation coverage but this applies only to work-related injuries, which tend to be under-reported. In most racing jurisdictions, health-related services have been initiated and supported through philanthropy, and these vary widely from racetrack to racetrack. In Illinois, the majority of health-related services are provided through the Racing Industry Charitable Foundation, Inc. (RICF), an endeavour that was seeded by Lucy Reum, a member of the Illinois Racing Board from 1976 to 1977. Peggy Goetsch, current Executive Director, has been working with this population for over 20 years. According to Goetsch, equine migrant and seasonal workers are isolated, with limited access to health resources (Barrett & Clippinger 1997). Services, particularly hospital-based services, for licensed horsemen may be funded through industry benevolent associations but benefits are limited and contingent upon available funds. Some, but not all, racing corporations contribute financial support and facilities for health-related endeavours. Given the nature of the backstretch community, the likelihood of pre-existing health disparities and the risks and exposure related to the work, there is greater need than existing services can address.

Over the past several years, specific research initiatives and funding mechanisms have been directed toward illuminating and eliminating health disparities, e.g. National Institutes of Health, National Center for Minority Health and Health Disparities. The rapidly accumulating literature affirms that health disparities are created or exacerbated by social, economic and behavioural phenomena. Disparities in health and access to quality health care disproportionately affect poor people of colour, poor women and their children, and people with disabilities (Smedley et al 2003). In turn, health status, social resources and overall wellbeing are inextricably related to the pursuit and execution of daily occupations (see also Chs 4, 5).

The workforce in the racing industry is a virtual microcosm mirroring the tensions and challenges inherent in health and health care in broader society. People involved in the industry are diverse and represent a continuum of attributes, resources and vulnerabilities that come to bear on health and quality of life. Partnering with academicians, and specifically occupational scientists and therapists, affords mutually beneficial opportunities to address health issues and improve health within the workforce to the mutual benefit of workers and employers and potentially yielding a more robust industry (see Chs 1, 2). Meeting health-related challenges may be best served by forging partnerships that entail systematic inquiry and analysis, culling wisdom from the health, social and behavioural sciences that yield conceptual models and relevant programmes.

Opportunities for occupational therapy to contribute to a better quality of life through meaningful engagement abound but must be culturally and contextually relevant. In addition to high-risk, low-paying work, backstretch workers live in a population-dense environment executing their daily routines while managing family life and forging relationships with others. Occupations related to work, self-care and leisure are delineated and adapted to fit the demands of the context. Backstretch workers learn to accommodate the prevailing culture while adhering to their own traditions. Exacerbated by its fluctuating nature and immigration issues, the backstretch community tends to be mistrustful and reluctant to gather, making some community participatory strategies unrealistic. Participatory observation and key community informants, including health service providers, have been invaluable for learning about the lives and needs of these workers and their families.

Stakeholders in the horseracing industry

To appreciate health-related challenges in the industry, understanding the interdependent component parts of the business as well as the characteristics of the population of interest is necessary. Unlike other forms of gaming, horseracing requires a plethora of agribusinesses and partnerships that culminate in sport and entertainment of patrons. Procuring stock, breeding and raising horses for racing is, in itself, a very complex business that entails an array of farmers, horsemen, bloodstock agents, veterinarians and farriers. Training horses generally begins at 2 or 3 years of age and involves another layer of industry personnel. Hay growers, feed companies, transport companies, farm supply companies and heavy equipment manufacturers all play their part in the industry's economy. All these stakeholders require workforce and all are affected by fluctuations in the industry.

The corporate entity that owns each racetrack facility hosts the racing stables, establishes the races and entries, and oversees the racetrack operations, including betting. State Racing Boards regulate the industry and issue licences to an array of horsemen. (In Illinois alone, the Racing Board customarily issues thousands of licences annually to horsemen, including owners, trainers, assistant trainers, jockeys, apprentice jockeys, exercise riders, pony riders, harness drivers, prospective harness drivers, stable foremen, grooms, hotwalkers and an array of service providers from veterinarians to feed salesmen (State of Illinois Legislature 1975, Illinois Racing Board 2005)). Owners of racehorses provide the capital that acquires and maintains the horses and their entourages. Trainers oversee the horses and the workers of the racing stable that they own or operate. The racetrack labour force is organized hierarchically and trainers generally have the most status and resources at their disposal. There are, however, many trainers whose small operations do not allow them luxuries such as health insurance.

In contrast to the owners and large-scale trainers, those who assume roles at the lower end of the hierarchy represent a good deal more diversity in terms of race, ethnicity and sex. Precise demographic data are unavailable and methodological challenges are similar to those encountered in collecting data for the US census. Although licences are required in each state, authenticity of documentation is sometimes questionable, impacting access to health-related services. Historically present in the racetrack environment, a small proportion of the backstretch population is African American. Over the years, women have become increasingly present, especially in the lower rungs of the labour hierarchy. More recently on the scene are Muslim men who are employed by racing stables owned by wealthy Middle Easterners. Today at least 50% of the people working and living on the backside of US tracks are Latino/Latina (more than 90% in Illinois) and a large number of them are new immigrants (P. Goetsch, personal communication, 2004). In Illinois in 2006, backstretch workers comprised 68.7% of the licensed horsemen who actually had responsibility for training and caring for the horses.

The setting

Caring for horses requires a 365-days-a-year commitment and the workers on the backside maintain the stable environment, the horses and the equipment. By dawn, stables are bustling with activity. Horses are fed and readied for their workouts, and exercise riders appear to condition them for their races. Between the hours of 5 am and 11 am, horses (upward of 2000 on major tracks) are fed, groomed and exercised. The work is physical and similar to that in other agricultural environments except that racehorses are sensitive, high-maintenance athletes. Not only must the animals' basic needs be met but they must also be carefully observed and tended. Grooms function much like athletic trainers, wrapping, rubbing, applying poultices or liniment and otherwise ministering to the elite equine athletes (Figs 18.1 & 18.2). After morning workouts, preparations are made for those entered in the afternoon's races. Consequently, days are long, and time off during a racing meet is rare.

The racetrack image more familiar to patrons invokes the pageantry of the bugler's call, the colourful silks worn by the jockeys and the parade to post. Most patrons are unaware of the array of people and hours of training devoted to the animals at the starting line. Those who live and work on the backside leave the track infrequently and any special needs, including health care, must fit into the ebb and flow of the racetrack routine. Since wages associated with these jobs are very low, many backstretch workers live meagrely, especially those who are supporting families. Most live in dormitories built to the prevailing standards for migrant and seasonal housing at the time of construction. When migrant housing is not available on the racetracks, workers tend to live in the immediate surrounding community. Given the expendable income of the workers, housing options are quite limited. Since the characteristics of the workforce have shifted to include couples and sometimes families, housing has been a source of increasing concern and controversy (Rozek 2004). Children are not allowed on the backside of the majority of racetracks but they are permitted in some of the venues in Illinois. High-spirited racehorses and impulsive young children sharing the same environment pose additional health and safety risks and housing challenges. Criddle (2001) reported that children who are bystanders are at risk of serious injury by livestock and horses when these incidents occur.

210

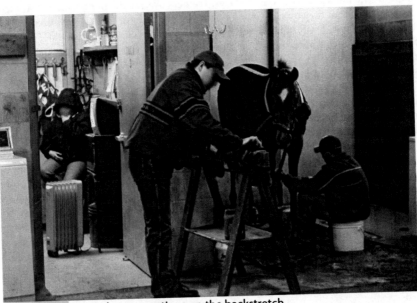

Figure 18.1 • Everyday occupations on the backstretch.

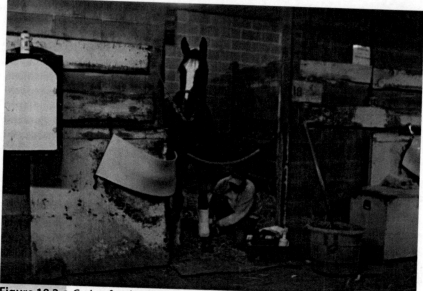

Figure 18.2 • Caring for the elite equine athletes.

The racetrack environment as a context for health

Risks and exposures relative to the work on the backside are similar to those encountered in other agricultural endeavours. A rural lifestyle entails strenuous, physical work and depends upon the physical abilities and determination of rural, agricultural workers, typically farmers. The racetrack, like the 'family farm', encompasses the workplace, the home and the playground for the workforce. Over the last 20 years, Department of Labor statistics indicate that farming has risen from the third most hazardous occupation in the US to the most hazardous (Petrea 2003, US Bureau of Labor Statistics 2003). The second highest number of fatalities of any industry was associated with farming in 2003, including an additional 110000 disabling injuries in that same year (National Safety Council 2004). Older workers, predominantly Hispanic migrant workers, and women are changing the nature of the workforce. These workers, with associated occupational risks for chronic health problems, work-related injuries and occupational exposures permeate traditional and non-traditional environments in agribusiness. In 1996, the National Institute for Occupational Safety and Health (NIOSH) defined such workers as populations of risk in agricultural settings, and they are among the research priorities set by NIOSH (National Institute for Occupational Safety and Health 1996). Backstretch workers share many of the same attributes and challenges and are thus likely to experience comparable problems and health disparities (Culp & Umbarger 2004).

Like other rural workers, most backstretch workers embrace an independent lifestyle with a strong work ethic. These personal characteristics, accompanied by a vulnerable position in the social hierarchy, make it very difficult for backstretch workers to take time from the workday for traditional health maintenance and chronic disease management activities. Lack of personal resources and health care insurance compound this problem (Patton 2005). Health status is also mitigated by stress, including housing instability, poverty and language barriers (Magana & Hovey 2003). Risk of occupational injury is a constant concern. Horses weighing as much as 550kg (1200lb) respond quickly to environmental stimuli, which sometimes cause them to behave in unpredictable ways. Canadian researchers Thompson and Von Hollen (1996) concluded that typical horse behaviour, including abrupt, unexpected movements, referred to as 'spooking', accounted for injuries in two-thirds of those injured by horses. Work-related occupational risk includes musculoskeletal strain, fractures, repetitive use injuries, inhalation of dust and other contaminants, and exposure to zoonotic infections.

Risk of injury is further amplified by alcohol and substance abuse, a reportedly common phenomenon (National Institute on Drug Abuse 2003). It has been conjectured that alcohol and drug abuse and other addictions appear to be more prevalent on the racetrack than in the general population (Oliveira & Silva 1996, Schefstad 1996, Erramouspe et al 2002). In addition to counselling services and 12-step programmes, a number of charitable organizations have emerged to address these needs. Examples of these agencies are the Winners Federation, Inc. and the Racetrack Chaplaincy of America. In 1989 the Ryan Family Foundation sponsored the first Conference on Alcohol and Drug Abuse Programs for the Horse Racing Industry in Louisville, Kentucky, and for several years afterwards that conference spawned new ideas and programmes (Barrett & Clippinger 1997). Nevertheless, chemical dependency persists and poses serious risks to both the horses and the horsemen.

The Illinois experience

Beginning with Reum's initiative in the 1970s, the Illinois racing industry has essentially established an alternative health care system. Through the Racing Industry Charitable Foundation, horsemen can access an array of medical, dental, mental health and social services on site that they would otherwise be unlikely to access because of eligibility criteria, transportation scheduling conflicts, and payment issues. Statistics indicate that the system is consistently heavily used but the need for services exceeds the system's designated resources. While specific patterns of usage cannot be extrapolated from the records, the data suggest that surprisingly large numbers of people working at the racetrack avail themselves of medical, dental, social services and mental health/addiction services when these are available.

Despite limited resources, the health agenda for the racetrack has met with some notable successes. Through community outreach efforts and education, 98% of the children have been immunized and increasing numbers of adults are getting inoculated. The Illinois Thoroughbred Horsemen's Association, in conjunction with the local school district, sponsors a successful summer day camp for children of workers, focusing on both recreation and education. During the school year children are now bussed to their home schools rather than being transferred when the venue moves to a different racetrack in the Chicago metropolitan region; however, continued funding for transportation is in jeopardy.

Project EXPORT and opportunities for partnering

In 2003, the University of Illinois at Rockford was awarded a 4-year $6.4 million grant authorized under the Minority Health and Health Disparities Research and Education Act of 2000 to establish an exploratory EXPORT Center at the Rockford campus. The acronym EXPORT stands for Excellence in Partnerships for Community Outreach and Research on Disparities in Health and Training. The mission of the EXPORT Center for Excellence in Rural Health is to identify, reduce and eliminate health disparities in rural and other underserved populations through research, education and community services. Themes recurring throughout EXPORT endeavours are collaboration, health disparities reduction, development of research scientists, development of health professionals, biomedical and behavioural science research interface, and interdisciplinary and multiprofessional approaches in education and programme development. The embedded rural communities on the backstretch manifest many of the issues and concerns central to EXPORT. Health and quality of life are issues that impact the workforce in all industries but the demands and characteristics of the racing industry and the people who contribute to it render some unique challenges and opportunities.

The US federal health agenda as stated in *Healthy People 2010* (US Department of Health and Human Services 2000a) reflects and supports EXPORT initiatives since the two overarching goals of *Healthy People 2010* are:

* to increase quality and years of healthy life
* to eliminate health disparities.

Healthy People 2010 includes 28 focal areas and specific objectives that 'focus on the determinants of health', including the physical and social factors that contribute to the health of the individual and the community. Both *Healthy People and 2010* and EXPORT emphasize the relationship between individual and community health and encourage forming partnerships, particularly non-traditional partnerships, to address health concerns. Achieving healthy communities requires new commitments, innovative approaches and collaboration, according to Shalala, who stated explicitly: 'It requires communities and businesses to support health-promoting policies in schools, worksites, and other settings' (US Department of Health and Human Services 2000b). This particular endeavour necessitates and exemplifies collaboration among academic, corporate and community partners.

Beginning the process of partnering

Academic partners can enhance industry health-related endeavours by collecting population data and information systematically using scientific methods. They can help to create models and programmes with demonstrable results and can pursue grants and funds for training, programme development and research. Ultimately, academic partnerships can inform industry in matters of health for sound decision-making.

Among the first activities conducted was a consensus building meeting that included representatives from three Illinois racetracks, racing-related agencies, health care providers, EXPORT representatives, backstretch representatives and other key individuals who participated in the 'Backstretch Brainstorm' hosted by Arlington Park. A total of 34 people associated with the racing industry and/or with health care attended. After a brief presentation pertaining to health disparities and the importance of a healthy workforce, each table became a small work group to discuss and prioritize health concerns and service needs. After the meeting, the results were reviewed for frequency and redundancy, and clusters of health-related concerns and perceived service needs emerged. Participants indicated an increased understanding of the importance of addressing issues of health and health disparities and the relationship of the health of the workforce to the industry. A meeting summary was prepared and distributed, and included potential partnership projects to address health-related needs.

Subsequently, new projects were launched, and others are in the planning stages. For example, Arlington Racetrack management identified a need for first-responder planning and a half-day workshop was presented to security and customer service personnel including relevant customized scenarios with culturally sensitive content. On a national level, links have been established with industry organizations, e.g. the Association of International Commissioners of Racing, a body of regulators, and the Jockey Club, an association hosting information accessible to horsemen and anyone interested in the thoroughbred industry. The Grayson–Jockey Club Research Foundation and the Jockey Club sponsored a strategic planning meeting (Welfare and Safety of the Racehorse Summit) in Lexington, Kentucky in October 2006, to address welfare and safety issues in the industry. A subcommittee was constituted to design and explore the feasibility of implementing an industry accident and injury surveillance system for both equines and humans, and preliminary work was reported at the meeting. Momentum for developing a national system is slowly building.

A pilot research project funded through the EXPORT Center, 'Determining Health Status and Health Disparities of an Embedded Rural Workforce', was initiated in 2005 and is still under way (Opacich & Lizer, in progress). The project seeks to query health status, health beliefs, health disparities and health-related needs for those working in the industry in Illinois, especially the cohort of backstretch workers. Phase I entailed a health fair strategy to collect an array of health indicators for comparison with national databases and prevalence statistics. During the planning for phase I, collaboration was established among 15 agencies and nearly 100 individuals representing health and social services, education and racetrack administration. Among the collaborating agencies and services were the village public health department, the community hospital mobile dentistry programme, local Rotarians, the county mobile mammogram team, the State mental health outreach programme, a Latino/a advocacy organization, the suburban tuberculosis public health agency, the Agricultural Safety and Health Network, medical students from the Illinois Health Education

Consortium participating in the Spanish immersion programme, SALUD (a grant-funded health literacy project) and more. Some are providing a service and others can potentially contribute to the care of this underserved population.

While the Horsemen's Health Fair was available to all Illinois-licensed horsemen and their dependants, the group of approximately 1200 workers and their families living in migrant housing on the racetrack were targeted. Approximately one-quarter of the backstretch workers participated in this event and results are thought to be representative of the community. Many of the findings were consistent with accumulating health disparities studies, while some indicators were even worse than comparable disparity populations. Racial and ethnic minorities, impoverishment and immigrant status are consistently associated with poorer health status and outcomes. Among the most dramatic findings were a high prevalence of untreated dental caries (Kaste & Opacich, in progress), childhood obesity, a higher risk of diabetes and higher risk of asthma (Opacich & Lizer, in progress). A high rate of exposure to tuberculosis and latent infections was also found, and many workers were enrolled in treatment. All these conditions have implications for occupations but especially for those associated with nutrition and food preparation, childhood activity and community living. As a result of their collaboration in the health fair, services have already been enhanced by outside organizations. SALUD installed health literacy software in the RICF clinic to enable patients to read or listen (in English/Spanish) to modules explaining a variety of health conditions. The local Rotarians donated materials to the children's summer camp to promote literacy. The mobile mammogram wagon has been scheduled for return visits, and 19 people identified with latent tuberculosis infection are receiving treatment on site.

Another area of concern pertains to the needs of ageing backstretch workers and potential strategies for role preservation and ageing in place. Given the business structure of the horseracing industry, there are no customary retirement programmes, resources or options for ageing racetrack workers regardless of status (Warr et al 2004, Saastamoinen et al 2005). Ageing backstretch workers are generally ineligible for federal and State-funded programmes. They work for low pay in a high-risk environment and are vulnerable to occupational injury, hazards and exposures, as well as more predictable decline, chronic illness, disability and infirmities associated with ageing. Many of these individuals age prematurely and, despite deteriorating health, continue to work past the usual retirement age for a variety of reasons, including financial necessity and attachment to place (Fulks & Fallon 2001). The intention of this line of enquiry is to investigate the feasibility of extending the self-sustaining work life of ageing workers that in turn supports coherent ageing and quality of life for a population with unique lifestyles and limited resources (Cutchin 2001).

Emerging needs and potential occupational therapy interventions

In light of a high rate of childhood obesity and a greater risk of diabetes, occupations associated with food procurement, selection and preparation as well as nutritional literacy, food habits and exercise routines beg an interdisciplinary approach. Cooking is prohibited in dormitory rooms because of the potential fire hazard. In good weather, some families barbecue outdoors but others rely on the track kitchen for their meals. While vending machines are readily accessible, grocery stores are not. Children can play in restricted areas for their own safety and that of the horses, but many of them lead sedentary lives. Because many workers lack childcare options, children may be confined in their dormitory rooms when not in school.

Occupations reflecting personal habits and routines that support health are amenable to intervention. Self-monitoring for those with existing chronic conditions such as diabetes and asthma can be addressed, as well as recognizing and responding to health-related emergencies. Both personal hygiene and community hygiene are challenged by the nature of the work and the built environment. Addressing these requires both health literacy and the establishment of routines that promote health and minimize transmission of infection to other humans, as well as to the horses.

Many other areas of occupation are yet to be investigated. Among these, childcare is a persistent problem that might be addressed by training/credentialling childcare workers within the community. Positive use of leisure time provides challenges for both children and adults. Both anecdotes and service usage reflect a high prevalence of alcohol and drug abuse. Although there are some resources for addressing these problems, establishing new routines and meaningful engagement is critical to maintaining sobriety. Additionally, occupational therapists might well promote agricultural safety and adapting worker roles for injured and ageing workers. Occupational scientists are well suited to illuminating and preserving the rich cultural traditions that are woven into daily life as well as developing strategies to facilitate acculturation and to promote cultural competency in this context.

Summary

The partnerships described are intended to be mutually beneficial, both contributing to the well-being of the racing industry and its workforce and accumulating wisdom and insights that can enhance the quality of life and ameliorate the health disparities in this and other populations. Potential benefits to the industry are: a healthier, more stable workforce, a safer racetrack environment, lower risk and concomitantly lower workers' compensation premiums, good public relations for the industry and attraction of new customers and, most importantly, a better quality of life for people working in the industry. Challenges and successes in the Illinois racing industry are thought to be relevant for other racing venues and may contribute to a more comprehensive national understanding of health-related issues in the industry.

Acknowledgements

This work was supported in part by the EXPORT Center for Excellence in Rural Health, which is funded by the National Center on Minority Health and Health Disparities, National Institutes of Health (grant no. 5 P20 MD000524-04).

References

Abu-Zidan F M, Rao S 2003 Factors affecting the severity of horse-related injuries. International Journal of Care Injury 34: 897–900

American Horse Council 2005 National economic impact of the US horse industry. American Horse Council Foundation, Washington, DC. Available online at: http://www.horsecouncil. org/statistics.htm: accessed 14 May 2006

Barrett C J, Clippinger D C 1997 The whole person. In: Winners! The story of alcohol and drug-abuse programs in the horse racing industry. Daily Racing Form Press, Highstown, NJ: p 62–70, 76, 129–135

Bateson M C 1996 Enfolded activity and the concept of occupation. In: Zemke R, Clark F (eds) Occupational science: the evolving discipline. FA Davis, Philadelphia, PA: p 5–12

Clancy C M, Chesley F D 2003 Strengthening the health services research to reduce racial and ethnic disparities in health care. Agency for Healthcare Research and Quality update (reprinted). Health Services Research 38(5): xi–xviii

Criddle L M 2001 Livestock trauma in Central Texas: cowboys, ranchers, and dudes. Journal of Emergency Nursing 27: 132–140

Culp K, Umbarger M 2004 Seasonal and migrant agricultural workers: a neglected work force. Journal of the American Association of Occupational Health Nurses 52: 383–390

Cutchin M P 2001 Deweyan integration: moving beyond place attachment in elderly migration theory. International Journal of Aging and Human Development 52: 29–44

Erramouspe J, Adamcik B A, Carlson R K 2002 Veterinarian perception of the intentional misuse of veterinary medication in humans: a preliminary survey of Idaho-licensed practitioners. Journal of Rural Health 18: 311–318

Frank A L, McKnight R, Kirkhorn S R, Gunderson P 2004 Issues of agricultural safety and health. Annual Review of Public Health 25: 225–245

Fulks J S, Fallon L F 2001 The older worker. Occupational Medicine 16: 501–507

Hansen E, Donohoe M 2003 Health issues of migrant and seasonal farmworkers. Journal of Health Care for the Poor and Underserved 14: 153–164

Health Resources and Services Administration 2004 The role of HRSA in elimination of health disparities. US Department of Health and Human Services, Washington, DC: p 9–14. Available online at:http://www.hrsa.gov/OMH/OMH/disparities; accessed 15 October 2007

Illinois Racing Board 2005 The year 2004 in review, the 2004 Racing Board Annual Report. Illinois Racing Board, Chicago, IL, p 6. Available online at: http://www.state.il.us/agency/irb/racing/reports/2003_Annual_Report.htm; accessed 17 December 2005

Kaste L M, Opacich K J (in progress) Oral health status and disparities for an embedded rural workforce. University of Illinois, Protocol #2006–0479

Magana CG, Hovey J D 2003 Psychosocial stressors associated with Mexican migrant farmworkers in the Midwest United States. Journal of Immigrant Health 5: 75–86

Marotta S A, Garcia J G 2003 Latinos in the United States in 2000. Hispanic Journal of Behavioural Science 25: 13–34

Mokdad A H, Marks J S, Stroup D F et al 2004 Actual causes of death in the United States, 2000. Journal of the American Medical Association 291: 1238–1245

Murdock S H, Hoque N, Johnson K et al 2003 Racial/ethnic diversification in metropolitan and nonmetropolitan population change in the United States: complications for health care provision in rural America. Journal of Rural Health 19: 425–432.

National Institute for Occupational Safety and Health 1996 National occupational research agenda. DHHS (NIOSH) Publication #96–115. NIOSH, Cincinnati, OH

National Institute on Drug Abuse 2003 Director's report to the National Advisory Council on Drug Abuse. National Institutes of Health, Bethesda, MD, p 1–16. Available online at: http://www.drugabuse.gov/DirReports/DirRep903/DirectorReport3.html; accessed 15 October 2007

National Safety Council 2004 Injury facts. National Safety Council, Itasca, IL

Oliveira M P, Silva M T 1996 Pathological and nonpathological gamblers: a survey in gambling settings. Substance Use and Misuse 35: 1573–1583

Opacich K J, Lizer S (in progress) Determining health status and health disparities for an embedded rural workforce. University of Illinois, Protocol #2006–0020

Patton J 2005 Wrong side of the track. Lexington Hearal-Leader 23–30 January

Petrea R E (ed) 2003 Using history and accomplishments to plan for the future: a summary of 15 years in agricultural safety and health and action steps for future directions. Agricultural Safety and Health Network, Urbana, IL

Press J M, Davis P D, Weisner S L et al 1995 The national jockey injury study: an analysis of injuries to professional horse-racing jockeys. Clinical Journal of Sport Medicine 5: 236–240

Purschwitz MA 2003 Creating a safer and healthier agriculture – are we asking the right questions? Journal of Agricultural Safety and Health 9: 87–89

Rozek D 2004 Arlington to improve dorms for track workers. Chicago Sun-Times 19 June

Saastamoinen P, Leino-Arjas P, Laaksonen M et al 2005 Socio-economic differences in the prevalence of acute, chronic and disabling chronic pain among ageing employees. Pain 114: 364–371

Schefstad A J 1996 The backstretch: some call it home. ProQuest Digital Dissertations, No. AAT 9608736. University of Maryland, Baltimore, MD: p 45–58

Smedley B D, Stith A Y, Nelson A R (eds) 2003 Unequal treatment: confronting racial and ethnic disparities in health care. Board on Health Sciences Policy, Institute of Medicine. National Academies Press, Washington, DC

State of Illinois Legislature 1975 Illinois Horse Racing Act 1975 (230 ILCS 5/). Revised 10/1999. Source: PA 79–1185

Thompson J M, Von Hollen B 1996 Causes of horse-related injuries in a rural western community. Canadian Family Physician 42: 1103–1109.

US Bureau of Labor Statistics 2003 Workplace injuries and illnesses in 2002. News USDL 03–913. US Department of Labor, Washington, DC. Available online at: http://www.bls.gov/iif/home.htm; accessed 18 December 2003

US Department of Health and Human Services 2000a Healthy people 2010, 2nd edn. With understanding and improving health and objectives for improving health. US Government Printing Office, Washington, DC

US Department of Health and Human Services 2000b Message from the Secretary. Healthy people 2010, 2nd edn. Understanding and improving health and objectives for improving health. US Government Printing Office, Washington, DC. Available online at: http://www.healthypeople.gov/document/html/uih/message.htm; accessed 30 October 2004

Villarejo D 2003 The health of US hired farm workers. Annual Review of Public Health 24: 175–193

Waller A E, Daniels J L, Weaver N L et al 2000 Jockey injuries in the United States. Journal of the American Medical Association 283: 1326–1328

Warr P, Butcher V, Robertson I, Callinan M 2004 Older people's well-being as a function of employment, retirement, environmental characteristics and role preference. British Journal of Psychology 95: 297–324

Occupational therapy with Native American youth

19

Maggie Heyman-Hotch

When developing a new occupational therapy programme where there have not been services in the past, it is essential for the therapist conducting a needs assessment to remain open to the many voices and opinions of everyone one may encounter. This includes the key stakeholders in the system itself, the administrators who inform policy and will make decisions and, most importantly, those who will receive direct services (see Ch. 1). When completing my capstone Master's project at Pacific University, I developed and piloted an occupational therapy programme at a federally operated boarding school for Native American high-school students. In reflecting on the development and subsequent evolution of this programme in the past 6 years, the concepts of occupational justice (Townsend & Wilcock 2004), occupational apartheid (Kronenberg & Pollard 2005; see Ch. 4) and occupational deprivation (Whiteford 2004) have applied on many levels. While it is not within the scope of this chapter adequately to explore the historical background for the current occupational situation of Native American youth both on and off reservations in the USA, I hope to tell the story of the youth that I have worked with as a means to illustrate the possibilities of occupational therapy to address the occupational needs of Native youth in the USA.

During the needs assessment process it became apparent to me that the occupational challenges of the students in Native boarding schools could not be considered in isolation. If occupational therapy services were to be effective for these students, it seemed that a programme truly holistic in nature must be designed to address the whole picture of the student beyond what traditional school systems provide. My undergraduate studies in anthropology had helped me understand that to do so would be to honour traditional Native philosophies of health and wellness. To accomplish this, interventions were designed that attempted to address the 'whole student' in context. This context included the occupational demands of the school environment, the effect and current influence of the students' home environment, the previous occupational experience of each student and the historical trauma of Native people both within and outside the boarding-school environment. In addition, the students quickly taught me that the sociopolitical environment of each student's particular tribe is also relevant to their occupational experiences.

For all students, the developmental stage of adolescence as it relates to their ability to develop their own personal identity is a critical time. For these students, the boarding-school environment provides a unique opportunity for this developmental task. Native youth from as many as 60 to 100 tribes in any given school year participate in occupations together that can help them collectively define their identities. For many, it presents the choice of different, healthier occupations than those engaged in on the reservation (i.e. gang activity, vandalism (starting fires, throwing rocks at cars, windows, etc., graffiti) and violence among youth, which appeared to be primarily the result of boredom, or occupational deprivation).

To provide occupational therapy services that are consistent with the philosophy of the profession in an occupation-based, client-centred manner seemed an opportunity to empower the students to connect the elements of their lives that had led to their boarding-school attendance in a manner that could help them find balance in their high-school experience. It was my hope that, if they could learn to experience balance and wellness at this high school, they could translate those skills to build a fulfilling and productive future of their choosing.

I started by conducting a needs assessment and developing a business plan that described in detail the ways that occupational therapy could holistically address the needs of the individual students and the school system as a whole. As a result, a full-time occupational therapist position was created using the school's existing federal funds. Initially the position was for half-time special-education-related services in accordance with the Individuals with Disabilities Education Act of 1997, which was reauthorized by Congress in 2004. The other half of my time was to provide transition services in the regular education programme aimed at helping students attend college or become gainfully employed. The focus in both programmes was on enabling students to pursue higher education through developing the skills sufficient to meet occupational performance demands.

The programme has since evolved as the needs of the students and the system have changed. Despite many changes I most highly value and appreciate the freedom that comes with developing an emerging practice programme where the occupational therapy services were not predetermined by what had traditionally been done in schools. I have been able to make sure that the role of the occupational therapist evolved to remain holistic in practice and demonstrate the contention that 'most people whose access to and engagement in meaningful occupation is at risk could benefit from occupational therapy services'. My experience in providing services to this population as teenagers and the obvious lack of services for these children in their younger years through the Indian Health Service and the federal and public schools systems supports many of the concepts presented by Kronenberg and colleagues in the book *Occupational Therapy Without Borders* (2005), in particular the contention that people who have experienced occupational apartheid or injustice are not in a position to seek the services of occupational therapists even if they have a referral.

The stories that follow will attempt to demonstrate how an emerging practice occupational therapy programme can holistically address the needs of Native students even in the traditional confines of a federally operated boarding school. Wherever possible the stories of the young people told in this chapter are the result of interviews and are told with permission from the individual, and in their own words to the closest extent possible. Identifying details have been removed for all students to reduce the effect of potential stigmatization of the young people through their participation in the programme.

Zac

The first story is that of a young man I met during my first year as an occupational therapist: a 16-year-old junior student struggling to stay in school at the boarding school. This young man, whom we will call Zac, came from a Plains tribe and had many challenges facing him. The son of an alcoholic mother, whom he was often required to care for while at home, he also had a significant cognitive deficit, dyslexia, and a drinking problem caused by several bouts of depression. School was very difficult for him even in modified classes, but he was successful socially and had many friends on campus. Zac was well liked by his peers but encountered difficulty in the dormitories with doing required chores such as cleaning, and hourly 'check-in' with dorm staff. He often got into confrontations with his dorm staff and was frequently written-up for violations related to his disability: he was unable to sequence the assigned tasks properly or remember to complete them. Zac hated to be in trouble and would get depressed when written-up, which usually caused him to leave the campus to drink, which often got him into more trouble.

As an occupational therapist I approached Zac trying to examine the whole picture of the student, and found the most pressing areas to be leisure skills, self-care and a need for adaptive strategies to overcome his cognitive and memory deficits. I hoped that this would assist him in avoiding further disciplinary action and improve his success in the classroom. He had so many strengths socially and I wanted to teach him to recognize how to use his strengths in meaningful and purposeful ways. I first tried to help him find occupational outlets for his leisure time that would replace the negative behaviour of drinking and build some confidence to help him overcome depression. I also found it necessary to educate his dorm staff, and even some of the other special education staff, who were often called on to serve as his advocate, as to how his cognitive delay affected his ability to follow the daily routine at the school.

We designed some memory aids together for him to use in the dorm so that he could remember to check in hourly. We made lists to help him sequence the steps required in the other self-care skills required in the dormitory such as cleaning his room, doing laundry and signing up to use the phone properly. I also invited Zac to be a part of a mentor programme I had started with a local elementary school, where he got the opportunity to be mentor to an emotionally challenged 4th grade student (age 9–10) each Tuesday morning. Zac really enjoyed this role, and taught the student he mentored to do Native crafts and told him stories of life on his reservation. Zac also recognized some of the behaviour he struggled to control for himself in this child – anger management, frustration tolerance with academic activities and low self-confidence. Helping this young student overcome the challenges that mirrored his own allowed Zac to identify his own challenges. This created the opportunity for us to work through those challenges in meaningful and purposeful ways in individual occupational therapy sessions.

Zac also liked animals and missed caring for his dogs and horses back home while he was at school. At that time I coordinated a volunteer programme at the local Humane Society, which I conducted on Friday afternoons – generally a high-risk time for drinking behaviour on campus. I invited Zac to attend each week and he became my most consistent volunteer. He loved walking the dogs and playing with them and was willing to give up going off campus to drink or being around for the Friday afternoons when his friends were planning their weekend and working out the details of how they would get alcohol and when they planned to drink. He found engaging in this occupation easier than resisting his peers' pressure to drink.

When working on anger management strategies to improve communication with his dorm staff during occupational therapy one day, Zac identified a strategy of listening to pow-wow music to calm himself when he was upset.

A pow-wow is basically a gathering of Native people to celebrate their culture. Such an event consists mostly of traditional drumming and singing by different drum groups and Native dancing in traditional regalia (their term for traditional costume). Some have a contest associated with them for best drum, best dancer in each category, but the ones we have at the school are celebrations of the school's birthday, Veteran's Day and a welcome back to school celebration. There are much larger ones nationwide and many people make their living travelling the 'pow-wow highway' going from one to another selling Native crafts or competing in the drumming and dancing contests. Some are more local to each reservation or community and not as large.

When I asked Zac if he liked going to pow-wows, he told me that he used to enjoy drumming and dancing at pow-wows when he was younger but he usually used the pow-wows at the school as an opportunity to drink. Even back home, he no longer drummed, sang or danced at pow-wows but spent his time partying instead of engaging in the occupations of dancing and singing in the traditional Native way. I asked him why he didn't dance at the pow-wows and he told me he did not have traditional regalia to dance in. The relative who had made his last grass dance outfit had passed away and the outfit no longer fitted him. I asked if he would like to make himself a new one and his eyes lit up. He needed assistance in requesting the funding from a local charitable organization that helped students financially with projects such as this, but was successful in obtaining the funding. We used the outings to purchase the materials as opportunities to work on skills such as community mobility and money management. The dormitories allowed him access to sewing machines in the family centre on campus and Zac began to spend a lot of his free time sewing his new grass dance outfit.

Adding the occupations of mentoring, dog walking and sewing to his routine outside of occupational therapy significantly reduced the number of disciplinary referrals for Zac within a period of about 2 months. Signs of depression were also reducing and he was more actively engaging in schoolwork and in the dormitory routine, now that he had memory aids and other adaptive strategies to understand what was expected of him, and staff who understood his needs better. While all these contributed to improved occupational performance, the most significant was Zac's decision to join the performing arts group on campus. This group performs Native songs and dances from a variety of tribal traditions in a variety of community settings, including the school's pow-wows. In most Native cultures there is a strict taboo against drumming and singing while under the influence of alcohol or drugs as it creates 'bad medicine' and can be harmful to the people present. Because of this traditional value and his commitment to the group, Zac remained virtually alcohol-free for the remainder of the school year. The following year, his senior year, Zac was elected president of the Performing Arts group. He also ran for and was elected Student Body President and did very well in his role to advocate for students' rights on campus, despite his low academic skills.

The use of occupations that were meaningful and purposeful to Zac allowed him to reconnect with his tribal culture and helped him to make the most of his strengths, his social and leadership skills, to overcome the depression he felt over his very low academic skills and difficult family situation. He graduated and was referred to his tribe's vocational rehabilitation programme, which offered a scholarship in a remedial reading programme at the local tribal college. The most I know at this point, 4 years later, is that he participated in this programme for a time. He is now 20 years old and still takes care of his mother, his sister and his sister's children, and recently became a father. He and his girlfriend plan to move out on their own soon and he currently has a job to save money to do so.

Being an open person

The second story is that of a young woman who was a freshman in my first year of service provision and participated in occupational therapy throughout her high-school years. It was from her that I learned the majority of what became the foundation for my current programme: specifically, how to tailor interventions to build the neurological skills necessary for the occupational demands of the classroom. Because she had the verbal skills to give me feedback on whether the adaptive strategies I had suggested to help her compensate for her learning disability were effective or not, I was able to ask relevant questions of the other students to get the information I needed to complete the analysis necessary to design effective interventions.

This student had impaired visual–motor integration skills as well as a sensory integration dysfunction. She enjoyed athletics but did not have confidence in her skills as a result of poor motor planning. She had an excellent academic work ethic and, although initially she was very shy, developed very good social and leadership skills over her high-school years. Despite her learning disability she was the valedictorian (the student chosen to give the address at graduation) of her graduating class.

After her first 2 years of intervention, which targeted the specific occupational skills and sensory supports she required for optimal classroom success, the focus of occupational therapy intervention shifted in her junior and senior year to facilitating access to transitional programming in a programme targeting at-risk students and those with disabilities at the local community college, which she attended and in which she maintained above-average grades. When as a senior I approached her with my plan to discontinue services for her, she asked me if she could still come to occupational therapy. When I asked her what she would like to work on she said, 'You just remind me to relax and balance everything out so I don't get so stressed.'

Her statement reminded me that I needed to look beyond the everyday successes as they are perceived by the administrators and the views of the dominant culture and remain holistic in my practice and address service needs that truly return to the roots of our profession and strive to enable students to maintain health and wellness through a balanced routine of self-care, productivity and leisure occupations.

The following quotes are transcribed from a telephone interview with this student, who was happy to help me give a more personal voice to the stories. This student says of her experience in her first 2 years, which was mostly sensory integration-based interventions with a focus on academic adaptive strategies for her learning disability:

> With the writing techniques that we did, I noticed that the way I used to write wasn't so comfortable but now I can write straight and it's a lot more comfortable. It helped me stay focused on what I was supposed to be writing about and keep up better in my classes. And then the whole going from left to right thing, because I would do the opposite before when I was drawing or doing other stuff, so when you had me draw the shapes and do the puzzles from left to right, that really helped me. And then sometimes the army crawling and the balance things really helped too. It helped me focus and pay attention more in class and also in sports I could have more confidence and pay attention more. I also got more confidence from talking to you, just personally talking to you, and all the stuff that was going on that year and you really helped me to find a way to sort it out and do something about it.

On her experiences in occupational therapy during her last 2 years, which were focused more on transitioning to college and balancing productivity, self-care and leisure, she says:

> You being an open person and letting us know it was OK if you don't know anything, like when we went to the colleges and visited. I wanted to see a lot of things above how I see it now and I had questions and you always made it OK to ask the questions. It would have been hard going to college not knowing where to go at the college and how to ask for help and that there are people there that can help me. I got into the TRIO disability programme [a federal grant to community college systems that identifies local high schools with significant populations of low-income students who may not go to college without an additional level of support for the transition process] there and that helped me out by meeting those people. They helped me out a lot to keep going in school just like you and everyone there did in high school.
>
> Physically and mentally it helped me a lot. All the techniques you had me do like interviewing other people, remember that when you made us do that? It helped me get more confident. Those things I had to work with you, there were a lot that I can't remember but it helped me to remember to relax too. We [students with disabilities] have to work a lot harder than everyone else and it really helped me to know I could take a break sometimes and that was good for me too.
>
> One day I was looking through my stuff and I found the card you gave me for graduation and that really helped me open up. You wrote in there that I need to be patient with myself and lately I haven't been very patient with myself when I have to take breaks from school because I don't have the money to go where I want right now. I'm working and saving up but it was good to read that I need to be patient with myself too and not feel bad that I'm not going to school right now. It really inspired me to know you and to know you were there to help me with my difficulties with learning disabilities and those things like that. I really liked going to school there and everyone helped me so much. Especially you, you helped me a lot physically and mentally, like I said before.

Being comfortable with ambiguity

Though providing services in any system has its own set of challenges and limitations, I have been mindful to modify the programme over time as the needs of the students and the overall system have changed. I believe it is because of this adaptability that I have so far successfully survived two rounds of staff cuts due to reduced funding. I believe that the reason my programme is still thriving is because in any emerging practice project one has to be comfortable with a tremendous amount of ambiguity and allow the process to lead you to the best service provision model from the bottom up, rather than taking control as the 'expert' and trying to force a top-down approach. By remaining aware of the political situation in which I practise at both the local and national level I have been able to serve a variety of needs, which I believe every occupational therapist who remains committed to the philosophy of our profession has the opportunity to do, even in a medical model system. While my duties at the Native boarding school have changed over time and may have looked to the administration more like the job of a teacher, counsellor, social worker or case manager, I have been careful to document and articulate why it is that my skills as an occupational therapist are unique to the approach taken *and the outcome generated*. It is my hope that this will document and demonstrate within the federal system that occupational therapy is effective for this population and that more positions can be created throughout Indian Country in schools, Indian Health Service clinics and community programmes where the holistic philosophy of occupational therapy and the traditional Native constructs of health and wellness can match up and improve the occupational, and therefore the social and political, situation of Native people. Even if there comes a time when I can no longer be employed by the federal system, my goal is to pursue the expansion of occupational therapy to Native communities across the country. I believe with passion and commitment it will be possible and that this will broaden the profession's scope as an agent of social change in the USA.

References

Kronenberg F, Pollard N 2005 Overcoming occupational apartheid – a preliminary exploration of the political nature of occupational therapy. In: Kronenberg F, Simó Algado S, Pollard N (eds) Occupational therapy without borders: learning from the spirit of survivors. Elsevier/Churchill Livingstone, Edinburgh: p 58–86

Kronenberg F, Simó Algado S, Pollard N 2005 (eds) Occupational therapy without borders: learning from the spirit of survivors. Elsevier/Churchill Livingstone, Edinburgh

Townsend E, Wilcock A 2004 Occupational justice. In: Christiansen C, Townsend E (eds) Introduction to occupation: the art and science of living. Prentice Hall, Thorofare, NJ: p 243–273

Whiteford G 2004 When people cannot participate: occupational deprivation. In: Christiansen C, Townsend E (eds) Introduction to occupation: the art and science of living. Prentice Hall, Thorofare, NJ: p 221–242

Postcolonial practice in occupational therapy:
the Tule River Tribal History Project

20

*Gelya Frank, Heather J. Kitching
with Allison Joe, Colleen Harvey,
Rani Bechar, Amber Bertram,
Jeanine Blanchard and
Jaynee Taguchi-Meyer*

Rudolf Virchow, the towering 19th century physician, anthropologist and statesman, noted that almost all problems of health and wellness are the result of politics (Waitzkin 1981, Eisenberg, 1984). Virchow was well versed in the new germ theories that took medicine into the modern age. He himself was a leader in the new science of cellular pathology (Ackerknecht 1953). But on a fact-finding mission to Silesia, where a typhus epidemic was raging, Virchow frankly blamed malnutrition, poor sanitation and, more basically, economic neglect and political oppression as causes. 'Medicine is a social science,' he asserted, 'and politics is nothing else but medicine on a large scale' (Rosen 1974, p. 65).

Occupational therapists today are coming to a similar conclusion. More than ever in the history of the profession, occupational therapists are harnessing the potential of meaningful and purposeful activities to build health and well-being in populations that struggle with the effects of colonization, racism, imperialism, war, violence, environmental degradation and economic exploitation (Watson & Swartz 2004, Kronenberg et al 2005). Occupational therapy has a track record in working with indigenous people at the individual level (such as managing diabetes and other chronic illnesses that disproportionately afflict Native people; Staples & McConnell 1993, Watts & Carlson 2002, McGarrigle & Nelson 2006). The profession is also beginning to engage with postcolonial projects at the level of the health and well-being collectively of the tribe, band or community.

The Tule River Tribal History Project is a postcolonial project based in occupational science and occupational therapy (Yerxa et al 1990, Clark et al 1991, Zemke & Clark 1996, Frank et al 2001). Designed in collaboration with an anthropologist consultant who has worked for over 30 years with a California tribe, the project made use of five meaningful, purposeful activities or occupations to facilitate an official goal of the Tule River Tribal Council since 1973, to preserve the history of the Tule River Reservation and its families (Frank 2007, Frank et al, submitted). The project was targeted for tribal elders, defined as age 55 or older ($n = 118$), but all tribal members were welcome to participate.

A full-time occupational therapy staff (one doctoral student and four level II master's field-work interns) from the Division of Occupational Science and Occupational Therapy, University of Southern California, developed methods and protocols for the history-making activities (described by Taguchi-Meyer et al 2005). They implemented the project over the course of 12 weeks in the summer of 2004. The activities included creating a digital archive of family photo collections, using computer software to construct family trees, one-on-one interviews beginning with the oldest of the tribal elders, video-recorded roundtable discussions of topics related to tribal history, and development of a website.

Five postcolonial occupations

Family trees
Learn to make your family tree. Use our tribal rolls from 1888. We'll help you get started on genealogy software even if you are new to computers.

Digital photo archive
Bring your old-time photos for scanning on to CD-ROM for the tribal archive. We'll help you index them and make a copy for your family.

Elders video interviews
Sign up for a video interview. Tell us about your parents, grandparents, uncles, aunts, sisters, brothers, husbands or wives, children, grandchildren. What were the old people like? What did they do? How did they – and you – survive?

Elders heritage roundtable talks
Reminisce with other Elders about Rodeo Days, Tripne Legends, Military Service, School Days, Life On (and Off) the Reservation. Food provided.

Tribal elders heritage website
Choose to have a portion of your family history on the website.

Postcolonial and indigenous views of health and well-being

Postcolonialism is a view of history and politics that gives 'equal weight to outward historical circumstances and, importantly, to the ways in which those circumstances are experienced by postcolonial subjects' (Young 2001, p. 58). Indigenous scholars and clinicians attribute many of the physical, mental and behavioural health problems among Native people to the disruptions or 'ruptures' caused by colonial domination.

These scholars and clinicians have begun to theorize and treat effects of colonization under the rubrics of *intergenerational trauma* and *historical trauma* (Duran & Duran 1995, Duran et al 1998, Duran 2006). Their work with indigenous patients and clients views the ruptures to Native societies caused by colonization as the root cause of high rates of alcoholism, drug addiction, addiction to unhealthful food leading to metabolic disorders such as diabetes, depression, self-destructive acts and violence against others that afflict Native communities.

Public health data for Native Americans support these assertions (Manson 2004). Ethnographic research on the Flathead Reservation in Montana and with Yurok tribespeople in northern California elucidates how some Native people have managed chronic depression or melancholy. Native people on the Flathead Reservation accord these symptoms specific cultural and ethical meanings with regard to how they should treat others. Native people interviewed among the Yurok of northern California engage in disciplined forms of ritual healing (O'Nell 1996, Buckley 2002). Such socially embedded remedies, like those of occupational therapy dating back to its moral treatment roots, are holistic (Ozarin 1954, Charland 2007).

Activities related to creating alternative histories are also important remedies. Postcolonialist scholar Linda Tuhiwai Smith (Maori) has proposed a set of 'twenty-five indigenous projects' that underscore the importance of creating alternative histories (Smith 1999). She names these projects: Claiming, Testimonies, Story-telling, Celebrating survival, Remembering, Indigenizing, Intervening, Revitalizing, Connecting, Reading, Writing, Representing, Gendering, Envisioning, Reframing, Restoring, Returning, Democratizing, Networking, Naming, Protecting, Creating, Negotiating, Discovering and Sharing.

These postcolonial projects are not simply ideas or topics for discussion. They must be experienced, performed or enacted. In other words, they are meaningful, purposeful activities or occupations. When enacted, such history-making occupations help to overcome the sense of disruption and loss that Native peoples tend to suffer as the legacy of genocide, forced acculturation and marginal living conditions. Importantly, postcolonialist approaches help to locate dysfunction in Native communities as having external causes rather than reflecting some inherent lack of ability or worth in the sufferers.

Never too late to begin cultural preservation projects

Indigenous museum planner Craig Howe (Oglala Sioux) notes that a common response of Native American tribal members to cultural preservation projects is that the project is 'too late'. Howe writes:

In many instances, the public meetings to which the entire community is invited are the first time that community members have gathered together to discuss tribal history. Aside from the political machinations that often accompany such gatherings, deep-seated issues within the communities are brought to these discussions. Questions concerning authority to speak, personal character, information dissemination, and loss of tribal knowledge are not uncommon. A recurring theme is that knowledge of the 'old ways' passed on with the last generation who were educated by the community instead of by formal schools.

Howe 2002, p. 175

The Tule River tribal elders initially expressed these kinds of concerns. But once the programme was up and running, the interest and participation of the tribal elders and their families grew steadily. In that case, as Howe (2002, p. 175) notes: 'The collective knowledge of the community is recognized. In discussing their tribal histories in public formats, individuals share stories and opinions that other community members are keenly interested in hearing.'

While parallels exist with narrative therapy and other mainstream treatments, postcolonial approaches explicitly focus on the colonization experience and work toward reconstituting a shared, viable cultural heritage (Epston & White 1992, Freedman & Combs 1996). Consequently, theorists and practitioners who use a postcolonial approach understand their work as operating at both the individual and collective levels, something that is not generally shared with mainstream Western or Eurocentric therapies.

The Tule River Tribal History Project was pitched precisely at the level of collective well-being rather than focusing on individual mental health. The project's activities were structured in the service of constituting a tribal legacy. It succeeded in promoting more cooperation and better communication among diverse generations and families within the tribe.

A brief history of the Tule River Tribe

The Tule River Tribe in central California comprises descendants of various local tribes who survived the genocide and social disruption that accompanied American colonization. These were mainly southern San Joaquin valley and foothill Yokuts and western Mono tribes, each with its own territory, dialect and hereditary leaders (*tiyas*) (Kroeber 1925, Gayton 1948, Latta 1977).

Native people in central California experienced three phases of colonial domination – Spanish, Mexican and American. However, the American occupation, starting in 1848, resulted in the most rapid and severe dispossession of land, cultural disruption and decline not only in California but in the history of North America (Rawls 1984, Hurtado 1988). It has been estimated that nearly 20% of the indigenous population was wiped out in the first 4 years, between 1848 and 1852, as a consequence of the Gold Rush (Cook 1976). But the genocide continued after statehood, which occurred in 1850. By 1880, only about 17% of the Native population remained (Cook 1976).

As anthropologist Gelya Frank and legal scholar Carole Goldberg recount in a forthcoming full-length history of the Tule River Tribe, federal policies resulted in successive ruptures to the inherent sovereignty or self-determination of the survivors (Frank & Goldberg, in press). Members of some local tribes were initially induced to move to the Tejon Reservation in the southernmost part of the valley in 1854. Two years later, others were defeated in a devastating war initiated by settlers and the local tribe ordered on to the first Tule River Reservation, near present-day Porterville. They became successful agriculturalists and viewed the reservation, established on a former village site, as their rightful permanent home.

A government employee fraudulently gained title to this tract of good agricultural land. He managed to force the government to pay an exorbitant yearly rental to keep the Native population there. Eventually, in January 1873, the federal government established a second Tule River Reservation in the remote foothills where the land was unsuited to agriculture without costly improvements. Troops on horseback brandishing swords eventually forced the tribe to move there in 1876.

While a few families who managed to gain the use of good land and plentiful water were able to live comfortably, many families lived a marginal existence and some left the reservation entirely. Although the size of the reservation had been doubled in October 1873 to include better land for farming, the government refused to allocate the funds needed to compensate prior settlers on the new tract. In August 1878, the boundaries were redrawn, returning the reservation to its original size.

The reservation population from the late 19th through the early 20th century remained at about 150 members. Some tribal members were able to get started in the cattle-raising business but, as the cash economy took over, most families had members who worked as seasonal labourers off the reservation. They earned a meagre living mainly caring for livestock, working in timber or picking fruit.

Federal policies in the 1930s and again in the 1970s have helped to restore a degree of sovereignty – i.e. self-government and self-determination – among federally recognized tribes on reservation land. The US Supreme Court decision *United States v Cabezon Band of Mission Indians* (1988) gave a huge boost to the sovereignty movement by removing impediments to the Indian gaming industry on tribal lands. While the Tule River Tribe's casino operation is comparatively modest, this new source of revenue made it possible for the Tule River Tribal Council to fund the tribal history project in 2004.

The Tribal History Project also received funds through the Owens Valley Career Development Center Tribal TANF (Temporary Assistance to Needy Families), a state–federal programme. Tribes may elect to administer funds earmarked for eligible members to promote culturally relevant services. The Owens Valley Career Development Center, in Bishop, California, represents a consortium of eight tribes, including Tule River.

The Tule River Tribe presently includes about 1500 members, who trace their membership to the original Indian families who moved on to the present Tule River Reservation pursuant to the executive orders of 1873. Constructing family histories has been pivotal to tribal members' survival because it is tied to the right to live on the reservation, inherit the use of tribal land and enrol children as tribal members. At the collective level, the use of non-indigenous consultants to write historical reports has been crucial for land claims and water rights, but a long-standing tribal goal to record family histories went mainly unresolved.

The Tule River Tribal History Project was innovative in offering another type of history making by the indigenous community at the collective level. Occupational therapy helped the Tule River tribal government to engage the tribe's members in creating together a legacy for cultural preservation and other nation-building goals. These activities are similar indeed to the 'indigenous projects' proposed by Smith (1999) and other contributors to postcolonialism.

An occupational approach with the Muwekma Ohlone

In his book *Abalone Tales*, anthropologist Les Field describes his work with the Muwekma Ohlone to provide historical documentation in support of their effort to gain federal acknowledgement for their tribe (Field 2008). Field helped to conceive and organize an abalone feast. Abalone, an endangered species, was formerly the staple food of the Muwekma Ohlone, a food that older members of the tribe would often mention nostalgically. The event helped trigger intergenerational sharing of new narratives about Muwekma Ohlone history and identity as part of ongoing revitalization efforts by the tribe. Field's work exemplifies that of anthropologists working collaboratively with Native Americans to achieve tribally defined goals (Lassiter 2005). At the same time, tribal governments are asserting their sovereign power to grant or deny permission to conduct research in Indian country, calling for more accountability to tribally defined needs (Champagne & Goldberg 2005).

Results of the Tribal History Project

The accomplishments of the Tribal History Project were impressive, especially given its short, 12-week, timeframe. About 2000 images dating from the early 20th century were digitally scanned and indexed, contributed by 25 elders and their family members. Some 40 tribal members of various ages created family trees using computers with genealogical software, often working in pairs across generations. Video interviews were recorded with nine of the oldest tribal members. Nine round-table talks were held and videotaped on topics related to tribal history. A tribal history website was launched (www.tuleriver.org).

A detailed set of evaluation data has been reported elsewhere, based on pre- and post-test surveys among a matched (but anonymous) sample of tribal elders ($n = 30$) (Frank 2005, Frank et al, submitted). The data indicate the success of the project across all measures, including:

- confirming an anticipated high level of tribal elders' interest in preserving tribal history
- increasing the tribal elders' confidence in the ability of the project to affect tribal youth's knowledge about the tribe's history (Fig. 20.1)
- drawing a strong and comparable level of participation across the project activities
- eliciting enthusiasm in participating in the specific activities regardless of gender
- eliciting enthusiasm regardless of whether living on or off the reservation
- eliciting high ratings of activities among tribal elders who actually participated in them
- improving relationships and communication between tribal elders and younger tribal members (Fig. 20.2)
- increasing the amount of communication between tribal elders and members of their own family, tribal youth in their family, and people in other families with whom they usually don't talk (Fig. 20.3)

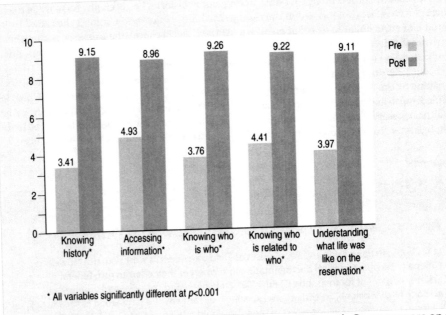

* All variables significantly different at *p*<0.001

Figure 20.1 Perceived future impact of the project on tribal youth. Responses are on a 10-point Hikert scale, where 10 is the most positive score.

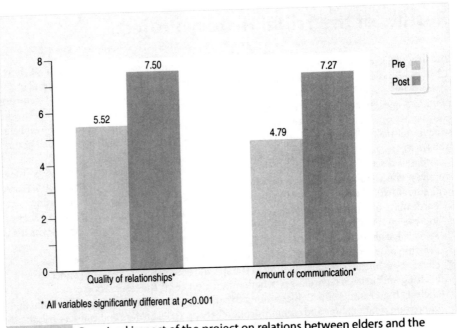

* All variables significantly different at *p*<0.001

Figure 20.2 Perceived impact of the project on relations between elders and the younger generation. Responses are on a 10-point Hikert scale, where 10 is the most positive score.

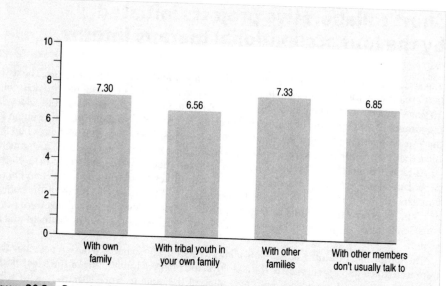

Figure 20.3 ● Perceived impact of the project on amount of communication between self and others. Responses are on a 10-point Hikert scale, where 10 is the most positive score.

- tribal elders' contribution of information and their sense that they could contribute even more
- tribal elders reporting that they had learned something new about their own family and that others had also learned something
- increase in pride in the tribe and hope for it (significant at the $p = 0.05$ level)
- no alteration of tribal elders' mood (already quite high) but a marginally statistically significant improvement in general health (at the $p = 0.07$ level):
- dramatic increase in tribal elders' overall assessment of the project's ability to achieve tribal goals (Fig. 20.4).

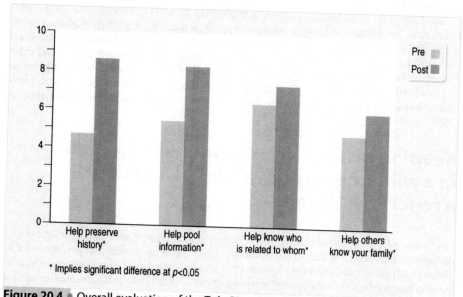

Figure 20.4 ● Overall evaluation of the Tule River Tribal History Project. Responses are on a 10-point Hikert scale, where 10 is the most positive score.

Short collaborative projects initiated by the four occupational therapy interns

The project director, Gelya Frank, was an anthropologist and occupational scientist. The assistant project director, Heather Kitching, was a registered, licensed occupational therapist with 10 years' experience working in a physical rehabilitation setting and enrolled in the doctoral programme at the University of Southern California. She provided guidance and supervision for the four occupational therapy advanced master's students. These four staff members had finished their coursework and were completing a final, 12-week, supervised fieldwork assignment.

Although none of the occupational therapy staff had worked previously in a Native American community, they drew effectively on their professional training to meet an important expectation of practice: to develop treatments suited to the specific needs of the patient or client, whether an individual or a community. The tribal elders as individuals were never considered 'cases' or 'patients', however. Rather, the client was the tribal government and its goals.

The professional training of the staff allowed them to construct and design activities that were well suited and appropriate to the cognitive and physical functioning of the tribal elders. Their sensitivity and knowledge base also allowed the staff to work effectively with tribal members of all ages, including teenagers and school-age children, adjusting activities to their developmental capacities and interests. The staff proved impressive in devising culturally specific protocols. The community, in turn, embraced them.

Three of the four interns had had extensive cross-cultural experience through family migration (India, Fiji, China), Peace Corps service (Turkmenistan) and extended travel abroad (Europe, Asia). The fourth came from a rural background in the USA and had majored in anthropology as an undergraduate. Her experience of the pace and style of rural life was an asset in relating to the tribal elders in the rural reservation setting.

As part of their level II fieldwork experience, the four occupational therapy interns were given the opportunity to initiate a short project in collaboration with a tribal elder. Postcolonial perspectives guided the design of each project in that the treatment or intervention had to focus on tribal goals of preserving history and indigenous culture through some form of occupation or 'doing'.

The four projects included: providing a wilderness survival workshop (Allison Joe with tribal elder Ruby Bays); offering a Western-style silversmithing workshop (Colleen Harvey with tribal elder Ray Flores Sr); creating an illustrated dictionary of the Wukchumne (Yokuts) dialect (Rani Bechar with tribal youth Evett McDarment and her grandfather, tribal elder Isidore Garfield); and reconstructing a traditional Yokuts story through narratives and dreams (Amber Bertram with tribal elder Luther Garfield). An account follows of the wilderness survival workshop by Allison Joe, from a presentation to the Occupational Therapy Association of California (Kitching et al 2004).

Keeping history alive through occupation in a wilderness survival skills workshop – a report by Allison Joe

The history of the California Indians is characterized by themes of survival in the face of the devastating effects of anti-Indian government policies, genocide, racism and poverty. Prior to contact with Europeans, California Indians lived and flourished on the land. Afterwards, people who remembered the old ways still relied on resources from the land to sustain themselves in hard times. History contributed not only to the limitations but also to the strengths of such people.

230

These skills of sustenance and survival were previously passed from generation to generation by doing them together. However, in the rapidly shifting times of today, the knowledge of survival and the land is not consistently passed on from elders to youth as it once was. I worked with tribal elder Ruby Bays to preserve the tribe's history of survival through the occupations of living off the land. My project sought to facilitate the sharing of the tribe's living history and ways of life from the elder generation to the younger generation through the doing of occupations that were meaningful both to the individuals involved and to the overall tribal community.

Ruby Carbajal Bays is a lively 71-year-old woman with a spunky smile and sparkling eyes. Ruby was born on the reservation and her family roots can be traced back to the time of the reservation's early years. She spent many of her adult years living in town and had just recently returned to a land assignment on the reservation. Ruby is known as an educator and an activist in her community. She attended Porterville College over a span of many years while travelling with her trucker husband and raising her 13 children. She was instrumental in starting the school for children on the reservation. She continues to teach as a master speaker in the tribe's Yokuts language programme. She has a reputation as a community activist, speaking up for issues such as water rights and reservation law enforcement.

My collaboration with Ruby began while working together on her family tree. As we entered the names of her husbands and children and traced her relations into previous centuries, she told stories of growing up, how they lived off the land and how in her adult life she became a community activist and youth educator. I could see that Ruby possessed not only a wealth of knowledge about outdoor skills but also an open willingness and generative desire to share her information with others. I wanted to work more with Ruby to develop ideas on ways to share her wilderness survival knowledge with the younger generation.

We arranged a time to meet at her home site at the top of steep Cow Mountain Road with a teenage project volunteer, Evett. Ruby toured us around her site and we stood on the hilltop, under an oak tree, overlooking the canyon. She spoke with joy about her plans for building a house on her assignment – 'not a house,' she clarified, 'but a shelter... in traditional Indian style'. She told me how she had lived all over but being on the reservation lands was where she was happiest, where she felt most at home and closest to the earth. As she spoke with us, she pointed out various plants and weeds around us and described their traditional uses. She told us about the ways of their people, 'the people of the earth', as she described them.

Ruby spoke with conviction about how, at some point, technology will not be able to meet all our needs and, for that reason, people need to know how to live off the land again. She felt that people nowadays are out of touch with the earth. Evett, a teenager, agreed that the kids of her generation did not learn these types of skill as the previous generations had. And Ruby was eager to share her knowledge with younger people. I explained the purpose of my project to add something meaningful to the Tribal History Project through the actions, or occupations, practised by their people for generations. Together we decided to do a wilderness survival skills workshop.

Ruby and I prepared for the workshop and promoted it throughout the community. We took a day to assess the site for the workshop, choosing the tribe's campground high in the mountains. We brought along Ruby's granddaughter, Kendie, who had never been up there. She was awed by the beauty of the area and fascinated by her grandmother's stories and knowledge. Here was Ruby's granddaughter learning directly from her grandmother about plants (medicines) and strengthening her connection to the campground as a secular place with sacred dimensions, where the Tribe's once-outlawed Bear Dance is now held each year.

The workshop took place on 4 August 2004 at the campground in the mountains. Nine people participated, including: three girls, ages 7, 9 and 10, who were not acquainted with Ruby and were seeing these activities for the first time; a young woman in her twenties who was active in Ruby's language revival class and basket-weaving group; Ruby's 35-year-old daughter-in-law with her baby; a middle-aged mother with her teenage daughter, niece and baby grandson; and a local man in his mid-fifties who described himself as a 'displaced Cherokee' who was looking to get in touch with his Native American identity.

Ruby brought samples of many of the plants and herbs in the area. The participants gathered around her as she demonstrated how to use mint, liniment, manzanita and bay leaves for medicinal use. She allowed them to experience the activities through their senses and their hands. They smelled the herbs. They tasted bites of acorn. They mixed mint extract with water to drink and spray on each other. They mixed up liniment extracts with mineral oil and petroleum jelly to use as lotion. They watched in fascination as she mixed up lemon rinds and moth balls to make a repellent for rattlesnakes. She showed everyone how flexible buttonwillow branches can be used to make a shelter and carved a fishing spear from one branch.

Together, we made Indian tacos for lunch. The kids rolled, pounded and stretched the pliable fry bread dough, then watched as they fried. We were visited by a bear and her two cubs. Very naturally, Ruby spoke with the animals, addressing them in her native language. It was a full day that helped to connect people who were interested in cultural preservation and sparked the interest of the children. Samples of medicinal plants were preserved with written descriptions in a poster format to display in the tribe's education centre. And the workshop was videotaped, photographed and recorded in audio for the tribal archives.

The outcomes from this project were expressed in multiple ways. The workshop itself met its objectives in that it created an opportunity for Ruby, as an active participant, to transfer some of the tribe's living history to younger generations via meaningful occupations and hands-on learning. The children had an opportunity for hands-on learning of cultural activities in a location that is meaningful to their tribe. The self-described 'displaced Cherokee' later expressed his enthusiastic appreciation for the workshop, which helped him to get in touch with his own Native American identity.

Similar to occupational therapy practice in a traditional setting, my short project involved the process of doing a needs assessment, defining goals and objectives, planning the project, implementing the project and evaluating outcomes. Where traditional treatment would focus on the individual client and the systems in which he or she lives, our approach required that I look at the community as a whole made up of individuals within it and the systems surrounding it.

The objective of our individual projects was to facilitate 'doing' with an elder in a meaningful activity that contributed to the tribe's history as well. We assessed the community's strengths and limitations based on input from members of that community and confirmed by our observations. We worked together with members of the community in order to facilitate creating change – by them and for themselves – using the strengths of their community to help ameliorate limitations associated with a history of oppression. The culture of the community becomes both the context and the means for the intervention. For indigenous people, the culture and land are intimately connected.

The Tule River Yokuts were forced to live on a reservation in a steep, rocky valley where their previously developed farming skills could not be fully exercised and they were far from opportunities for employment or education. However, that land is what they have survived on for generations and it continues to be a source of historical identity (e.g. Painted Rock), recreation (the Tule River), spiritual renewal (the campground) and recent economic opportunity (Eagle Mountain Casino).

As fieldwork students, we took the principles of occupational therapy and postcolonial approaches and implemented them in a non-traditional practice setting. As we grappled with framing this new kind of project as a legitimate practice of occupational therapy, we connected with the people we came into contact with by being present in their daily lives and through acts of sharing and 'doing together'. In the process we were blessed to know the people of the Tule River Indian Reservation. They brought to light my own understanding of the long-term impact of California's own history on its Native peoples as well as how much kindness and goodwill is offered in return when you share some of your own time, hard work and genuine concern.

> ## What Tule River tribal elders said about the Tribal History Project
>
> *This programme should be an ongoing project. We need this as long as we are Indian people. This gives a lot of people pride in themselves, knowing they have a background. We need this programme. – A prideful Elder of Tule River Reservation*
>
> *Female, born 1933*
>
> *I believe the Project needs to stay for a while longer, because the youth seem very interested in learning of their Ancestry.*
>
> *Male, born 1940*
>
> *I would like to thank you for all your effort and professionalism with making this project turn out the way it has. Hopefully we will have some more time to be with and share some laughs, smiles and wonderful company. Hope your path in life takes you on a journey in a good way. A-Ho.*
>
> *Male, age 51*
>
> *I'm truly happy. Talking about our families is the greatest. Some pictures our other relatives have of great-grandma were awesome. We could have had others come forward. The rewards of knowing your true family.*
>
> *Female, born 1943*

Conclusion

The occupational therapy profession appears to be entering a new phase, finding more expansive ways to work than typically available under the regime of Western medicine and its emphasis on the individual organism. This does not mean that occupational therapy should reject its ties with medicine but, as a leader of the occupational therapy profession Charles Christiansen suggests, the profession must use science and medicine to help validate occupational therapy's holistic treatments.

Postcolonial and indigenous thinkers are pointing the way for occupational therapy to help restore health and well-being to people whose lives have been disrupted by political domination and oppression. Indigenous projects involving history making call for the thoughtful application of everyday activities.

In the Tule River Tribal History Project, occupational therapists worked with a postcolonial approach. The Tule River tribe has suffered losses and disruptions – not only in the lives of today's tribal elders but over the course of many generations. Just as occupational therapists traditionally work with individuals to support independence, the Tule River Tribal History Project worked with the Tule River tribe to support its collective goals of tribal sovereignty and nation-building.

References

Ackerknecht E H 1953 Rudolf Virchow: doctor, statesman, anthropologist. University of Wisconsin Press, Madison, WI

Buckley T 2002 Standing ground: Yurok Indian spirituality, 1850–1990. University of California Press, Berkeley, CA

Champagne D, Goldberg C 2005 Changing the subject: individual versus collective interests in Indian country. University of Minnesota Press, Wicazo Sa Review 20: 49–69

Charland L C 2007 Benevolent theory: moral treatment at the York Retreat. History of Psychiatry 18: 61–80

Clark F A, Parham D, Carlson M E et al 1991 Occupational science: academic innovation in the service of occupational therapy's future. American Journal of Occupational Therapy 45: 300–310

Cook S F 1976 The conflict between the California Indian and white civilization. University of California Press, Berkeley, CA

Duran B, Duran E, Yellow Horse Brave Heart M 1998 Native Americans and the trauma of history. In: Thornton R (ed) Studying Native America: problems and prospects. University of Wisconsin Press, Madison, WI: p 60–76

Duran E 2006 Healing the soul wound: counseling with American Indians and other native peoples. Teachers College Press, New York

Duran E, Duran B 1995 Native American postcolonial psychology. State University of New York Press, Albany, NY

Eisenberg L 1984 Rudolf Ludwig Karl Virchow: where are you now that we need you? American Journal of Medicine 77: 524–532

Epston D, White M 1992 Experience, contradiction, narrative and imagination: selected papers of David Epston and Michael White 1989–1991. Dulwich Centre Publications, Adelaide, South Australia

Field L W 2008 Abalone tales: collaborative explorations of sovereignty and identity in Native California. Duke University Press, Durham, NC

Frank G 2005 Final report of the Tule River tribal history project, Phase I. Tule River Tribal Council, Porterville, CA

Frank G 2007 Collaborating to meet the goals of a native sovereign nation: the Tule River tribal history project. In: Field L W, Fox R G (eds) Anthropology put to work. Berg, Oxford: p 65–83

Frank G, Goldberg C (in press) Defying the odds: one California tribe's struggle for sovereignty in three centuries. Yale University Press, New Haven, CT

Frank G, Fishman M, Crowley C et al 2001 The New Stories/New Cultures After-School Enrichment Program: a direct cultural intervention. American Journal of Occupational Therapy 55: 501–508

Frank G, Murphy S, Kitching H J et al (submitted) The Tule River Tribal History Project: evaluating a California Tribal Government's collaboration with anthropology and occupational therapy to preserve indigenous history and promote tribal goals. Human Organization, submitted.

Freedman J, Combs G 1996 Narrative therapy: the social construction of preferred realities. W W Norton, New York

Gayton A H 1948 Yokuts and Western Mono ethnography, I: Tulare Lake, Southern Valley, and Central Foothill Yokuts. Anthropological Records 10:1. University of California Press, Berkeley, CA

Howe C 2002 Keep your thoughts above the trees: ideas on developing and presenting tribal histories. In: Shoemaker N (ed) Clearing a path: theorizing the past in Native American studies. Routledge, New York: p 161–180

Hurtado A L 1988 Indian survival on the California frontier. Yale University Press, New Haven, CT

Kitching H J, Frank G, Bechar R et al 2004 Direct cultural interventions: meeting the needs of communities. Paper presented at the Annual Conference of the Occupational Therapy Association of California, Pasadena, CA, 7 November

Kroeber A L 1925 Handbook of the Indians of California. Bureau of American Ethnology Bulletin 78. Smithsonian Institution, Washington, DC

Kronenberg F, Simó Algado S, Pollard N 2005 Occupational therapy without borders: learning from the spirit of survivors. Elsevier/Churchill Livingstone, Edinburgh

Lassiter L E 2005 The Chicago guide to collaborative ethnography. University of Chicago Press, Chicago, IL

Latta F F 1977 Handbook of Yokuts Indians, 2nd edn. Brewer's Historical Press, Exeter, CA

McGarrigle J, Nelson A 2006 Evaluating a school skills programme for Australian indigenous children: a pilot study. Occupational Therapy International 13: 1–20

Manson S 2004 Meeting the mental health needs of American Indians and Alaska Natives (report to the National Technical Assistance Center). US Department of Health and Human Services, Washington, DC

O'Nell T D 1996 Disciplined hearts: history, identity and depression in an American Indian community. University of California Press, Berkeley, CA

Ozarin L 1954 Moral treatment and the mental hospital. American Journal of Psychiatry 111: 371–378

Rawls J J 1984 Indians of California: the changing image. University of Oklahoma Press, Norman, OK

Rosen G 1974 From medical police to social medicine: essays in the history of health care. Neale Watson, New York

Smith, LT 1999 Decolonizing methodologies: research and indigenous peoples. Zed Books, London

Staples A R, McConnell R L 1993 Soapstone and seed beads: arts and crafts at the Charles Camsell Hospital, a tuberculosis sanatorium. Provincial Museum of Alberta, Edmonton, Alberta

Taguchi-Meyer J, Kitching H J, Frank G 2005 A community-based level II fieldwork in direct cultural intervention: Tule River Indian Reservation. Paper presented at the 88th Annual Conference of the American Occupational Therapy Association, Long Beach Convention Center, Long Beach, California, 14 May

Waitzkin, H 1981 The social origins of illness: a neglected history. International Journal of Health Services 11: 177–183

Watson R, Swartz L (eds) 2004 Transformation through occupation. Whurr, London

Watts E, Carlson G 2002 Practical strategies for working with indigenous people living in Queensland, Australia. Occupational Therapy International 9: 277–293

Yerxa E J, Clark F, Frank G et al 1990 An introduction to occupational science: a foundation for occupational therapy in the twenty-first century. Occupational Therapy in Health Care 6: 1–18

Young R J C 2001 Postcolonialism: an historical introduction. Blackwell Publishing, Malden, MA

Zemke R, Clark F (eds) 1996 Occupational science: the evolving discipline. F A Davis, Philadelphia, PA

Facing the challenge:
a compass for navigating the heteroglossic context

Nick Pollard, Dikaios Sakellariou

In part, the fuzziness of the phenomenon of human occupation arises from its universality (Wilcock 1998). Because it is everywhere, it is taken for granted; it is not really appreciated as a social need. Although social action and explicitly social practices are central to the origins of occupational therapy they have not always been the focus of the environment of practice (Hocking 2007). Now, however, occupational therapy is reclaiming its interest in social contexts and interventions, whether through social occupational therapy in Brazil (Barros et al 2005, Galheigo 2005), transformational approaches and community-based rehabilitation (Watson & Swartz 2004, Fransen 2005, Whiteford & Wright-St Clair 2005) or through service learning and an attention to the contextual nature of occupation, for example recently in Australia (Hunt 2005), South Africa (Joubert et al 2006) and the USA (Wood et al 2005). Not all of these are new directions: some have been slow-burning developments; social occupational therapy, for example, has been part of Brazilian occupational therapy education since the 1970s (Barros et al 2005), while the antecedents of current practice and service-learning initiatives in South Africa were established in the mid-1990s following the fall of the apartheid regime (Joubert et al 2006).

Occupational therapy bodies, professional and government agencies and other social actors frequently apply a top-down, policy-driven focus to community needs. Even where consultative measures are employed by public health bodies these often operate to a predetermined agenda that does not identify or serve real needs so much as obtain answers that fit a corporate purpose (Coney 2004, Hammell 2004, 2007). As allied health professionals, occupational therapists need to explore other forms of alliance beyond the medical professions if they are to address the social and environmental aspects of disability experiences.

There are many other stakeholders, most importantly the people who face disabling situations themselves, clients and carers. Paradoxically, the people who are least able to access services are those who perhaps are best placed to inform challenges to the allocation of health and social care resources. The pursuit of evidence-based practice through a positivist hierarchical framework does not allow for a particular experience to be expressed, or individual needs and diversity in context to be addressed. The evidence hierarchy needs to be able to deal with the complexities that arise from variable data that are difficult to systematize. Occupational therapy needs to develop a *moving viewpoint* (Good 1994) in order to allow for a diverse perspective on the realities it encounters. In order to be responsive to a diversity of needs, a variable focus is required, rather than one that provides a narrow and false objectivity.

Therapists continuously learn through the stories told them by the disabled people and the relatives and carers with whom they work, and in the process of developing their own narratives of experience and reflection. This set of narratives, with multiple perspectives according to who has told the story and the number of times it has been told, is often revealed gradually. It is often interpreted through the medium of their professional knowledge, the monoglossic lens of occupational therapy culture, but this provides only one perspective. While such narratives may be framed with the occupational therapist as the intended audience, they may also serve a purpose for the narrator, and other people who may be present. Through the course of intervention the therapist and other professionals can often enter the story as protagonists themselves. A complete understanding of disability and restriction of access to occupation can be achieved only through a synthesis and culturally sensitive interpretation of the heteroglossic discourse within which these phenomena are structured (Good 1994). Of course, a therapeutic understanding of disability is different from the client's experience of disability; the interpretation that mediates this depends on the formation of a rapport with the people therapists are working with and the development of effective responses to immediate practicalities. The same embedding in practicalities can also encourage the adaptation of assessments and standard tools to fit local needs, making comparisons between different sources of evidence difficult.

Bannigan (2007) argues that if clinicians consider the problems clients face rather than the mechanistic application of a small range of solutions such a diversity need not present a difficulty. Although there are many models for practice, none has emerged as an overarching meta-framework that is informed by a heterarchical approach and thus offers a multi-dimensional perspective (Ch. 3). Instead, each framework deals with some of the issues of human occupation but not others. As a consequence, occupational therapists may have missed opportunities to address occupational choices that clients may prioritize over the interventions they are being offered (Ch. 5). Clearly, more than one discourse is in operation if the client determines different prime needs to those that have been identified by the clinician. Occupational therapists may need to engage in a process of critically reassessing their values and beliefs, but their response to the diverse and divergent discourses related to access and engagement in meaningful and dignified occupation should be carefully negotiated. Complexity can easily slip into confusion.

This divergence is the subject of Fernandez-Armesto's (1997) attack on the fragmentation of truth through such philosophical movements as postmodernism and relativism. He argues that the individual interpretation arising from such movements makes the possibility of shared interpretation impossible: nothing can be real. All language is like 'a serpent biting its own tail' (Fernandez-Armesto 1997, p. 229): it does not refer to other things but to other words, yet none the less words are what we use, along with our senses and actions, to describe the world. Language therefore hovers between the tangible and the intangible but is the means by which we describe truth and untruths. The idea of truth thus remains a possibility that is bigger than the individual; it requires a consensus to establish some idea of a shared objectivity, even though the perceptions of that objectivity may ultimately be individual experiences. Fernandez-Armesto's position, since he refers to his Catholicism, is particularly interesting, as the validity of early accounts of the Gospel and the higher truth it purports to reveal are based on claims of personal testimony, and the practice of Catholicism involves reflection and personal confession, a process of validating experience through repetition. In the formation of ideas of truth, the living witness is of especial importance. Morley and Worpole (1982), Ragon (1983) and Worpole (1983) have described the importance of personal testimony in working-class writing, a 'gospel' of the vernacular that aims to counter the 'higher truth' mediated by literary narratives and sociohistorical discourses of the classes of privilege. It is this same personal testimony through which therapists aim to identify the components of occupational lives, the search for the lived experience of people and their communities, the individual meaning of illness or the individual narratives of community values from which a notion of occupational justice can be established (Garro 2000, Mattingly & Garro 2000, Simó Algado & Burgman 2005, Simó Algado & Cardona 2005).

While this potentially presents a client-centred occupational therapy based in the individual occupational narrative of an expert patient, earlier discussion in this book (Ch. 6) shows it to be in tension with other elements of social and health contexts. If the client's experience has to be considered against a biomedical framework of objective, empirically determined truths, it also has to contend with a range of organizational and policy imperatives. These offer a separate set of truths based on economic and commercial data concerning the affordability of treatments, the market for medication, health insurance or access to facilities. If the complexity of occupational therapy is underestimated in the clinical arena (Creek 2003, Whiteford et al 2005), any difficulties in articulating its values are complicated further by the pressures that arise from this. Hammell (2007) has suggested that economic self-preservation may produce a therapist-centred professional approach, concerned with survival and justifying its existence in a competitive health and social care market but in the process distancing itself from negative experiences of its clients.

A history that relies on personal testimony, or perhaps occupational narrative, is something that is remembered, reconstructed and therefore partial. We may think that a better picture can be obtained only by gaining more viewpoints but these further accounts may reveal many differences, confusions and distractions. One narrative, as recorded in the client's notes, more often reflects the therapist's interpretation of this negotiation of need than that of the client. In interactions with therapists the client may attempt to seek resolution for problems or to understand them but often has to accept the clinicians' conceptualization of them in order to obtain treatment. Disabled people find they have to admit all kinds of people into their lives in order to receive care, obtain continued benefits and be observed to be complying responsibly with their treatments. Even when these processes are necessary, they remain an imposition that arises from the way in which disability is negotiated. To argue against this can be interpreted as a refusal of treatment (Kirmayer 2000). The experience of disability, then, may be seen as being occupied or perhaps colonized by the treatment process. The progress of treatment becomes a period of time that no longer belongs to the client but is determined by the way it is broken into usable segments through treatment, appointments for further assessment and the demands for compliance in following up exercises. The narrative recorded in clients' notes will not indicate the experiences of waiting rooms or of journeys to hospital, or much of the anxieties of families waiting to hear treatment outcomes. While each stage of the intervention and assessments between are recorded, the intervening spaces experienced by the client form no part of the clinical story and the truth of the client experience may differ from the truth of the professional or organizational experience.

Consequently the search for knowledge is an occupation of making successive approximations, each sufficing until a new proposition appears to replace it. It is sometimes important to attend to the intervening spaces to find out why treatments are not working according to plan, clients have not followed advice, or progress is interrupted. Kirmayer (2000) suggests that it can sometimes be difficult for clinicians to think outside their professional focus to accommodate these circumstances into a course of treatment. When the search for new means of uncovering truths runs into a cul-de-sac it can be necessary to return to traditions, or earlier paths, in order to make progress (Fernandez-Armesto 1997, Garro 2000), just as the occupational therapist seeks to enable the rediscovery of previous abilities or the development of new ones, or the profession seeks to develop perspectives for the future by returning to its root values.

In the quest for new occupational territories this also produces difficulties. Johnson (1997) describes how the search for new lands to conquer led to the creation of fantasies and myths. Real geographical features such as the southern tip of Greenland or Iceland were misplaced through error, myth, mirage and the experiences of being lost and identified as new lands. These substantial cartological formations continued to show up on maps for centuries. Although they shifted in position and reduced in size, lack of knowledge maintained such islands through successive generations of navigators and cartographers.

The perception of truth is relative to the amount of access we have to knowledge, education and experience. This is why the early literatures valued personal testimony and supplied reasonings in terms of these experiences to describe phenomena that could not be directly explained. Personal narrative is often a stronger force than the rational written word because it relates the testimony of direct experience. Those who practised the traditions of oral literatures have sometimes described the writing down of ballads and other pieces as destructive. The written variant has sometimes been described as dead because it is fixed in the page and not in the memory, and the process has often involved the introduction of editorial 'improvements', which may either be untrue or even bring in elements alien to the oral tradition (Buchan 1997).

Heteroglossia is therefore a product of a living process of language, the means by which human contiguity is expressed. On the one hand the written tradition may present a spiritual line of communication from the dead to the living, but in daily life we often value the spoken word, the sense of a real personal connection conveyed orally, even if memory proves more unreliable than text. The power of the word that the ancient poets possessed in many cultures was not so much to do with the word itself but the lasting representation of the actions of individuals, their deeds, to others. To the individual who might be the subject of a verse, however, the important and disconcerting issue of encountering a bard or poet was that they might make your deeds immortal by setting them out in a way that would become more true, and more widely known, with every repetition.

Repetition was the authenticating tool of testimony, and, in fact, in the recording of the key legends of Celtic culture, the early scribes sometimes offered several versions of a myth despite the contradictions it might produce, rather than refining one clear narrative (Nagy 1997). During a similar drive an attempt has been made to capture the last vestiges of an oral culture in Europe during the 19th and 20th centuries through the search for different versions of folk songs. The several versions underpin the verity even though they contradict each other, just as, perhaps, the New Testament has several accounts of the Gospel. Thus, while language is important, speaking together is about achieving not a common language but a common understanding of occupation, its meanings and importance, so that interactions can take place from a common basis.

Successful navigation

This multiplicity of similar but different narratives produces an incomplete understanding or lack of clarity, which in turn makes it necessary to share readings. An occupational literacy is centred in a polyphonous exchange of interpretations (Ch. 3). It entails a process of navigating the space between parallel dimensions in the separate universes of experience expressed by diverse voices. Through the recognition of differences it is possible to close some of the gaps between theory and practice and between theory and the commonplace experience. Through a process of mutual and cooperative facilitation achieved by such processes as the pADL framework it is possible to identify actions that can be jointly owned by the participants. It may also be appropriate to identify and explore points of conflict, in order to determine to what extent they will obstruct the agreed interventions, or can be circumnavigated by consensus.

Occupational therapists are learning to 'speak the language' and navigate effectively through moving vantage points in a polyphonic social world focusing on access to and engagement in meaningful and dignified occupation. Our awareness as health professionals needs to be critically informed or raised in an analytical response to these issues as clients experience them. Recently introduced terms such as occupational apartheid (Kronenberg & Pollard 2005; see Ch. 4), occupational deprivation (Whiteford 2004) and occupational justice and injustice (Townsend & Wilcock 2004) can be helpful in broadening up the focus of occupational therapists, encouraging them to look at the underlying and interconnected reasons for restriction from access to and engagement in occupation. These terms point to realities faced by people all around the world and act as a reminder to occupational therapists that occupation is not restricted to an occurrence within a rehabilitation setting but happens within a network of interrelated factors. As concepts they are all very well, but they lack any force unless they are accepted as having validity beyond the professional discourse of occupational therapy.

As suggested by Good (1994), phenomena need to be named before they can be recognized. Indeed, to engage with situations such as occupational apartheid or occupational deprivation occupational therapists first need to acknowledge them. Learning new terminology, a new language, is not simply about learning new words but about constructing new worlds of meaning. As a medical student noted: 'learning new names for things is to learn new things about them' (Good 1994, p. 74).

Examples from practice indicate a range of diversity and polyphony in practice and culture (Chs 17, 19). Polyphony is inevitable when occupational therapy is applied across a widening range of practice contexts and where the profession itself begins to take full account of its complexity. The emergence of a polyphony in expression of occupational therapy perhaps signals a stage in its maturity as a profession. In order to achieve its goals and meet the challenges put before it, the profession has to take account not merely of the problems directly before it but also of the underlying factors or conditions in which they are based. Occupational therapists have to build new capacities or acquire new frameworks in order to facilitate their participation in processes that serve as important preconditions for meeting the problems they want to address. One area of this has been the recognition of the political implications of occupational therapy. Polyphony centres on negotiation and discussion with other actors in community-based interventions. This is an important aspect of gaining permission and establishing a rapport with people in order to be able to work with them, and at the same time valuable for conveying an idea of the humanistic principles that occupational therapists might employ. For people to accept the input of professions in a way that is participatory, it is necessary to get them to understand what is being offered so as to make informed decisions about it as fellow citizens (Duncan & McMillan 2006).

Humanism derives from a stance in which 'human' values are respected over 'barbarian' mores, in other words the exclusion of others' viewpoints (Clarke 1996). A belief in the therapeutic value of occupation and ideas about equality and social justice have all contributed to the development of occupational therapy and still remain the main tenets of our profession, but the narrow association of occupation with 'work' or of occupational justice with 'occupation' might also present problems in recognizing diversity. Many societies place a higher value on community than work or materialist activities. Even those societies that formed on a communal or cooperative basis during some of the social experiments of the 18th and 19th centuries appeared to value community activities over the work and production upon which they depended for their income (Nordhoff 1965).

Conclusion

Mattingly (1994) suggested that occupational therapists view clients in a holistic way and value both the 'lived body' and the 'body as a machine' (Mattingly 1994, p. 37). Unfortunately, intentions for holistic practice do not always lead to holistic practice and the three-track-mind therapists, as described by Mattingly and Fleming (1994), often end up having a rather one-sided view of occupation and disability. Reasons for this include the monoglossic processes of occupational therapy, which lead to incomplete and biased perspectives, a theory–practice gap, the disempowered position of occupational therapy as a health profession and the perceived arbitrary nature of holism, as suggested by McColl (1994). Indeed, holism has been found to mean different things to different people (Owen & Holmes 1993, Finlay 2001, Schmidt et al 2005).

Occupational therapy is constructed and operates within a complex context (Whiteford et al 2005) made up by diverse and interconnected elements. The political practice of occupational therapy is essentially about developing a holistic understanding through a synthesis of these elements and learning to navigate effectively in the social world in ways that enable the realization of an occupationally just society. But if holism is to present some form of occupational truth, occupational therapists need to be cautious in laying claim to it. Given its variety and its intangible nature, for no-one can claim an objective and perfect 360° vision of holism, it seems more appropriate to recognize the theory–practice gap than to assume possession.

This is a complex and paradoxical position to adopt, counter to the empirical tradition in some ways in that it is not about the possession and occupation of facts but the identification of a lack of knowledge. This is the basis of complexity, an understanding that it is impossible to know everything. This does not imply that research cannot take place, rather it demands that the person you are working with, who has the experience of disabling situations and the knowledge of their meaning, is enabled to inform the process as part of the continuous demand for evidence and a critical examination of the purpose that evidence serves in terms of the client's experience. Occupational therapists have been advocating for political engagement to face the challenges of functioning in a complex context (Kronenberg et al 2005, Whiteford & Wright-St Clair 2005). They have been urged to become 'agents of social change' (Wilcock 2002, Sinclair 2005). Access to and engagement in occupation is highly influenced by the physical, social, cultural and political environment within which it takes place. Laws, policies, societal attitudes, cultural norms, as well as individual characteristics, wills and needs, work together to shape the occupational trajectory of individuals. Being holistic entails recognizing these parameters (Ch. 4; Kronenberg & Pollard 2005).

It is important to implement a moving viewpoint approach to develop a synthesis of experiences of occupation and restriction from access to it, and to identify the origins of such restriction in order to develop appropriate strategies to negotiate solutions and maintain the outcomes of intervention. Without an understanding of the underlying causes of problems therapists will be unable to provide effective solutions. However, in a complex world with too many factors to isolate, no permanent solutions or formulae are available. What occupational therapists can work for is achieving effective context-specific approaches informed by the people they are working with and their communities.

References

Bannigan K 2007 Making sense of research utilisation. In: Creek J, Lawson-Porter A (eds) Contemporary issues in occupational therapy, reasoning and reflection. John Wiley, Chichester: p 189–216

Barros D D, Ghirardi M, Lopes R E 2005 Social occupational therapy: a socio-historical perspective. In: Kronenberg F, Simó Algado S, Pollard N (eds) Occupational therapy without borders: learning from the spirit of survivors. Elsevier/Churchill Livingstone, Edinburgh: p 140–151

Buchan D 1997 The ballad and the folk. Tuckwell Press, East Linton

Clarke B 1996 Deep citizenship. Pluto, London

Coney S 2004 Effective consumer voice and participation for New Zealand: a systematic review of the evidence. New Zealand Guidelines Group, New Zealand

Creek J 2003 Occupational therapy defined as a complex intervention. College of Occupational Therapists, London

Duncan M, McMillan J 2006 A responsive curriculum for new forms of practice education and learning. In: Lorenzo T, Duncan M, Buchanan H, Alsop A (eds) Practice and service learning in occupational therapy: enhancing potential in context. John Wiley, Chichester: p 20–35

Fernandez-Armesto F 1997 Truth: a history and a guide for the perplexed. Thomas Dunne, New York

Finlay L 2001 Holism in occupational therapy: elusive fiction and ambivalent struggle. American Journal of Occupational Therapy 55: 268–276

Fransen H 2005 Challenges for occupational therapy in community based rehabilitation. In: Kronenberg F, Simó Algado S, Pollard N (eds) Occupational therapy without borders: learning from the spirit of survivors. Elsevier/Churchill Livingstone, Edinburgh: p 166–182

Galheigo S 2005 Occupational therapy and the social field: clarifying concepts and ideas. In: Kronenberg F, Simó Algado S, Pollard N (eds) Occupational therapy without borders: learning from the spirit of survivors. Elsevier/Churchill Livingstone, Edinburgh: p 87–98

Garro L C 2000 Cultural knowledge as resource in illness narratives. In: Mattingly C, Garro L C (eds) Narrative and the cultural construction of illness and healing. University of California Press, Berkeley, CA: p 70–87

Good B 1994 Medicine, rationality, and experience. Cambridge University Press, Cambridge

Hammell K W 2004 Dimensions in meaning in the occupations of everyday life. Canadian Journal of Occupational Therapy 71: 296–305

Hammell K W 2007 Client-centred practice: ethical obligation or professional obfuscation? British Journal of Occupational Therapy 70: 264–266

Hocking C 2007 The romance of occupational therapy. In: Creek J, Lawson-Porter A (eds) Contemporary issues in occupational therapy, reasoning and reflection. John Wiley, Chichester: p 23–40

Hunt S 2005 Participatory community practice: a community-based rehabilitation curriculum in occupational therapy and lessons learned through partnerships with undergraduate students. WFOT Bulletin 51: 14–18

Johnson D S 1997 Phantom islands of the Atlantic. Souvenir Press, London

Joubert R, Galvaan R, Lorenzo T, Ramugondo E 2006 Reflecting on the contexts of service learning. In: Lorenzo T, Duncan M, Buchanan H, Alsop A (eds) Practice and service learning in occupational therapy: enhancing potential in context. John Wiley, Chichester: p 34–49

Kirmayer L J 2000 Broken narratives, clinical encounters and the poetics of illness experience. In: Mattingly C, Garro L C (eds) Narrative and the cultural construction of illness and healing. University of California Press, Berkeley, CA: p 153–180

Kronenberg F, Pollard N 2005 Overcoming occupational apartheid: a preliminary exploration of the political nature of occupational therapy. In: Kronenberg F, Simó Algado S, Pollard N (eds) Occupational therapy without borders: learning from the spirit of survivors. Elsevier/Churchill Livingstone, Edinburgh: p 58–86

Kronenberg F, Simó Algado S, Pollard N 2005 Occupational therapy without borders: learning from the spirit of survivors. Edinburgh, Elsevier/Churchill Livingstone

McColl A 1994 Holistic occupational therapy: historical meaning and contemporary implications. Canadian Journal of Occupational Therapy 61: 72–77

Mattingly C 1994 Occupational therapy as a two body practice: body as a machine. In: Mattingly C, Fleming M (eds) Clinical reasoning: forms of inquiry in a therapeutic practice. F A Davis, Philadelphia, PA: p 37–63

Mattingly C, Fleming M 1994 Clinical reasoning: forms of inquiry in a therapeutic practice. F A Davis, Philadelphia, PA

Mattingly C, Garro L C 2000 Narrative as construct and construction. In: Mattingly C, Garro L C (eds) Narrative and the cultural construction of illness and healing. University of California Press, Berkeley, CA: p 1–49

Morley D, Worpole K 1982 The republic of letters. Comedia, London

Nagy J F 1997 Conversing with angels and ancients. Cornell University Press, Ithaca, NY

Nordhoff C 1965 The communistic societies of the United States. Schocken, New York

Owen M, Holmes C 1993 'Holism' in the discourse of nursing. Journal of Advanced Nursing 18: 1688–1695

Ragon M 1983 Histoire de la littérature prolétarienne de langue française. Albin Michel, Paris

Schmidt K, Rees C, Greenfield S, Wearn A 2005 Multischool, international survey of medical students' attitudes toward 'holism'. Academic Medicine 80: 955–963

Simó Algado S, Burgman I 2005 Occupational therapy intervention with children survivors of war. In: Kronenberg F, Simó Algado S, Pollard N (eds) Occupational therapy without borders: learning from the spirit of survivors. Elsevier/Churchill Livingstone, Edinburgh: p 253–268

Simó Algado S, Cardona C E 2005 The return of the corn-men: an intervention project with a Mayan community of Guatamelan retornos. In: Kronenberg F, Simó Algado S, Pollard N (eds) Occupational therapy without borders: learning from the spirit of survivors. Elsevier/Churchill Livingstone, Edinburgh: p 347–362

Sinclair K 2005 Foreword. In: Kronenberg F, Simó Algado S, Pollard N (eds) Occupational therapy without borders: learning from the spirit of survivors. Elsevier/Churchill Livingstone, Edinburgh: p xiv

Townsend E, Wilcock A 2004 Occupational justice and client centred practice: a dialogue. Canadian Journal of Occupational Therapy 71: 75–87

Watson R, Swartz L 2004 Transformation through occupation. Whurr, London

Whiteford G 2004 When people cannot participate: occupational deprivation. In: Christiansen C, Townsend E (eds) Introduction to occupation: the art and science of living. Prentice Hall, Thorofare, NJ: p 221–242

Whiteford G, Wright-St Clair V 2005 Occupation and practice in context. Elsevier/Churchill Livingstone, Marrickville, New South Wales

Whiteford G, Klomp P, Wright-St Clair V 2005 Complexity theory: understanding occupation, practice and context. In: Whiteford G, Wright-St Clair V (eds) Occupation and practice in context. Elsevier/Churchill Livingstone, Marrickville, New South Wales: p 3–15

Wilcock A 1998 An occupational perspective of health. Slack, Thorofare, NJ

Wilcock A 2002 Occupation for health volume 2: a journey from prescription to self health.

British Association and College of Occupational Therapists, London

Wood W, Hooper B, Womack J 2005 Reflections on occupational justice as a subtext of occupation-centered education. In: Kronenberg F, Simó Algado S, Pollard N (eds) Occupational therapy without borders: learning from the spirit of survivors. Elsevier/Churchill Livingstone, Edinburgh: p 378–388

Worpole K 1983 Dockers and detectives. Verso, London

Index

NB: Page numbers in **bold** refer to figures and tables

Lightning Source UK Ltd.
Milton Keynes UK
UKOW020304060413

208719UK00002B/32/P